Since Owen

A Parent-to-Parent Guide for Care of the Disabled Child

CHARLES R. CALLANAN

THE JOHNS HOPKINS UNIVERSITY PRESS
BALTIMORE AND LONDON

© 1990 The Johns Hopkins University Press
All rights reserved
Printed in the United States of America

The Johns Hopkins University Press, 701 West 40th Street, Baltimore, Maryland 21211
The Johns Hopkins Press Ltd., London

The paper used in this publication meets the minimum requirements of American
National Standard for Information Sciences—Permanence of Paper for Printed Library
Materials, ANSI 239.48-1984.

Library of Congress Cataloging-in-Publication Data
Callanan, Charles R., 1925-
   Since Owen: a parent-to-parent guide for care of the disabled child/Charles R.
Callanan.
      p.   cm.
   Includes bibliographical references.
   ISBN 0-8018-3963-7 (alk. paper).—ISBN 0-8018-3964-5 (pbk.   :   alk. paper)
      1. Handicapped children—Home care—United States. 2. Parents of handicapped
children—United States. I. Title.
   HV888.5.C34   1990
   362.4'083—dc20   84-24678
                                                                              CIP

Through a grant from the Joseph Meyerhoff Fund, 1,000 copies of *Since Owen* were
distributed to organizations that provide support to the families of children with
severe disabilities.

Contents

PART FOUR

The Promise of Education for All Handicapped Children

PART FIVE

Life in the Adult World

Note to the Reader

This book is intended to provide helpful information about the many areas that affect the child who has a disability, but reading it should be seen as only a first step toward understanding and competency: parents, too, need continual education. Furthermore, in no way should this book be considered a substitute for professional consultation. It is written from the background and experience of a family, seen principally through the eyes of a father.

My decision to use the masculine pronoun "he" was made for the sake of simplicity and to avoid mind-numbing repetitions of "he and she" or "him and her." It does not reflect a sexual bias, and occasionally I have thrown in a "she." Also, I have used the terms *handicap* and *disability* interchangeably.

This book is addressed to parents who are responsible for their children's care and who often make decisions for them. In many instances, however, youngsters with physical handicaps or mild mental impairment are capable of making their own decisions and can and should play a prominent if not decisive role in the decision-making process as they grow older. When this is the case, the suggestions that I make to parents are applicable to their children, with the parent playing only a supportive role.

To make this book as understandable and comprehensive as possible, I have drawn upon many resources, although I realize no parent should or could make use of every resource or follow every suggestion. It would be impossible and most certainly counterproductive. (Do the best you can and try to relax. If you get uptight, your child will, too. There's always tomorrow.) For the reader who wishes to obtain additional information about specific areas, the "Resources" section at the end of the book is designed to point you in the right direction.

Although the information in this book is presented in roughly chronological order, key events may not follow the same progression for all readers nor will all readers face similar problems. In addition, information on a specific subject may not be limited to one chapter but spread over many. I have tried to keep to an absolute minimum interruptions of the "for additional information, see Chapter X" variety, so if you encounter a subject in the text that interests you—respite care, for instance—and you want additional information, look it up in the index or Resources section.

Dozens of professional disciplines are involved with care of the disabled population. Since professional jargon is often unintelligible to those of us who inhabit the world of the disabled child, several dictionaries dealing with some of the fields with which you may be involved are listed in the Resources section. If professionals won't speak a language we understand, and some won't, it's up to us to learn their "lingo." If you don't understand a term, don't be intimidated; ask for an explanation or look it up.

How to Use This Book to Get Information in a Hurry

Refer to

- the **Contents** (pages v–vii)
- the checklists of **Dos and Don'ts** (located at the end of each of the five major parts of the book), which summarize key practical suggestions
- the **Resources** section (pages 427–49), which tells you where to find other sources of help and information
- the **Index** (pages 451–466), which locates topics alphabetically
- **Aids to Basic Competency** (Chapter 8 and Appendix B), which list other sources of general information.

Acknowledgments

More people helped me with this book than I can name here, but a few made significant contributions of their time and I wish to thank them: Gladys Hager, teacher and intuitive organizer, Kathleen Powers, an authority on human services and research associate at the University of Southern Maine, and Snowden Stanley, a Baltimore attorney particularly knowledgable about the law's impact on handicapped persons, since one of his children has a disability.

The suggestions of Bruce Mallory, Chairman of the Department of Education of the University of New Hampshire, were invariably helpful, and Mark Batshaw, Professor of Pediatrics at the University of Pennsylvania School of Medicine, offered me both advice on the manuscript and help with Owen's medical problems. Another professional, one of whose children has a disability, who gave me unsparingly of his time despite an overwhelming workload of his own, is Carl Cooley, a developmental pediatrician at the Dartmouth Medical School.

Jean Toll, a professional editor and neighbor, helped shape up the book during the last stages and gave me support when I faltered. Betty Schmidt of the Department of Education in Washington was always available on the phone when I needed impossible-to-get information. And, perhaps most of all, Alan Guttmacher, pediatrician and geneticist at the University of Vermont, proved himself a loyal friend during the many long days we spent together on the manuscript with nothing to sustain us but thoughts of Owen, discussions of heredity, and chocolate chip cookies.

Finally, there is my family, whom you may get to know just a little through the pages of the book. My wife, Mary, and daughter, Miss Mary, helped more by what they didn't say or do than by what they did, particularly when my writing dragged on and on and friends began to look thoughtful and to ask if I were still working on "that book" and was I all right.

I thank all—experts, friends, and family—for their help and for their patience. And, I also thank the wonderful staff of Stewart Home School for giving our son the finest gift of all—a warm and loving second home.

Introduction

Mary and I named our fifth child Peter Owen Callanan, but we've always called him Owen. As babies go, he was quite presentable, apparently normal, and, for a Callanan, not that bad looking.

Today, twenty-nine years later, Owen lives in a school for severely handicapped people near Frankfort, Kentucky. Among other things, he can neither speak nor understand language. No one knows for sure what went wrong or why, but his problems have been extensive. The experts call him "unique," and we have realized that "unique" is something you don't want to be.

During the period between Owen's birth in Albany and his placement in the institution in Kentucky, our whole family found itself increasingly set apart. Not that our altered life was always bleak; on the contrary, we shared many things that others may live a lifetime without knowing. Even during dark times, unexpected moments of laughter would pop out of nowhere and draw us together, because Owen, despite his quirkiness, has a contagious smile, and hidden deep inside his mind is a delightful sense of humor, as if he's always known something that we weren't in on, something that tickled him enormously.

The fact of the matter is, "since Owen," our family began a new, fundamentally different existence. Many of the problems we faced confused and frustrated us, leaving us little confidence either in ourselves or in the professionals who bobbed in and out of our lives. We had no body of experience upon which to draw, as if we had been pushed into the middle of a strange and crazy game in which we knew neither the names of the players nor the rules. As Owen's behavior grew more unusual, our isolation increased. The old world didn't know how to handle us, and neither did we.

Since Owen, our new existence has been a continuing struggle to cope, a search for answers, a need to make decisions without sufficient information. Throughout the years, we have often felt the need for one comprehensive source of information, instead of the out-of-date pamphlets we found in agency waiting rooms or scholarly articles written by and for professionals. We needed a how-to manual that would give us the information required to make the decisions for which we felt inadequate, information that would cover all the bases, from genetic counseling to final institutional placement. We knew that such a book would have more meaning if it were compiled by someone who had struggled through the same experiences, someone who, like us, knew what it means to be "unique." In important ways it would have been comforting in moments of isolation to know that others had been there before and had survived, to know that we were not alone.

What follows is our attempt to meet this need. Although it comes nearly thirty years too late for Owen, it is to him and to his unique and wonderful band of friends that this book is dedicated.

A Thumbnail Sketch

1960

Owen was born at 3:50 P.M., January 3, 1960, in the Albany Hospital, Albany, New York. He weighed seven pounds and eleven ounces, was fair, blue-eyed, and bald—a typical baby. His siblings, Reid, Tom, Martha, and Sarah, were normal kids and "cool" when it came to new babies. (His third sister, Miss Mary, also normal, made her appearance when Owen was eleven, giving Owen his turn to be "cool.") Rh blood differences between Mary and me, and Martha's bout with German measles during Mary's pregnancy with Owen, had caused us some concern, but tests indicated that there was no problem. In later years, however, rubella was often cited as a logical source of Owen's many disabilities.

1960–1961

Owen's development was surprisingly slow, but he was so quiet and so good it never occurred to us to worry. He was temporarily a bit jaundiced, but that rapidly disappeared. He turned over at eight months and crawled using his elbows at eleven months. However, he showed no signs of the beginnings of speech or even normal baby babble. We began to feel uneasy.

1961: Owen at One

At Owen's one-year checkup our family doctor recommended a specialist. The specialist's diagnosis: "possible hearing loss; massive mental retardation." We were crushed. The specialist, the first of many, proved to be wrong.

1962: Owen at Two

Owen still couldn't speak, didn't react to hot and cold sensations, rocked in his crib, banged his head, and rolled his eyes in an unusual fashion. He didn't walk, but he struggled along upright on his knees. Mary and his grandmother sewed countless knee patches on his overalls. He ate only baby food (couldn't seem to chew) and began sleeping on the floor. We were desperate to find out what was wrong. Our doctor scheduled a complete work-up at the Hearing and Speech Center at Johns Hopkins Hospital, in Baltimore. Some comments we heard from the experts: "average to bright-average ability level," "evidence of central nervous system abnormality," "whatever else his multiple problems may turn out to be, this is certainly not a classic picture of deafness," and "what can be done to aid and abet his capacity and willingness to cooperate remains an open question."

1963: Owen at Three

Owen finally began to walk, a kind of awkward amble. He required orthopedic shoes to correct a low instep and toeing-out problem. We began looking for local special schools. Owen would eat only puréed food, and he loved applesauce. (He still does.)

1964: Owen at Four

Owen was admitted to the Albany Hospital because of a bowel impaction, the first episode in what was to become a chronic and distressing problem. Unable to find a local school for special children, we sent him to a "play school" for normal kids conducted in a friend's home. He sat cross-legged, he watched and smiled, but he didn't participate.

1965: Owen at Five

We moved to Baltimore to enroll Owen in the Gateway Pre-School for children with "communication disorders." Owen's brothers and sisters didn't want to move, and Tom hid in his secret cave at the top of our hill the day we were to leave. Mary held the family together. Owen's year-end report at Gateway said that he'd made progress in his "ability to work in a group without distraction." He still had no spontaneous speech but he imitated some sounds.

1966: Owen at Six

Owen was admitted to the Children's Hospital of Baltimore, where he had an operation for a "wandering eye." Another year at Gateway yielded only slow progress. He still ate only soft food and didn't chew. We wondered whether it was a case of "couldn't" chew or "wouldn't" chew. Owen's biting and swallowing reflexes were tested, and no physical explanation for his abnormal behavior was found. His toileting problems—constipation, soiling, and wetting—continued, to the consternation of the school staff.

1967: Owen at Seven

Our family moved again, the second time in one year, this time to Baltimore County, so that Owen could attend the Woodvale School, a well-regarded public school for "special children." There he would have a jar of applesauce at juice and cookie time, but he declined the cookies (since he couldn't/wouldn't chew). Suddenly, under the guidance of an inspired teacher, he began to make great strides. By year's end he could write and read the number symbols 1–10. His writing was neat and legible; his speech, although never spontaneous or in complete sentences, was intelligible. He loved his teacher and going to school. He loved being successful. This proved to be the high point in his speech development.

1968: Owen at Eight

Owen spent six weeks at the John F. Kennedy Institute (for habilitation of mentally and physically handicapped children) in Baltimore. A behavior-changing technique called operant conditioning was used in an effort to improve his language and social behavior but met with no success.

1969: Owen at Nine

Owen still wouldn't eat solid foods, and he still wet his bed regularly. A second year at Woodvale with a new teacher showed little progress. Elation turned to disappointment. Since Maryland could no longer offer appropriate schooling, we made the agonizing decision to send Owen away to a residential school and enrolled him at the Devereux School in Pennsylvania. The school's initial evaluation stated, "He appears to have conceptual abilities but is handicapped at present with a communication disorder that is not clinically totally comprehensible at this time." "Not clinically . . . comprehensible" is jargon at its best, meaning that no one really knew what was wrong.

1970: Owen at Ten

Eyeglasses were prescribed. Owen wore them for three years but lost or repeatedly broke them. (Perhaps he didn't like what he saw.) After a while we gave up on glasses.

1971: Owen at Eleven

Owen's years at Devereux were relatively happy, with frequent home visits. He progressed slowly in all areas except language, in which he didn't progress at all. Although he still didn't chew, he did "choke down" some semisolid food. His constipation had become a way of life, requiring ongoing medication and weekly suppositories, the intended results of which Owen resisted by standing with one leg so far crossed over in front of the other that we wondered how he managed to maintain his balance. This stance has become habitual.

1972: Owen at Twelve

Due to his "poor expressive and receptive abilities," Owen began having difficulty adjusting to the more advanced school program. Professionals at the Audiology Department at Temple University Health Services Center found a "moderate sensori-neural learning impairment" and recommended a hearing aid and placement in the Elwyn Institute (a much larger school) in a program that stresses speech and learning development. For the first time Owen lived in a dormitory. Over the next four years he was moved four times. He kept losing or breaking his hearing aid. (Perhaps he didn't like what he heard.) Finally he began to eat solid food in earnest by mashing it against the roof of his mouth with his tongue, a process that interested his tablemates.

1973: Owen at Thirteen

Owen was enrolled in the language program at Elwyn and finally began to learn signing, but he was unhappy and after vacations never wanted to return to school. We had to hide his packed bag the night before he was to leave or he would unpack it and put his clothes back in the drawers. It was a difficult time for all of us.

1974–1976: Owen from Fourteen to Sixteen

Owen made no real progress in schoolwork and, although generally healthy, began to become withdrawn. (One of his earliest evaluations mentioned the possibility of autism, perhaps because of his bizarre habit of flapping his hands when excited.)

1977: Owen at Seventeen

In 1977 Elwyn's yearly evaluation stated: "*Impression:* 1. Healthy 17-year-old adolescent male. 2. Organic Brain Syndrome with borderline intelligence. 3. Bilateral sensori-neural hearing loss, severe. 4. Communication disorder (limited expressive speech) with withdrawal reaction." A psychiatric evaluation was recommended. We reluctantly agreed, and an appointment was scheduled with a psychiatrist and a sign-language interpreter for the doctor (although Owen couldn't sign). The diagnosis: "Emotional withdrawal: an ego deficit should not be ruled out." Part of the recommendation was that "Owen is in need of some type of psychotherapy to help him out of his emotional withdrawal." Before a decision could be reached on this recommendation our family moved to Maine, to be nearer our New England roots, and Owen was admitted to the Baxter State School for the Deaf. The people whom we had contacted at the Vocational Rehabilitation Department arranged a vocational evaluation and a four-week "work adjustment" period for Owen at Goodwill Industries, a sheltered workshop, to see if he could develop necessary work habits and manual skills.

This was a difficult period. Owen's bowel-control problems upset the dormitory staff, and he really didn't fit into the academically oriented program at Baxter, which was geared for deaf children, not children with communication disorders and other problems. At Goodwill he went through a period when he patted female bottoms to get attention. He definitely did get attention and was discharged from both programs with dispatch. The administrator at Baxter and I had a falling out about the way he expelled Owen. He apparently thought I was an unreasonable parent. I thought he was uncaring.

1978–1980: Owen from Eighteen to Twenty

After the joint expulsions I spent weeks scouring Maine, searching for a combination residential/day program for Owen, but found that appropriate programs had waiting lists and available placements weren't appropriate. State agencies were of little help. At home everyone got on everyone else's nerves; then, just in the nick of time, a private educational consultant located a small combination home/school called Seven Elms on a farm in a rural section of Maine. Only two students were enrolled when Owen arrived, but the population eventually swelled to twelve. Owen made great strides during his two-year stay there. Again an inspired teacher made the difference. Owen opened up and tried to communicate. He appeared happier than he had been in years, especially when he helped with farm chores and became involved with outdoor activity. The emphasis on pure academics that had been so much a part of his former schooling was replaced by a realistic, balanced program. We, as his parents, became very involved: we started a parents' support group, wrote and published a parents' newsletter, helped organize parents' work days at the school, etc. Everything was going well. Our local school system was extremely helpful and supportive of our experience at Seven Elms and in all our relationships while Owen was within its jurisdiction.

1980: Owen at Twenty

For reasons never specifically disclosed to the parents, Seven Elms was shut down with practically no notice by a state agency. I tried to help the proprietor defend herself in the courts, but time and expense wore us down. With no school, Owen was home for six weeks, and our family structure almost buckled under the impact of his crazy behavior. Finally, in desperation, we tried a respite home. It and a brief work experience for Owen at another sheltered workshop helped us maintain our family's collective mental health.

1980–1986: Owen from Twenty to Twenty-six

We had exhausted state-agency help in our search for a suitable placement for Owen. Through a girlhood friend of Mary's, we heard of a marvelous institution for handicapped people in Kentucky. It was, and is, our dream come true. Owen is happy. Stewart Home School, located on a lovely rolling campus, is staffed by people who obviously have affection for the residents. We no longer have to hide Owen's bag the night before he returns to school. As a matter of fact, after a week or so at home, he's usually bored with us and wants to get back to his friends. Owen's problems remain the same. A biopsy has been performed on his colon in an unsuccessful attempt to diagnose his digestive problem.

1987: Owen at Twenty-seven

Mary and I have finally become reconciled to the fact that there will be no more improvement in any of Owen's problems. As a result, we have adjusted our goals and are content if he is well cared for. But as grandchildren have begun to appear, we are reminded of the indefiniteness of Owen's diagnosis, and the focus of our attention has shifted from concern for him to concern for the other children and their children yet unborn. What if Owen's problems were hereditary after all? We have undergone genetic counseling, and preliminary findings indicate that rubella may not have been responsible for his birth defects. A recently discovered chromosomal condition called fragile X syndrome was also suggested as a possibility, but after a series of complex tests and a long wait, the results proved negative. Owen continues to remain a sometimes happy, sometimes sad, puzzle to all of us. We may have to reconcile ourselves to the fact that he's just "not clinically comprehensible."

1988–1989: Owen from Twenty-seven to Thirty

Just when all our children seem to be doing smashingly well and Mary and I have begun to think about trips with Elderhostel and sleeping late on the weekends, we receive a phone call from Stewart Home. Owen's bowel-control/soiling problem is getting worse, and the staff at his sheltered workshop are near the end of their collective rope. We know what they mean. We can only hope that this will turn out to be just one more alarm and that it, too, shall pass. We ask for another examination by a specialist in digestive disorders. The thought of having Owie home with us on an ongoing basis as Mary and I launch into our golden years is sobering. This characteristic, ongoing tentativeness and lack of closure is typical of the lives of many parents of severely handicapped children. What it boils down to is that, as long as the three of us live, our fortunes are tied inextricably to one another.

PART ONE

"Where shall I begin, your Majesty?" he asked.
"Begin at the beginning," the king said gravely,
"and go on till you come to the end: then stop."
LEWIS CARROLL, *Alice in Wonderland*

Before: From Family Planning to Birth

Prologue

From Owen's Mother

Although this story is told by my husband, as Owen's mother I know better than Chuck how it all began. He and I always wanted to have a large family. Chuck was an only child and had often felt alone and isolated. I, on the other hand, although the youngest of three, was never close to my brother and sister. Chuck and I both felt that having a lot of kids close together would bring us the best of all possible worlds.

When I found I was pregnant with child number 5, I was pleased, but pregnancy was getting to be routine, so I decided to wait a while before telling the other children or even going to see my obstetrician. As in most families with many small children, someone always seems to be sick, and our family doctor, Ike LeFevre, was a regular visitor to our rural home. (In time he became a close friend.) When Martha came down with German measles, it seemed to be just another in a string of childhood diseases, but when Ike, who had come to check her high temperature, finished his examination and was about to leave, he turned at the door and asked if there was any chance I might be pregnant.

I don't remember any feeling of foreboding or alarm at Ike's question, but I was embarrassed to have to tell him I was more than three months along with our next child and hadn't yet been to his office. He chuckled and congratulated me but said that, although we shouldn't worry, German measles could cause problems. He prescribed large doses of gamma globulin. With earlier pregnancies we had been concerned about our Rh blood incompatibilities and nothing had ever come of that, so I dutifully went each month for my gamma globulin shots and thought no more about it. I had complete faith in modern medicine and in my own good luck and invincibility.

Owen was born on a cold January day. It was another easy delivery for me, so easy in fact that I almost didn't make it to the hospital. The nurses didn't even have time to "prep" me before I was wheeled into the delivery room for the final pushing stages of another miraculous natural childbirth. Owen was a handsome, chubby, healthy baby.

Owen was the first of my children I didn't breast feed. With four other youngsters to care for, we had hired a live-in nurse to help out for the first six months. I decided she could get up in the middle of the night to feed him his bottle, and for a change I would get some sleep. I did go through a bit of a "guilt trip," but Owen thrived on his bottle and grew fat and happy. He was good natured, forever smiling and gurgling joyful baby sounds. I was so busy tending all five children that I was relieved and delighted to have such a passive and cooperative addition to our family. I remember saying to envious friends, "Owen is a perfect fifth child. He *has* to be good: I don't have time for a difficult baby." I could pop him into his playpen after breakfast and he would stay there contentedly all morning, watching the action swirling about him, even falling asleep for short naps.

The fact that Owen was slow to crawl or to pull himself up to his feet never bothered me. I was happy not to have to chase him around the house or to worry about his falling down the stairs. The other children loved to push him around in his stroller. They would race up and down the driveway with Owen, and he would laugh with joy. There were many arms willing to hold and rock and carry this smiling child. I didn't worry that he wasn't getting about under his own power; he was just lazy, that was all, and it was easier to let others do everything for him.

When I took Owen for his one-year checkup, it was a terrible shock to see a look of puzzlement and concern come over Ike's face; I was so accustomed to see him smile and kid me about my healthy, growing family. He said he was worried about Owen's slow reflexes and his inability to hold himself upright. Ike urged us to see a pediatrician for a more comprehensive examination and sophisticated testing. With fear and trepidation we made an appointment with a doctor in town, who, after a brief examination, abruptly told us we had a "seriously retarded son."

I was holding Owen in my lap; when I heard the doctor's words my arms tightened about my baby's body as if to shut the world out. I listened to the doctor's suggestions for future tests, but my mind went blank and my heart welled with an overpowering sense of love and a desperate need to protect my little boy from the words I was hearing. I almost ran as we left the office, and once in the car I burst into uncharacteristic tears. How could that awful man tell us Owen was retarded? Anyone with eyes in his head or any sense at all could see that my beautiful child was perfectly normal.

And so it began—anger, denial, fear, but most of all, fierce love. It has been this fierce, sometimes unreasoning love that has carried us through the many years since Owen.

1

What Causes Birth Defects?

Alice eventually awoke and left Lewis Carroll's topsy-turvy Wonderland behind. Other children, like our son Owen, aren't so fortunate. As many as 4 percent of all pregnancies result in children with severe birth defects, while abnormalities of some nature occur in more than 7 percent. Each year more than 250,000 American babies are born with physical or mental problems of varying severity. Did you know that, on average, 30 percent or more of the children in pediatric hospitals are there for conditions wholly or partly genetic in origin? Did you know that there are approximately 3,000 hereditary disorders? Such statistics are particularly important if you are part of them—and you may be. Again, being a statistic, like being unique, is no honor.

However, it is important to keep things in perspective, to remember that only a small percentage of newborn children suffer from a genetic disease, a major birth defect, or mental retardation. The overwhelming majority are born sound and healthy. Yet, since percentages and chance are central to the understanding of genetics, it is equally important to be wary of any figures quoted. The *probability* of something happening has significance to an individual only to the extent that he understands exactly what mathematical probability means. The same mathematical considerations govern probability in a Gallup Poll and in a poker game, but its consequences assume a life-or-death significance when it is used as the basis for family-planning decisions.

In recent years science has made remarkable progress in solving the mysteries surrounding birth defects, but much remains to be learned; for example, our son's problem is still a mystery. Today prospective parents can obtain information not dreamed of a generation ago—information about prenatal development and the cause, detection, and probability of a particular problem's being present at birth. As more knowledge is gained, increasingly effective methods are being developed either to eliminate these problems entirely or to reduce their severity. But this new knowledge carries with it a serious responsibility for the modern parent: an obligation to take advantage of it and to use it wisely.

The central point is to keep yourself informed. The subject of genetics is complex; knowledge is expanding every day, and questions involving governmental intervention, human rights, and religious beliefs further complicate the situation. By itself knowledge will not set handicapped persons free or make them normal, but ignorance or complete dependence upon the judgment of others will often lead to frustration and sometimes despair. Truth (or information or knowledge—whatever you call it) is worth working and fighting for.

This section is written not only for those parents who already have a handicapped child and who are considering expanding their family but also for those with a higher-than-average risk of bearing a child with a birth defect. There are many: the older mother, the couple with a high-risk ethnic background or a genetic problem somewhere in their family background, the pregnant teenager, and the mother with a health problem, such as hyperthyroidism, hypothyroidism, phenylketonuria, diabetes, galactosemia, or a sexually transmitted disease. The father over fifty may be a candidate, too. Information on heredity is also vital for siblings of handicapped children once they, too, reach childbearing age.

Birth abnormalities are often the result of not a single cause but a combination of factors that influence one another. For our purposes, birth abnormalities can be viewed as the result of three general influences and their interaction: heredity (what is inherited from our ancestors), the maternal environment (the mother's condition during pregnancy), the overall environment (factors from the outside world), and a combination of heredity and the environment.

What Is Heredity?

When birth defects are discussed, heredity is often the first culprit blamed. Included in this broad term are characteristics passed on to the child at conception by the father through his sperm or by the mother through her egg. Indeed, the tendency toward certain disorders can be inherited in somewhat the same way that we inherit other physical characteristics. It's not important here to examine the details of this marvelously complicated biological process, but if you are to evaluate your own situation, a general understanding is helpful.

A few basic terms lay the groundwork:

- **Genetic:** Hereditary or inherited.
- **Birth defect** or **congenital disorder:** An abnormal physical or mental condition present at birth that may or may not be hereditary in origin.

- **Birth injury** or **birth accident:** An injury that occurs at birth and is not hereditary.

A congenital problem, even if hereditary, will not *necessarily* be passed on to one's descendants. That potential depends upon the nature of the problem. Some will; some won't.

The human body is made up of billions of cells. Each cell contains *chromosomes*, which are inherited from parents and determine in the most minute detail exactly what characteristics a body has. The chromosomes are messengers linking generations together. Chromosomes are made of thousands of tiny subunits, called *genes*, which actually do the work of passing on characteristics from parents to offspring.

Ordinary human cells contain a total of forty-six different gene-carrying chromosomes arranged in twenty-three pairs. Each pair of chromosomes contains one chromosome contributed by the father and one from the mother. Twenty-two of these pairs are called autosomal chromosomes. The two chromosomes making up the twenty-third pair are called the sex chromosomes because they determine, among other things, the sex of the individual. For identification purposes a female's two sex chromosomes are each labeled X; a male has one X and one Y.

Most traits are the result of the interaction of many pairs of genes, with half of each pair received from one parent and half from the other, but for some traits only a single pair of genes is involved. (I'm using the term *traits* fairly loosely here. I mean visible or functional characteristics of an individual.) The good news is that most of our millions of genes miraculously work in a perfectly normal fashion. The bad news is that a few are always abnormal. Every one of us—your boss, Miss America, the president of the United States—carries some "faulty" genes. It is impossible to say how many. Some experts estimate four to eight. Fortunately, in most cases, these abnormal genes are harmless and we are never aware that they exist. (Actually, when you consider it, it's remarkable that so many people are born *without* defects, not that a relatively small percentage have problems. Even in our family, we had five healthy, normal children.)

Dominant Genes

Some genes are called *dominant*, meaning that one gene in a given pair takes precedence. Many dominant genes and the traits they pass on are harmless, such as the ability to roll your tongue into a U shape (see who can do it sometime at a party) or having a cleft chin, like the actors Kirk Douglas and Cary Grant. However, some dominant genes can be destructive, since they cause a disease. The parent having one of these rare destructive dominant genes will, according to the laws of probability, on average, pass the disease it causes to half of his or her children, regardless of the sex of the child—a 50 percent probability of trouble. The other 50 percent of the time, fortunately, the child will receive the harmless gene.

Be careful how you interpret these odds. A 50/50 risk does not mean that, if your first baby is born with the defect carried by a dominant gene, your next child will necessarily be free of the disability, any more than, after flipping a coin and watching it fall heads, you can be sure that the next toss will come up tails. The second child conceived in such a family, like the second toss of the coin, will still have a 50/50 chance of falling one way or the other—not having or having the disease. Professionals put it this way: "Chance has no memory."

Hundreds of diseases, most of them rare, are known or suspected to be caused by dominant genes. They are called *autosomal dominant disorders*. Some examples are:

- **Achondroplasia:** A bone disorder causing a form of dwarfism.
- **Marfan syndrome:**[1] A disease affecting the skeleton, heart, and other tissues. (Abraham Lincoln may have had this disease.)
- **Huntington disease:** Progressive degeneration of the nervous system. (Woody Guthrie had it.)
- **Noonan syndrome:** A syndrome often characterized by short stature, congenital heart defect, and mental retardation.
- **Polydactylism:** Extra fingers and/or toes.

Recessive Genes

Some genes are called *recessive*, meaning that *both* genes in a given pair have to carry instructions for the same trait in order to cause the person to be affected. Such recessive genes can cause a variety of conditions, which are called *autosomal recessive disorders*. In such disorders, a parent, either a mother or a father, who has a potentially dangerous recessive gene would not actually have contracted the disease or even necessarily know that the gene is in his or her body if the *other* gene of the pair is normal. In this case, he or she is what is called a *carrier* (he or she carries the potential to pass on the disease to the next generation). Thus the gene causes no trouble for the carrier; however, if the person's spouse also carries a similar recessive gene transmitting the *same* disease, in each pregnancy there is a 25 percent likelihood that their baby will actually have the disease, a 50 percent likelihood that it will be only a carrier, and a 25 percent chance that it will be completely normal.

1. Until recently, syndromes named for individuals used the possessive, i.e., "Marfan's syndrome" and "Down's syndrome." Current practice is to eliminate the possessive; hence "Marfan syndrome."

In summary, if an abnormal gene inherited from either parent is dominant, then the child who receives that gene will definitely be affected in some way, no matter what kind of matching gene is inherited from his other parent. On the other hand, for a person to actually have a trait or disease carried by a recessive gene, both genes in his body that control that characteristic must be abnormal. An individual who has only one recessive abnormal gene is a carrier; a carrier will not have the disease and will appear perfectly normal, but two carriers may pass the disease on to some of their children if they carry the same recessive gene.

Some autosomal recessive disorders are:

- **Cystic fibrosis:** A serious and common disease that significantly shortens life due to its respiratory and digestive complications.
- **Phenylketonuria** (commonly called PKU): Deficiency of an essential liver enzyme, which, if untreated, can lead to mental retardation.
- **Sickle-cell anemia:** A disorder of the red blood cells that primarily affects blacks.
- **Tay-Sachs disease:** A condition that causes fatal brain damage.

These disorders illustrate an important concept in genetics: a child's condition can be genetic even if the disease has never before been obvious in the family of either father or mother. Think of it this way: If one of your ancestors was a carrier of PKU and married another carrier, there was a 25 percent risk in each pregnancy that their child would have PKU. However, the chance, in the first place, that a PKU carrier would happen to marry another PKU carrier is only 1 in 60, and many generations could easily pass without this happening. The first case of PKU in such a family would be completely unexpected and could be incorrectly viewed as nonhereditary if no one realized that for generations the gene for the disease was being silently carried forward. In addition, an individual can inherit a disease that no one knew the family was carrying because all the ancestors who suffered from the disease exhibited unusually mild, and therefore unrecognized, symptoms. This individual might incorrectly believe himself to be the first in the family to have the disease and have no concern that future generations of his family will be at risk for the problem.

X-Linked Inheritance

Genetic defects may be passed on by women to their sons only through so-called X-linked recessive inheritance (not to be confused with sexually transmitted diseases, which are discussed later in this chapter). For example, sometimes a mother will have a faulty gene on one of her X chromosomes (remember, normal women have two X chromosomes). When this happens, each of her sons will run a 50/50 risk of inheriting that faulty gene and manifesting (showing the characteristics of) the disorder carried by that gene. Each daughter has a 50/50 chance of being a carrier like her mother and is usually not affected by the disease, but she may pass it on to her sons. No father-to-son transmission is possible for X-linked defects, since a father gives his sons a Y and almost never an X chromosome. Some disorders passed on in this fashion are:

- **Hemophilia:** A defect in the blood-clotting mechanism.
- **Muscular dystrophy** (some forms): A weakness and wasting away of muscles.
- **Color blindness.**

Fragile X syndrome is a condition that has been only recently identified. In it, an abnormal X chromosome can result in varying degrees of mental retardation. (It is called "fragile" X because of the tendency of the arm of the X chromosome to break.) This syndrome is more commonly found in males, although females sometimes show milder symptoms, and it is often found in families, where there can be several affected males. It probably accounts for a significant percentage of heretofore undiagnosed cases of mental retardation and autism. Indeed, something like one in every 1,200 males has fragile X syndrome. Although the affected male's physical appearance is apt to be generally normal, prominent ears, a high forehead, and enlarged testicles are typical of some cases. Much remains to be learned about this disorder. Although it clearly involves the X chromosome, geneticists do not yet know exactly how it is inherited. We were concerned that fragile X might be the cause of Owen's problem, particularly since we have three daughters, whose children might then have also been affected.

Chromosomes

Unfortunately, chromosomes are no more perfect than any other part of the human body, and a variety of errors can occur in the complicated process of their formation. How the error occurs can determine whether that error will be limited to a single individual and his offspring or whether it will affect his siblings and their offspring as well. While there are several ways that an error may occur, only the two most common patterns are discussed here.

The first pattern occurs when a parent with normal chromosomes produces a sperm or egg that for some reason contains a chromosomal abnormality. This occurrence is called a *mutation*. (Although not much is known yet about how or why mutations occur, chance, radiation, and the action of certain chemicals are known to be among the culprits.) The child formed by the changed sperm or egg will be affected and will have a significant chance of passing on the mutation (harmful or not) if he has any children. However, the chance that his parents will have another similarly "abnormal" child is usually quite small, since the abnormality was caused by an accident and the chance that the same accident will recur is slight.

In the second pattern, one parent, the mother or the father, already has a chromosomal abnormality as part of his genetic makeup and may pass it or a related abnormality on to a descendant. The hereditary picture can be complicated by the fact that in some instances individuals can carry a chromosomal abnormality in their body and yet be unaware that they have it, since they show no symptoms in their outward appearance or ability to function adequately. They are said to have a "balanced translocation." Such individuals have substantial risk of passing on chromosomal defects of varying degrees of severity to some of their offspring, who in turn could pass them on to their descendants, and so forth. This phenomenon can cause parents who give birth to a child with a hereditary disorder to insist that there has been no chromosomal abnormality in their family, since up to that point the symptoms were hidden.

For reasons not completely understood, the possibility of a chromosomal abnormality of the first pattern increases dramatically toward the end of a woman's reproductive years. In women under thirty, less than 1 pregnancy in 1,000 results in a baby with Down syndrome, but the risk increases significantly for this syndrome and some other chromosomal errors as the woman grows older. Evidence is accumulating that older fathers (over age forty or fifty) may have an increased risk of having children with a few genetic disorders, especially autosomal dominant ones.

The following chromosomal conditions can, under certain circumstances, occur in any of the patterns described above:

- **Klinefelter syndrome:** A condition affecting males and usually characterized by infertility.
- **Cri-du-chat syndrome:** A disorder named for the catlike cry of affected infants; the symptoms also include mental retardation and a small head.
- **Trisomy 21:** The most common form of Down syndrome. It occurs because the child has three, rather than the normal two, copies of the twenty-first chromosome. Because of a characteristic slanting of the eyes, children with this condition were in the past referred to

as Mongoloid, but this is an inappropriate term and should not be used. Abnormalities often found in Down syndrome are: defects of the heart, eyes, and ears, and mental retardation from faulty brain development.

- **Trisomy 13** and **Trisomy 18:** Usually fatal conditions involving mental retardation and a variety of malformations.

The Maternal Environment

The Mother's Health

Birth defects can also be introduced through the maternal environment during pregnancy. What goes on inside the mother's body, what she eats, drinks, or smokes, the drugs and medication she takes, or a disease she may have (diabetes, for instance)[2] all can have a significant effect on her baby. The fetus is an innocent fellow-traveler, completely dependent on the mother's good sense. The entire period between conception and birth is important, but the critical first weeks, during which a baby's basic body parts are being produced, one by one in regular order, are of primary concern. The heart, the central nervous system, the limbs, the eyes, teeth, ears, and the palate are all particularly vulnerable during the first eight weeks of fetal development.

It is particularly important that mothers who may be at risk in any way be careful to learn about and faithfully follow basic good health practices suggested for all pregnant women. Suggestions for such practices are readily available in every community from an obstetrician or a public health nurse. Moderation and care are minimal precautions concerning everything that a pregnant woman introduces into her system. Certain substances commonly encountered and currently thought to be *teratogens* (agents causing birth defects) are particularly important to avoid.

Alcohol

A woman who drinks alcohol heavily during pregnancy definitely places her fetus at risk. Children of alcoholic mothers are susceptible to *fetal alcohol syndrome* (FAS), a combination of physical and mental defects, including growth deficiency, heart defects, and malformed facial features (see Resources: Disabilities: Fetal Alcohol Syndrome). Some suggest that women who consume six drinks per day (6 oz) run a

2. A diabetic mother is twice as likely to have a malformed child as a nondiabetic mother. Lewis B. Holmes, "Congenital Malformations," in *Manual of Neonatal Care,* 2d ed. (Boston: Little, Brown, 1985), p. 128.

40 percent risk that their fetus will to some extent be affected.[3] FAS is particularly dangerous because of its potential for widespread damage: there are an estimated one million alcoholic women of childbearing age in the United States today. The effect of even moderate drinking is unknown, but once again, the lesson for the pregnant woman is "Moderation in all things."

Smoking

Women who smoke heavily tend to give birth to small babies, and low birth weight is a major cause of death during the first year of life. Many doctors consider low birth weight to be in itself a birth defect, since babies of low birth weight are more apt to encounter health problems in early infancy. In addition, a significant number later experience learning problems in school. Some doctors suggest that nicotine may even deprive the fetus of adequate nutrients. Smoking is not good for the unborn child, and women should stop smoking before they become pregnant or at least should cut down during pregnancy.

Drugs

Any medicine that a pregnant woman takes "treats" her unborn baby as well as herself, but the baby's tiny, immature body may not react in the same way hers does. Unfortunately, it is not always known what drug quantities, taken over what period of time, can be harmful. Drugs, both over-the-counter and prescription, may comfort the mother but they may also interrupt her unborn baby's development. A woman must be sure that the doctor who prescribes for her knows that she is or may be pregnant.

Aspirin and other pain relievers used occasionally in early pregnancy should not be harmful, but frequent use later in pregnancy may disrupt a baby's blood-clotting mechanism and/or cause bleeding problems for the mother at delivery. Heavy use of aspirin may even delay the normal labor process.

What about antibiotics? Like alcohol, these infection-fighting drugs cross the placenta quickly and can affect the unborn child. Actually, some new medical techniques purposely introduce drugs into a mother's system to treat the fetus. On the other hand, drugs carelessly used by the mother or prescribed by a doctor ignorant of a woman's pregnancy may damage the fetus. Tetracycline, for example, may result in discoloration of the child's permanent teeth and affect bone growth,

3. John W. Larsen, Jr., and Karen Greendale, "Teratology," *American College of Obstetricians and Gynecologists* (ACOG), Technical Bulletin no. 84 (Feb. 1985): p. 494, Table 1.

and some sulfa drugs taken late in pregnancy might disturb the baby's liver function.

Like prescription drugs, vitamins should not be taken except as prescribed by a medical caregiver, for under certain conditions excessive vitamin use can harm the unborn baby. The only nutrients that are often inadequately furnished by a normal diet during pregnancy are iron and folic acid.

Narcotics, hallucinogens, cocaine, and amphetamines, as well as drugs that cause physical addiction and lead to psychological dependence, can, as you would expect, have a devastating effect on both mother and unborn child. For example, heroin use in pregnancy may cause the baby to undergo withdrawal symptoms soon after birth. Even if scientists can't yet evaluate the full effect of drugs on the unborn, a pregnant woman should, without question, for her baby's sake if not her own, avoid every street drug.

Sexually Transmitted Diseases

Sexually transmitted diseases (STDs), which include gonorrhea, syphilis, herpes, and Chlamydia, are examples of the potential for harm that an unfavorable maternal environment can exert. For example, gonorrhea and Chlamydia can lead to sterility in both mother and father and can cause a serious eye infection in the newborn that can lead to blindness if untreated. (Because of this danger, babies born in hospitals today receive eyedrops soon after birth to prevent this infection.) A pregnant woman suffering from active herpes can transmit the disease to her baby during delivery, causing severe infection and physical and/ or mental damage. (Caesarean sections are sometimes performed in this case to bypass the birth canal and avoid infection.) If a baby is infected with syphilis in the womb, he will enter the world with a congenital case of the disease.

Although presently there are no vaccines against STDs, they can be prevented. Even if contracted, most STDs can often be cured by early treatment, but positive action must be taken to protect both mother and baby. If you believe you have an STD or have been exposed to someone who has, see a doctor! Don't take chances, and don't try to treat yourself. You are taking an unnecessary risk for both yourself and your child.

Little is known about AIDS and nothing I know to say is helpful. The fact is that infected infants are being born today in ever-increasing numbers; if the trend continues, within 5 years the AIDS virus will be the leading infectious cause of mental retardation and brain damage in newborns. Currently there is no cure for AIDS. All we know is that parents who have consistently practiced safe sex and who have not used contaminated hypodermic needles are at far less risk of having infected children than those who haven't.

The Influence of the Outside World

Another potentially dangerous influence, the larger environment beyond the mother, can act in unknown ways, often with unexpected consequences. It's difficult, sometimes impossible, to avoid its effects, a fact that is particularly significant for the pregnant woman, since these negative influences can have a much more serious effect upon her unborn child than upon her own system. She can control her use of alcohol, drugs, or nicotine; outside forces, however, can harm her fetus without her knowledge or active participation, with devastating results.

Infections

Like sexually transmitted diseases, other infections contracted by the mother during pregnancy can be important causes of birth defects. A significant percentage of all mental retardation can be traced to infectious diseases. Perhaps the classic example is rubella (German measles). Although we still don't know for sure what part, if any, rubella played in creating Owen's multiple disabilities, we do know that it can have a disastrous effect upon a fetus. Maternal rubella can cause severe defects in the fetal heart, eyes, brain, and ears, leaving the child both physically and mentally disabled.[4]

Other infections that attack the mother can also harm the fetus. For example, a viral infection called cytomegalovirus is also a cause of birth defects and/or mental retardation. As is true for rubella, the mother usually suffers only misleadingly mild symptoms. In the child, however, mental retardation, eye defects, and infection of the heart, liver, and other organs may occur separately or together. Fortunately, blood tests are now available to determine if a woman is susceptible to cytomegalovirus, and a vaccine is being developed.

Similarly, an infection called toxoplasmosis can damage an unborn baby's brain and eyes and cause mental retardation. Mothers can

4. I have included rubella and similar viruses with environmental forces, although an argument can be made to group them with the maternal influences. Today, there is an immunization available that will eliminate the possibility of a woman's bearing a rubella child. If a woman never received a rubella shot as a child, or can't remember whether she did or not, she should consult a doctor before contemplating pregnancy so that steps can be taken to protect both her and any future children she might have.

pick up this disease from cat feces or undercooked meat and may have an unnoticeable, mild infection. To avoid toxoplasmosis, a pregnant woman must wash her hands after handling the family cat, have someone else empty the cat's litter box, and eat only thoroughly cooked meat.

It is only common sense that a pregnant woman, as part of ordinary prenatal health practices, should protect her baby by protecting herself from disease and possible contagion. The best precaution is for the mother to discuss with her doctor her own particular situation and local conditions at the time of pregnancy and to follow his advice.

Radiation

The average person is most frequently exposed to radiation (X-rays) in diagnostic procedures. It has long been known that radiation exposure early in pregnancy can lead to serious abnormalities of the fetus, including bone defects, small head (microcephaly), and retardation. In spite of popular belief, the relatively small amounts of radiation involved in routine diagnostic procedures, such as chest X-rays, have not been shown to cause abnormalities in the fetus. Nonetheless, to be prudent, a woman should advise her doctor, dentist, and X-ray technologist if she thinks she may be pregnant, and, if feasible, she should postpone any X-rays until after her child is born.

Some jobs may involve repetitive exposure to small amounts of radiation. Women who believe they are pregnant should meticulously follow applicable job safety guidelines.

Chemicals

Much less is known about the possible genetic threat posed by the thousands of chemicals used in modern society. Various chemical wastes and pesticides can cause birth defects in laboratory animals, although such effects usually result from a much higher exposure than is common in the environment. Only a few pollutants, including PCBs and methyl mercury, have been shown to cause birth defects in humans, but there is concern that in some instances humans may be more vulnerable than the animals used in testing chemicals. Furthermore, it is difficult to link defects to specific pollutants with certainty, since other variables are almost always present to influence the outcome of a pregnancy.

Cerebral Palsy

Another problem that may have serious consequences for the affected child is cerebral palsy (CP), which may be caused by lack of oxygen during the birth process itself.

Heredity and the Environment

As noted earlier, few birth defects can be attributed to a single cause. The majority are thought to be the result of a combination of environmental forces (including the mother's health) and heredity. The severity of their effect will depend upon inherited susceptibility, the stage of the pregnancy at exposure, and the degree of environmental hazard. Some geneticists have estimated that approximately 20 percent of birth defects are caused by abnormal genes, 10 percent by faulty chromosomes, and 20 percent by environmental factors. That leaves a whopping 50 percent that are thought to result from unknown forces or from the interaction between environmental and genetic factors. While figures vary widely, there is agreement that the specific causes of a significant percentage of birth defects remain unknown.

The Interaction of Genes and the Environment

Some genetic problems occur as the result of an interaction among large numbers of genes (polygenic disorders) or between genes and environmental factors (multifactorial disorders). How environmental factors can influence our genes is not always well understood, but there is obviously a connection between many common diseases and geographic, economic, and social conditions. Some birth defects are more common at certain times of year and occur more frequently in specific countries. The incidence of spina bifida, for instance, is dramatically higher in some countries than in others.

The numbers of birth defects caused by multifactorial conditions are not yet known. Some such conditions are:

- cleft lip and/or palate
- congenital dislocation of the hip
- spina bifida—incomplete closure of the spinal column
- pyloric stenosis—narrowed opening from the stomach into the small intestine.

Much is still to be learned, but it is reassuring to know that the probability of recurrence of these disorders within the same family is reasonably low. However, there is an eightfold increase in the occurrence of open-spine defects among the first cousins of affected individuals. Research may eventually explain these occurrences, but communication within a family about any history of birth defects can be vitally important to other family members.

Another important condition in which heredity plays some role is epilepsy. While the exact cause of most cases of epilepsy is still unknown, fortunately most children who have epilepsy can be given medication or treatment and will lead fruitful and happy lives.

Rh Blood Condition

Rh blood condition, in which differing parental blood types create problems, was a cause for alarm in all of my wife's pregnancies. It is an example of potentially dangerous interaction of maternal and other factors, including:

- The blood characteristics of both parents. (Problems can occur when the father is Rh positive and the mother is Rh negative.)
- The reaction of the mother's immune system. (If she is Rh negative, she may develop antibodies in her blood that can destroy the red blood cells of future Rh-positive babies.)
- The order of the pregnancy. (Is this the first? Second? Third? The likelihood of problems increases with each pregnancy. Owen was our fifth child, but prenatal tests indicated no problems.)

In Owen's case, since his patchwork quilt of defects includes only a few characteristics of the typical rubella child, it is possible that hereditary or environmental forces combined with the disease, or that the Rh blood problems interacted with rubella to create his uniqueness, or, what is even more likely, that some completely unknown factor was involved. The interaction of the environment with heredity is perhaps the area in birth defects where the least is now known and where the most should be learned in the years ahead.

2
Genetic Counseling

How much knowledge of genetics should you seek? Parents who know something about their genetic background have a better chance of avoiding or alleviating certain serious medical problems. You may drive your doctor batty with questions, but that's better than agreeable ignorance. In the past, patients and their families were expected to leave matters entirely in their doctors' hands. Today, doctors know more than ever before and have available the most sophisticated techniques imaginable to alleviate illnesses, and patients can get more involved. Genetics is such a complex area, however, that the average general practitioner will often refer patients to another professional: either a physician with advanced training in genetics (a medical geneticist) or a nonphysician with a master's degree in genetics (a genetic counselor).

In fact, genetic counseling may be as old as medicine itself. Centuries ago, Jewish scholars, although unaware of the nature of heredity, recognized that a certain blood disease (hemophilia) followed a distinct family pattern. They dictated that if a male baby bled unusually after circumcision, any sons born later to that child's mother should not be circumcised. This is an instance of early seat-of-the-pants genetic counseling that came as the result of careful observation.

What is new about genetic counseling now is that we have options that never existed before. Utilizing the basic principles governing heredity and their knowledge of the characteristics of specific birth defects, genetic counselors can sometimes predict the probability that a certain abnormality will recur in a certain family—your family, perhaps. Every year new techniques are discovered to help couples who are planning a family to make intelligent decisions about their future. These techniques can include tests before conception or during the prenatal months to determine the presence or absence of one of a growing list of inherited defects. Sometimes, knowing that a certain defect will not occur is as important as determining that it might.

Many couples whose first child had a birth defect give up the thought of having other children of their own. Other couples hesitate to start a family because a relative has suffered some devastating disease. Depending upon the circumstances, the geneticist or genetic counselor may be able to assure such people that there is no unusual risk of recurrence at all, or advise them how to lessen their risk.

As I have said, early in her pregnancy with Owen, my wife, Mary, was exposed to rubella, which has intermittently been blamed for Owen's troubles. Genetic counseling, in its infancy at the time of Owen's birth, would have told us that rubella influences only the pregnancy concurrent with the mother's infection and not future children. It is an infection, an environmental factor, and since no change occurs in parental ova or sperm, it affects only that one pregnancy. Such knowledge would have placed our minds somewhat more at ease as we waited for our sixth and last child, Miss Mary, who was eventually born healthy and normal.

It's important to remember that even when a birth defect is diagnosed as being genetic, it does not necessarily follow that another sibling will inherit the problem or that future generations will be affected. Therefore, it's important for parents to know whether the risk that the disorder will recur is high, moderate, or negligible.

Genetic counseling, then, attempts to provide an accurate diagnosis of an existing disorder and to help the family understand the implications of the diagnosis. The objective is definitely not to make decisions for the parents, but to offer counseling that will provide background information from which the parents themselves can make informed judgments. Genetic counseling can also help parents make informed decisions about the care of a child already affected and can reinforce the family group in its efforts to cope with the typical emotional problems encountered. Since there is no immunization against hereditary disease, counseling is one of the few means of insulating the family from tragedy. Unfortunately, many who need such counseling do not receive it, often because they are unaware of its potential.

Can Genetic Counseling Help You?

If you fall into any of the following categories, you may be at risk and therefore should consider genetic counseling. (To be "at risk" is to be more susceptible to a particular condition than would normally be expected.)

- If there has been, or you think there might have been, a genetic problem in your family, or if the cause of a family member's handicap is still unknown.
- If any two relatives—your parents, children, brothers, sisters, grandparents, cousins, aunts, uncles—have the same disorder, whether you believe it's genetic or not.

- If you already have a child with a problem and you're thinking about another pregnancy.
- If you belong to an ethnic group that is considered to be at increased risk for certain genetic disorders.
- If you are a woman over thirty-five or a man over fifty and you hope to have a child.
- If you marry a close relative.
- If for *any* reason you are worried that you might have an abnormal child or grandchild, speaking with a genetic counselor can be reassuring. (Typical of such worries is a concern that you have been exposed to some harmful environmental factor.)

Some racial, religious, or national groups are particularly susceptible to certain genetic diseases (examples include sickle-cell anemia in blacks, Tay-Sachs disease in certain Jewish populations, and thalassemia in localized Italian and Greek populations). Why? Most disorders originally came into existence through genetic mutation, and once introduced into a closely knit population, they tend to remain concentrated in that population. A genetic counselor can tell you what implications, if any, your own background might have for future children.

In some cases, laboratory tests may be necessary to establish or confirm a diagnosis. They may, for example, determine the level of certain critical substances in your body fluids, or a small sample of blood may be drawn so that chromosomes can be studied.

Here are five questions that genetic counseling might answer:

- What help can you get for a child with an existing disorder, and where is the nearest source of such help?
- What may the future bring for you or for a family member with a genetic disorder? Can anything be done about it?
- Are you a carrier? Do you, or does your child or another relative have a truly genetic disease? What are the risks for future generations? (This can be a real concern for older people like Mary and me, approaching grandparenthood, who have never found out if their disabled child's condition is hereditary and are concerned about the health of future grandchildren. More people should consider genetic counseling.)
- What assistance is available if you have to make decisions about prenatal diagnosis, the use of a sperm bank, or abortion?
- Is a diagnosis of your own or your child's condition that was reached years ago when genetics was in its infancy still a correct one?

The Family Tree

What kind of information will the geneticist or counselor need before he can be of help? Basically, he must have as many facts as possible about you and your relatives. If there is an existing problem with one of your children, it's important to review the family histories of *both* father and mother.

Draw up a complete family history. The technical term is *pedigree* (yes, high-class dogs and horses have them, too). You can construct your own pedigree chart. Ask your doctor or the diagnostic center (discussed later in this chapter) where you can get a form, or the March of Dimes Birth Defects Foundation (see Resources: Associations) may have available, free of charge, a form called the "Family Health Tree," which contains a list of resources to help obtain family information. (Many of the foundation's pamphlets have been extremely helpful in the preparation of this book. Contact them to see what material is available.)

To fill in a pedigree chart, start with brothers or sisters (siblings) and parents. Be sure to include every birth and miscarriage. Note who is alive, who is dead, and what caused a death. Record any significant illnesses or disorders experienced by either the living or the dead. After you have recorded your immediate family, try to check back another generation. Account for aunts, uncles, cousins, grandparents. See how far back you can go. You may find yourself hooked on the study of families (genealogy). It can be enjoyable and enhance your local public standing, especially if you stumble on a founding father or a bootlegger in your pedigree.

Most of us are not sufficiently motivated to gather this information systematically. One helpful method is to talk to relatives. Recording such conversations can be fun (you may even develop an oral family history as a legacy for your children). Try to discover if there are any family secrets, any skeletons in the closet that could be attributable to genetic disease. If you're trying to track a particular illness, the search is easier because it is targeted, but even so, it sometimes takes some detective work. Your doctor or genetic counselor can help you, as ours did. We found the entire process easy, painless, and valuable. Once you have collected the other information mentioned in this section, don't lose it. Keep a notebook to contain all this material. Although it may not seem important to prospective parents, it is critical from the beginning to keep a record of *all* significant events that may affect your future child.

It's human nature to allow your notebook to get lost or become outdated. We did. You shouldn't. It is sometimes impossible to recapture lost information—yet recapture it you must. You will find, if worse comes to worst and your child proves to have a handicapping condition, that each succeeding doctor and every new institution will ask for identical facts and figures over and over again. (Mary and I are on a first-name basis with every quick-print operator north of the Mason-Dixon line.) Appendix A contains a suggested format for your notebook.

It may take longer than you expect to gather the sometimes sensitive information needed from relatives (who may not answer the phone if they know what you want). The ideal time to begin is before a family is planned or even before marriage, although it might tip your hand to your sweetheart's family. Faithfully kept, a family history can be a useful diagnostic tool not only in genetic counseling but also for all subsequent medical consultations. Although it may seem premature, carefully retain for future reference all information about your genetic concerns, including your family tree. Be frank about your family background. Innocent people can be hurt when a medical history is withheld or distorted. The days when a handicapped relative is the source of embarrassment or feelings of guilt should be over. One final word of advice. Some parents may avoid counseling because they fear the answers they might get. They are living in a fool's paradise. Don't!

Counseling

Locating a Genetic Counselor

Where can genetic counseling be obtained? Some counselors prefer to have patients and families referred to them by physicians or other health professionals, but many readily accept self-referred patients. There are now genetic diagnostic centers in every state, and their numbers are growing. Your logical source of information is the medical professional whom you normally consult, that is, your family doctor, pediatrician, obstetrician, gynecologist, nurse practitioner, physician's assistant, or midwife. If, however, you choose not to work through these channels, the local hospital, public health department, or nearest medical school should be able to provide information specific to your region. Help may be as close as your nearest library; it is remarkable how much information is at the fingertips of a reference librarian.

The telephone directory, especially the yellow and blue pages, is another source of helpful information about many health-related areas with which you should become familiar. Nearly all directories have a section called "Community Services Numbers" (or some similar phrase). Start there. Then look up Social Service Organizations, Health Services, Health Maintenance Services and Clinics, and particularly Genetic Counseling, Family Planning, Reproductive Health Care, Pregnancy and Counseling. In addition, most states and larger cities have a Human Services Department or, listed under the city's name, a Department of Health that can be helpful. Don't overlook such listings as the Nursing Division, Health Bureau, Hospital Service Division, and Public Health Nursing. I'm giving you many alternatives because experience has taught me that it is often necessary to try a wide range of possibilities before getting the answer you seek. Also, resources differ from one location to the next, even in the same state.

The March of Dimes is an excellent source of information and can be particularly helpful in providing information about recent developments in genetic counseling; their nearest branch office should be able to supply up-to-date information. At least two other national organizations are knowledgeable in this field:

- The National Center for Education in Maternal and Child Health. They publish some excellent materials. (See Resources: Clearinghouses.)
- The National Genetics Foundation. This organization coordinates a network of genetic counseling and treatment centers throughout the United States and Canada (see Resources: Clearinghouses). I have drawn upon some of this foundation's excellent pamphlets for background information in this book.

Before you call an organization for information, rehearse in simple words what you want to say. It usually helps to write it down, particularly if you are intimidated (as I am) by switchboard operators. Here are examples of the facts you may want to get across in such a phone conversation:

> I live in southern Illinois and am looking for information on genetic counseling. Can you give me the name of the nearest organization that might be helpful? [All states belong to one of ten regional genetic networks. Your own center should help you get advice. Ask about it.]

> Do you have any printed information you could send me explaining services your organization offers? I'm particularly interested in such topics as the cost of counseling, setting up appointments, and the exact location of centers.

Have paper and pencil ready to record answers, and always be sure to express your thanks.

The telephone is one of the primary information-gathering resources available to you; I mention it many times in various contexts throughout this book. Use it effectively. Although the specifics vary depending upon circumstances, a few general rules always apply:

- Keep dated records of all important calls; include the names of people with whom you spoke.
- Follow up all vital understandings reached in phone conversations with a confirming letter.
- Be courteous. Try to make the person on the other end a confederate, not an antagonist.
- Try to make every conversation accomplish some goal, no matter how minor.

The Genetic Counseling Interview

It's important that you go to a counseling session well prepared, not only with information about your family but also with specific questions that you want answered thought through beforehand. In addition, it's extremely important that you and your spouse go together; that you schedule a return visit some weeks later, if necessary, to re-explore all the issues, questions, and answers discussed in the first session; and that you get a written report from the counselor (retain this with your valuable papers). Selecting a genetic counselor is like choosing any specialist to work with you in a sensitive area. Be sure that you find someone in whom you have confidence, with whom you feel comfortable, and who understands your needs.

Seek a second opinion if you have a serious question about or dissatisfaction with the results of your first consultation. Never be embarrassed to seek another professional evaluation. (Suggestions for getting the most out of sessions with professionals and on obtaining a second opinion are discussed in specific chapters later in the book.)

The Costs of Genetic Counseling

Charges for genetic counseling vary from one center to another and are often based upon ability to pay (a sliding scale). If an organization happens to be engaged in research on a particular disorder, some charges may be reduced or eliminated. Some public and private third-party payers (Medicare, Blue Cross, and insurance companies, for example) will reimburse for many genetic services (ours did), and their numbers are increasing. However, concern about cost should not stop you from obtaining genetic counseling if you feel you need it. Don't hesitate to discuss finances with the organization providing services. Most will try to help you with your financial concerns (see Resources: Finances).

Read, But Read Thoughtfully

Part Three of this book deals in depth with developing your own basic reference (survival) library and offers suggestions about how specific written material may be obtained and used. However, since some parents begin their search for information early during the prenatal months when questions first begin to pop up, a few preliminary observations are in order.

Don't assume that any book or article necessarily contains material that is authoritative, up to date, and comprehensive: publication does not guarantee reliability. Read with caution and with the guidance of a competent professional, and double-check facts upon which you base important decisions. Sometimes the popular press oversimplifies a problem in its effort to cater to the interest of its readership. An article you pick up at the checkout counter of the supermarket will have a different approach to a subject from that of a professional journal, although it will probably have pictures and be easier to read. (It also may be misleading.)

It's true that "scholarly" journals are often difficult for a layperson to understand, but most scholarly articles contain what is called an *abstract*, which summarizes the findings. Read the abstract and check the date of publication. Research on handicapping conditions changes rapidly, and a ten-year-old article can easily be outdated and inadvertently misleading. Also remember that, in research, the more cases examined, the more reliable the study. Therefore, beware of conclusions drawn on the basis of a small number of cases. Finally, if you are interested in the information presented in the article, discuss it with your doctor.

3
Testing before Birth

It's important for a family genetically at risk to become aware of its situation through genetic counseling before the conception of a baby. It is equally important to learn as much as possible about the baby's development during the pregnancy. Often, genetic counseling will uncover facts that make the collection of additional information from the fetus crucial. Did you know that virtually every recognizable chromosomal abnormality can be diagnosed through prenatal testing? What procedures are currently available? When should such procedures be used? How can they be helpful? What are their limitations?

Prenatal Tests

Amniocentesis

Amniocentesis is perhaps the best-known prenatal diagnostic procedure. It is based upon analysis of the amniotic fluid (the liquid surrounding the fetus in the uterus) to determine whether the fetus has a chromosomal or other abnormality. Currently, amniocentesis is usually performed between the fifteenth and eighteenth weeks of pregnancy. Until the fifteenth week, there may not be enough amniotic fluid to support such a test; after the eighteenth week, there may not be enough time to act on the test results obtained. However, research suggests amniocentesis will soon be safely performed earlier in the pregnancy, and some medical centers are performing the test earlier. The test is usually done on an outpatient basis in a hospital with qualified staff and specialized laboratory facilities. Occasionally, the test is performed in the doctor's office.

Amniocentesis requires a relatively painless surgical procedure in which a needle is inserted through the mother's abdominal and uterine walls to extract (tap) a small amount of fluid. A special technique called ultrasound (or sonography), which utilizes sound waves to produce an image, is usually used to locate the placenta and outline the fetus to avoid damage by the needle. During the weeks after the tap, the sample of fluid, which contains cells naturally shed by the fetus during development, is examined biochemically and the fetal cells are analyzed, usually to determine if there is a chromosomal abnormality. Although the actual fluid tap takes only a few minutes, several hours are often required for the entire process, which includes taking the family's health history and the ultrasound exam. Time can be saved if you already have prepared a pedigree, as described in Chapter 2.

Chromosomal analysis of amniotic fluid is over 98 percent accurate when performed by competent laboratories. In rare instances, the results can be difficult to interpret, and the effects of certain chromosomal abnormalities difficult to predict. In a twin pregnancy it may not be possible to obtain amniotic fluid for both fetuses, and therefore the chromosomal analysis may show the results for only one twin. The best-known chromosomal disorder identified by amniocentesis is Down syndrome, but amniocentesis and related tests may also be helpful in detecting other chromosomal abnormalities, identifying such biochemical disorders as Tay-Sachs disease and beta-thalassemia, and predicting certain developmental abnormalities, such as open neural tube defects.

If the fetus has spina bifida (an opening in the spine) or anencephaly (a severe defect of the head), the amniotic fluid often contains high levels of a substance called alpha-fetoprotein (AFP), which can be identified by testing the same sample of fluid withdrawn for the chromosomal analysis. A low AFP level can be indicative of an increased risk of Down syndrome in the fetus. Another common method of testing for AFP is to measure its level in the mother's blood. This technique is known as maternal serum AFP (MSAFP) testing.

Amniocentesis is relatively safe for both the mother and the unborn child. Nevertheless, the risks involved should be considered. Approximately 1/2 percent or less of the tests may result in miscarriage or injury to the fetus. In addition, there is a 2 or 3 percent chance that such relatively mild maternal complications as cramping, bleeding, and leakage of amniotic fluid may occur. Women with Rh negative blood may need medication after the procedure to prevent Rh complications.

Although the risks involved with amniocentesis are small, only some of the women who might benefit from the testing actually take advantage of it. You might consider using the test if you fall into any of the following categories (partially drawn from the National Genetics Foundation's pamphlet *Should You Consider Amniocentesis?*):

- Pregnant women who are over thirty-five (their offspring have an increased risk of chromosomal abnormalities, so amniocentesis is frequently recommended for these "older" mothers).
- Women who already have a child with Down syndrome or some of the other chromosomal abnormalities, such as trisomy 13 or 18.

- Women who already have a child with an inherited biochemical or developmental disorder for which there is a reliable prenatal test available.
- Women who have found that both they and their husband carry a recessive gene for a disorder for which there is a prenatal test.
- Women who know that either they or their husbands are carriers of a chromosomal rearrangement.
- Women who are known to be carriers of certain serious genetic disorders that can be transmitted only from mother to son (X-linked disorders). Duchenne muscular dystrophy and hemophilia fall into this category. Although the test may not always detect the disease, it will determine the sex of the fetus. A male child has a 50 percent risk of being affected, while a female will have no risk whatsoever of having the disease.
- The Rh-sensitized mother whose husband is Rh positive.

Over 95 percent of the results of amniocentesis prove negative, that is, do not show any abnormality. Don't underestimate the value of such information, since it can spare some couples many weeks of anxious waiting. In the small percentage of cases where the fetus is found to be affected (the test is positive), parents have the option of either continuing the pregnancy or terminating it. For those who choose not to terminate the pregnancy, the test results provide families time to adjust to the difficult fact that their child will in all probability have a congenital defect and may alert the medical team to a situation in which advance preparation can benefit the newborn.

Ultrasound

Ultrasound, in addition to its use in amniocentesis, is now used for diagnostic purposes. It can produce pictures sharp enough to identify such fetal abnormalities as enlarged or missing kidneys, hydrocephalus, forms of dwarfism, spina bifida, and even some types of congenital heart disease. The determination of the amount of amniotic fluid present in the sac can also be important.

Although there have been no indications to date that ultrasound adversely affects either mother or fetus, it is recommended that the procedure be used only for specific medical reasons.

Chorionic Villus Biopsy

A technique called chorionic villus biopsy (CVB) or chorionic villus sampling (CVS) is being developed to obtain a biopsy of the placenta. It offers the possibility of obtaining, early in the pregnancy (usually by nine or ten weeks), information that is critical (such as the fetus's chromosomal pattern), particularly if a therapeutic abortion is to be considered. This procedure offers many advantages but is currently available in relatively few locations, can be expensive, does not obtain any amniotic fluid for use in other tests, and may pose a greater risk to the fetus than does amniocentesis.

In some as yet rare instances, it is possible to treat the fetus before birth. Already disturbances of the unborn baby's heart rhythm have been treated by giving appropriate drugs via the mother's bloodstream, and some surgical procedures have been successfully completed in utero (in the womb). Medical and surgical procedures can, with time, become more effective, and birth defects for which there is currently no remedy may in the future be treatable while the baby is still in utero. At the present time, however, such prenatal treatment is extremely limited and is applicable to only a very few types of defects.

Because of the information provided by prenatal diagnosis, important therapies can be started either at the moment of delivery or immediately after birth. For example, with spina bifida, a planned Caesarean delivery may reduce risk to the newborn. In some instances, alerted by test results, a pregnant woman can schedule her delivery at a medical center that offers sophisticated personnel or equipment unavailable at smaller institutions, thereby avoiding dangerous delays.

Be Forewarned

It's important for parents who are considering any kind of prenatal diagnosis to realize that such advance information can have profound medical, financial, emotional, and ethical implications for the entire family, since under certain circumstances its results can raise the possibility of an abortion. The decision to undergo a therapeutic abortion is difficult and should come only after much thought and perhaps discussion with physicians, relatives, and others. Specific information should be obtained from the family's doctor, lawyer, a legal aid organization, or a local family-planning service. You might consider discussing the situation with parents who are raising an affected child in order to benefit from their insights.

The risks and benefits of gaining information that can lead to the necessity for such decisions must be carefully weighed beforehand. You should ask yourselves, "Do we really want to seek this knowledge, and will we be able to cope with the difficult decisions that may be required when we're given the answers?" On the other hand, prenatal diagnostic tests have allowed many couples who are willing to consider abortion and who might not otherwise have risked having children to plan a family with almost the same confidence as other couples. Your regular health professional, public health clinic, or nearest hospital will be able to direct you to a doctor or medical center in your vicinity where such prenatal diagnostic procedures may be performed.

Legal Counsel

Although it is unlikely that parents will need a lawyer's consultation during the prenatal period, such issues as therapeutic abortion or an insurance carrier's responsibility to cover certain procedures may require an expert opinion. (Legal matters are discussed frequently throughout this book along with the problems that cause or involve them. See "Law" in the index.) Some organizations that may be able to direct you to free or reduced-cost legal aid if you qualify economically are:

- Your state's congressional delegation. Usually, a staff member will be knowledgeable about such help, particularly if the assistance is funded by federal monies.
- The law school nearest you. Often, the telephone switchboard operator, Title IX officer, or law librarian knows who in the school has such information.
- The American Bar Association or your state's or city's bar association. Occasionally these groups sponsor various types of free legal aid or know where it is available. (See Resources: Law.)
- The legal staff of such state agencies as the Department of Human Services or the Department of Mental Health and Hygiene.
- Members of local parents' support groups.
- The social worker at your local hospital.

You can usually find the phone numbers of these organizations in your telephone book, either in the white pages (e.g., University of Kansas School of Law, Cumberland Legal Aid Clinic) or in the Yellow Pages under Lawyer Referral Service. Refer to the "Community Services Numbers" section in the front of your phone book for such listings as Health and Legal Services. Although the phone-directory listings may and probably will differ across the country, all directories should provide this information one way or another.

Here is an example of what you may want to ask over the phone:

> I have a question concerning certain legal aspects of abortion, insurance carrier's responsibility, etc. [fill in others], and would like to know how I can get free or reduced-cost legal advice. Can you tell me the name of an organization or individual who can help me, and the telephone number, if possible?

Ethical Questions

Advances in medical science have remarkably increased our understanding of the causes of birth defects and provided us with some of the tools needed to combat them.

- Genetic counseling can often predict the probability that certain parents may have children with birth defects.
- Screening tests are able, in some instances, to identify parents who may be carriers of certain genetic disorders.
- Many birth defects can be diagnosed prenatally.
- In an increasing number of cases it is now possible to lessen the severity of or correct unfavorable conditions while the baby is still in the womb.
- It is possible, through the control of maternal health, to decrease a child's risk of having a birth defect or congenital disease.

Like the fruit of the tree of knowledge in the Garden of Eden, however, these developments and their consequences pose complex moral issues. Is abortion justified to save a child from a life of pain and indignity, parents from the sometimes crushing burden of caring for the handicapped child, or society from the often excessive costs of institutionalization? Should adverse genetic factors influence a person's choice of a mate? Do doctors have a moral obligation to tell patients about the potential of prenatal diagnosis? Should they be legally required to do so? Is it desirable for the state to require postnatal screening (for sickle-cell anemia, for example)? Should parents who are known carriers of a disease decide not to have children, or should they consider using a sperm bank or some other form of conception? For example, utilizing techniques currently available, we could virtually eliminate a disease like Tay-Sachs: Is society willing to pay the price?

The heart of many of these issues lies in the relationship of the individual to society. What responsibility, if any, does a parent of a handicapped child have to society in caring for that child, and what reciprocal responsibility does society have to participate in that care? Even the decision to seek genetic counseling involves a moral judgment.

It is not the province of this book to make moral judgments. However, these ethical questions are facts of today's world, and parents and those concerned about the handicapped population have to wrestle with them if they are to make informed decisions about the prenatal options discussed in this chapter. Both as parents and as citizens, we must remember not to ask a question unless we are prepared for the answer.

Dos and Don'ts
for Parents Potentially At Risk

(Some of these guidelines apply to both parents, others specifically to the mother.)

1. *Learn all you can about birth defects, both how they are caused and how they might be avoided, but be sure your information is up to date and correct.*

2. *Determine if you might be at risk.*

If you believe there is any possibility, see a genetic counselor before starting a pregnancy.

3. *If you believe you are pregnant, let your professionals know.*

To protect yourself and your baby, notify all consulting doctors or dentists so that drugs and X-rays may be prescribed accordingly.

4. *When you know you are pregnant, consult a doctor immediately and regularly.*

Research has shown that women who visit their doctors infrequently tend to have babies with lower birth weights than women who have regular and frequent checkups.

5. *If you are worried, speak with the doctor.*

If you have any concern about the possibility that your unborn baby may have a problem, consider with your doctor the pros and cons of prenatal diagnosis.

6. *Be persistent when you seek information or services during the prenatal period.*

Don't be apologetic. You can usually be sure that the agency you are contacting is being paid to provide this information; they would be out of business if it weren't for you.

7. *Record keeping is vital.*

Begin keeping a notebook (see Appendix A) with all the information you can collect. Even if all goes well, as it probably will, this recorded history will be useful to you in the future in many ways.

PART TWO

How many desolate creatures on the earth
Have learnt the simple dues of fellowship and
social comfort in a hospital

ELIZABETH BROWNING

The Hospital: Sometimes It's the Best Place to Be

Prologue

Our first grandson, Peter Thomas, was born after what seemed to me to be an extremely long labor. But Mary, the new grandmother and my live-in consultant on matters obstetrical, informed me that fourteen hours "wasn't long at all for a first pregnancy." It just seemed long to me, since I had been abandoned at home sitting by the telephone with our dog, Piper, waiting for news.

Our daughter Martha, a single parent, had chosen natural childbirth with a midwife. She used the birthing room at the hospital, with all its equipment, and an obstetrician was close by to offer help if necessary. The birth was "routine," Mary assured me, although our new grandson Peter had progressed through the involved process "sunny side up," which had caused the back of his head to be molded by the birthing canal into what seemed to me to be a very unusual looking cylindrical knob. My consultant coolly assured me not to worry, that it would shape up in a day or two, which surprisingly it did. But I remember thinking, "If this is 'routine,' I want no part of the unusual."

In comparison, the birth of our second grandson, Tom's son Bapu, made the earlier experience, cylindrical knob and all, seem a ho-hum affair. His mother had decided she wanted an even more natural childbirth—under water. No matter how one looked at it, it wasn't routine, and I looked at it from the point of view of a jittery, fifty-year-old Victorian. No hospital birthing room, no hovering covey of attendants were on tap for this youngster's entrance: He made his transition into this world submerged in the briny waters off a tiny Bahamian key chosen because of its warm waters and gently sloping white sand beach. His was one of the early underwater births, with only mother, father, and some willing but unprofessional family attendants splashing around to help out. The baby emerged wet and salty, with a well-shaped head and everything intact. (Today he swims like a fish.) Fortunately, there were no problems, unless you consider disoriented grandparents a problem.

But there's another side to this coin. Occasionally, natural processes run into trouble and require outside help. The grandson of friends of ours was born in a small community hospital in the South-east. Their family wasn't as fortunate as ours. A routine birth became an emergency when a complication in the delivery process caused some amniotic fluid to enter the baby's lungs. A Caesarean section was performed and an ambulance rushed the baby to a major medical center, where sophisticated equipment and highly trained specialists were required for his unexpected complications. His condition was eventually diagnosed as cerebral palsy. The child's life was saved, not by good fortune but by good transportation, good medicine, and quick action.

The differences among these births are profound, but one point is clear. The dividing line between a normal and an abnormal birth can be narrow, and although the birthing process is usually wonderfully natural and spontaneous, occasionally things go wrong and often without warning. When they do, you need help and you need it fast.

4

The Hospital

A hospital stay can become necessary for reasons other than the birth of your child. You may go to the hospital for tests and treatment, and the hospital may be the place where you learn there is something wrong with your child. Your visits may be frequent and prolonged, or quick, unexpected, and traumatic. Despite the tensions and worries that usually accompany our thoughts about this institution, the hospital is still the best, safest place to be at certain moments. Making the most of a hospital visit is important for all patients. It is especially so for the handicapped or chronically ill youngster, whose exposure is apt to be more frequent and complicated.

This chapter gives an overview of the hospital's buildings, labs, and offices, as well as the men and women who occupy them. It does not consider the administrative details of how and by whom hospitals are run, financed, and evaluated, except to point out that each hospital is required to have a state license to operate, to meet certain standards, and to be evaluated regularly. The patient is protected in many ways by both state and federal laws and regulations, and this section deals specifically with the rights and responsibilities of the hospital–patient relationship. It also looks at the special language and common abbreviations used and the routines, such as admissions, discharge, and billing practices, that make possible the hospital's daily operation. The goal is to make your stay both medically effective and more comfortable. The hospital is an institution, a system. It has to be highly organized and structured to operate and to fulfill its mission, but it need not be cold and impersonal.

An adult almost always feels more comfortable and functions best in a place he knows and understands. The unknown can be scary and reduce our resilience. How much more true this is in the case of a child! The best way to help a child cope with the fears associated with a dark, frightening room is to go in with him, turn on the lights, and, together, see what's there. If you can help your child understand what goes on in a hospital, the chances are he will feel more comfortable mentally and eventually do better physically than he would otherwise.

Be aware of the complex relationship between the mind and the body. A good general principle in all our dealings with the people and institutions to whose care we consign our children is to remember that medical results are invariably influenced by the attitude and receptivity of the patient. In your travels with your child, you may hear the terms *psychosomatic* or *holistic* used when speaking of this interrelationship between mind and body.[1] Remember, too, that young children almost invariably sense and assume the attitudes of their parents. Be sensitive to this relationship between mind and body. Careful planning will help maximize its potential.

Selecting a Doctor

In most instances, except in emergencies, the hospital your child will enter is determined by the health professional you select, since to practice at a particular institution and to admit patients there, the doctor must be on its staff. Therefore, when you select a doctor, you also may select a certain hospital. If you have a strong preference for one particular hospital in your area, ask your prospective physician if he practices there.

Choosing your health professional can be simple or complex, and requires different approaches depending upon circumstances. By the time it becomes necessary to choose a doctor for your child, you will probably already have established medical contacts who can offer appropriate possibilities. Your family doctor or visiting nurse should be familiar with both your needs and the local situation. Consult with one or more professionals, and be sure you are given a minimum of two alternatives. Often your network of family and friends can provide feedback and recommendations. Members of parents' support groups have a wealth of practical experience with physicians in the area and are usually eager to share their views with other parents. The final decision, however, must be yours, and to make this choice wisely, you should first decide what qualities are important to you. Other parents may have different priorities.

The medical profession has a tongue-in-cheek theory that explains how patients choose their doctors. It is sometimes called the "triple-A maxim" because it suggests that affability, availability, and pure and simple ability (in descending order of importance) are the key factors. (I

---

1. Both terms are used to describe the philosophy that considers the entire (whole) individual and not just one particular aspect. Many approaches to healing employ the holistic medicine concept, practiced by individuals with a wide range of background and training, running all the way from the licensed physician who utilizes it as an everyday part of his approach to medical practice, to individuals with neither license nor formal training.

would make it a "quadruple-A maxim" and add "affordability" to the list.) The implication is that a doctor's personality and his attitude about medicine—the characteristic once called "bedside manner"— exert a greater influence upon the patient's choice than does a doctor's professional competence. As frivolous as the theory seems on the surface, there is valuable substance beneath the humor. Serious thought about how you, yourself, view the "A's" may clarify your own thinking and help you decide which professional best meets your needs and what characteristics are important to you.

In the literal sense of the word, *affable* means "friendly," "pleasant," or "at ease." In the broadest and most positive sense, affability can promote a doctor–patient relationship in which the patient, your child, and his family feel that the physician cares about them as people and that he understands their burdens and their pain. (I deal with the patient–doctor relationship in Chapter 9. The complaint, "My child's doctor really has no idea of what we're going through; he just doesn't understand" has been a refrain running through many of my dealings with other parents. Actually, the doctor probably did have a good idea and did understand, but failed to communicate.) If a doctor's approach to his patients is of key importance to you, before beginning what may be a long-term relationship, schedule an appointment with him to get to know one another and to discuss your child. If he doesn't welcome this kind of preliminary session, that in itself may tell you something about his attitudes and priorities.

Some physicians—surprisingly enough, even some pediatricians —have difficulty relating to children. Other doctors, like some non-professionals, are not at ease with serious birth defects or chronically ill children, youngsters who can't be cured. However, there are physicians who obviously enjoy all kids and are able to communicate their affection. The parents' perception that their doctor is comfortable with handicapped children, in general, and likes their child, in particular, can positively affect a family's attitude and, I suggest, the child's chances for effective treatment.

The importance of a physician's sex is another topic for parental discussion. Some mothers feel a female doctor understands them better, particularly the workload they carry and the everyday emotional pressures they're under. This issue is significant to the extent that it matters to you. Ask yourself the question before you make the decision.

Physician "availability" can be viewed in two ways. First, some doctors, particularly surgeons, are so busy that they either are not available at all or are available only after a long waiting period. Whether the wait is worth it will depend upon your evaluation of the particular doctor in comparison with others. Availability can also mean "accessibility"—how easy it is to reach the doctor when it matters. Does he make house calls? (The currently increasing doctor surplus seems to be reinstating this practice.) Is the doctor a member of a group practice in which others may routinely cover your case? Is he so busy that appointments must be made months ahead? Will he call you to find out how your child is responding to a change in medication? The availability of a doctor should be ascertainable. A few questions put to his secretary should give an indication of the way his practice is run.

Professional ability is much more difficult to evaluate. Even professionals themselves have difficulty judging one another's competence. Because of licensing requirements, much of the evaluation of basic professional competence has already been done for you. If a doctor has passed the national boards in his area of specialization, you know that he has successfully met a test of competence. Sometimes a certain doctor will have a reputation for particular technical excellence among hospital staff or parents, but beware, such evaluations are not always objective, particularly if voiced by one or two vocal supporters. Although a physician's knowledge and technical ability are always of prime importance, they may be of controlling importance when you need specialized consultation in a highly complex and rapidly changing field. When evaluating professional ability it's prudent to rely on a health professional in whom you have confidence to suggest doctors who possess the necessary credentials. Then, you can make your final decision on the basis of the other criteria. Perhaps the inability of prospective patients to evaluate professional competence explains why we may sometimes give it lower priority in our selection process.

My own fourth "A," affordability, is important even to that portion of the public who are fortunate enough to be covered by third-party payers (insurance, Medicaid, etc.) because many doctors do not accept the fee schedules established by these organizations and patients must foot the remaining cost of their medical bill. A physician who accepts the schedule and requires no additional payment will certainly have appeal. (Practical day-to-day considerations in your dealings with your doctor are discussed in Chapter 9.)

Evaluating the Hospital

Your choice of a hospital may follow inevitably from your choice of a doctor, or you may choose a hospital before selecting a doctor. In either case, you should evaluate the hospital to be sure it meets your needs and concerns.

The Size and Location of the Hospital

In general, the smaller community hospital is more convenient for a parent, since it is by definition closer to home and may seem more friendly and less institutional. Also, it may charge less. Costs generally are related to facilities and services available, even if they are not all utilized by the patient, and large urban hospitals must provide a wider variety of facilities. Although expenses, as a result, are often higher, a major medical center might still be preferable, since the sophisticated equipment needed for diagnosis or treatment may be available only there. (One advantage of prenatal diagnosis is that the knowledge gained allows a mother to arrange her delivery at a location where appropriate help is available to face any anticipated emergency. Sometimes, however, an unanticipated birth defect occurs. This is a time when everything rests in the hands of Providence and the technical skill of your doctor or midwife. When my son Tom, miles away from any medical help, "knew" that everything would be all right in the underwater birth of his child, the chance that something unexpected would happen, that there would be a complication, was slim, but it was the chance he took. The reality of this gamble, a significant factor for the high-risk mother, should be reason enough for any vulnerable couple to ensure that qualified medical assistance be quickly available at delivery time.)

If a prospective mother or the parent of a youngster whose handicap requires specialized treatment not available locally has been in regular touch with the doctor, hospital selection will be easier. The doctor, in consultation with the parent, can make medical arrangements, but parents will still be faced with the problems involved with moving a child to a strange city while maintaining tranquility at home.

Money should not normally be a factor in hospital selection, but it is prudent when choosing your health professional to discuss candidly not only his charges but also estimated hospital costs and miscellaneous expenses. Discussing money matters can be difficult for many people, but the best time to face the facts of hospital costs and your means of handling them is before you have become involved and while you have time to plan. Prospective patients should realize that hospitals do differ in their approach to billing. For instance, in past years most not-for-profit institutions received various types of federal assistance and were obligated by statute to provide free or reduced-cost medical community service. Although most of this funding has now been eliminated, many not-for-profit hospitals still continue some form of this practice for low-income patients. Hospitals that operate for profit generally do not receive any public funding and are not under a similar obligation. Costs and conditions of billing for both profit-making and not-for-profit hospitals vary, so check your local situation.

Natural Childbirth and Home Delivery

The pregnant woman who desires natural childbirth and wishes to use a special birthing room may find it available locally at only one hospital, and in this case hospital selection may influence physician selection. It should be easy, however, for her to choose a professional from the many on that hospital's staff. Usually she chooses a doctor or midwife because she is sympathetic to, and knowledgeable about, the natural childbirth approach and has privileges in a hospital with appropriate facilities.

For a variety of reasons—some economic, some personal—a woman may decide to deliver her baby at home. Plans for a home birth, however, should be made only in consultation with a professional who is up to date on developments in the field and is aware of any reason why the woman and/or her child might be at risk. The mother-to-be should clearly understand the kinds of problems that might be involved in home delivery, such as the delay that often takes place when specialized help is needed for mother or baby in an emergency. Parents should also know which hospital they will go to in the event of a birthing crisis.

The Ideal Hospital

Although parents often have few alternatives in hospital selection, it is still important to know what attributes an "ideal" hospital would have to serve your child's needs, whether he be a newborn or an older child returning because of a chronic condition. Your hospital may not have some of these advantages. If it doesn't, ask why they aren't available. If the answer doesn't satisfy you, see if you can work with other parents and the institution to assist in making them available. Work constructively toward this goal without allowing your efforts to degenerate into an adversarial relationship that can prove counterproductive.

What makes a good hospital? If you're a hardened campaigner with a chronically ill child, you will have formed your own ideas. Here are some characteristics that can be important. Are these points important to you? Each hospital with a separate pediatric service should have the following:

- A preadmission program for the young patient and his family that provides a thoughtful yet sensitive explanation of what hospital life consists of and an opportunity to ask questions and to visit before admission.

- Arrangements for simple discharge and readmission procedures for chronically ill children.
- Health teams organized so that *one* person is responsible for all aspects of a child's care and can speak for the team.
- Flexible visiting hours: twenty-four-hour privileges for parents and siblings whenever possible as well as a rooming-in arrangement for one parent.
- Educational, emotional, and concrete support for parents and patients that sees to it that they are informed of surgical and medical procedures, that they receive help getting in touch with resources to address their needs both in the hospital and at home, and that they are put in touch with support groups if desired.
- A pediatrician on call at all times.
- A professionally staffed child life program. A child life program is the provision the hospital makes to care for the normal emotional and nonmedical aspects of a child's life during his hospital stay. The program's goal is to minimize stress and to maintain normal living patterns as much as possible. You hope staff are sensitive to the special needs of the special needs/chronically ill patient.
- A well- and creatively equipped playroom.
- Coordination with schools to provide continuing instruction while the youngster is in the hospital and planning for his re-entry into the school.[2]

Many of these points are discussed in detail later in this section.

From my own experience, gained while serving as a volunteer in a pediatric playroom, I emphasize two more criteria. In addition to the staff mentioned, the pediatric service should also be augmented by such skilled volunteers as foster grandparents, individuals who are able to spend time with sick youngsters in their parents' absence, when it is often impossible for busy professionals to be available. Second, an active social work staff should assist the parents in such matters as financial planning, coordinating the transition to home (sometimes called "discharge planning"), and parent counseling. One word of caution: Hospitals are not all alike and may do things differently. Don't get in a blue funk if you encounter new ways of doing things. Get to understand what's going on before you criticize.

Can you think of areas where you can pitch in and help fill a need —little things that could improve the hospital experience for others? For example, we all know how important it is, on occasion, for a parent

2. Some of the suggestions here are drawn from two pamphlets of the Association for the Care of Children's Health, *Your Hospital: Meeting the Special Needs of Children* (1981), and *Preparing Your Child for Repeated or Extended Hospitalizations* (1982).

to get away from her youngster and the pediatric floor, even if it's just to go down to the cafeteria for a cup of coffee. I have often seen other parents on the floor pitch in and take over respite duty for a beleaguered mom. Even more telling is the parent who acts as a surrogate parent for a sick child whose real mother or father is rarely, if ever, there. These are the kinds of things you can do to make the hospital a better place for others.

The Hospital Manual

Once you know to which hospital your youngster will be admitted, learn as much as you can about how it functions. Write or call the hospital and ask for their patients' guide. This guide, published in some form by almost every hospital and often routinely sent out to all prospective patients in a preadmission packet, is designed to offer miscellaneous information about such subjects as finances, admissions, policies, visiting hours, cafeteria use, and TV rental. In addition, many hospitals offer a guide designed especially for parents that specifically covers the pediatric department. Look over this material carefully. Consider it a preadmission homework assignment.

The Hospital Staff

Sometimes in addition to describing hospital policies and practices, a parents' manual will introduce you to the people who work there. Explaining hospital life to a child and explaining it in terms he will understand is like making sense out of an athletic contest. To understand what's going on, the child should know the jobs of the various participants, the names of their different positions on the team, and the layout of the area where the action takes place. Knowing who does what and why can make the people in their strange uniforms much less threatening. Even familiarity with little bits of hospital trivia can help your child feel more at home. For example, one hospital's brochure explains why nurses wear different caps (although more and more nurses are dispensing with caps altogether). Did you know that it's often possible to tell where a nurse did her training by the kind of cap and pin she wears? Many of the hospital staff wear uniforms or badges reflecting the jobs they do. Make a game of it. Keep track of how many different jobs you and your child can identify. You may even want to involve other kids on the floor in spotting the following people who may be involved with their care.

Doctors

A medical doctor (M.D.) is someone who has graduated from an accredited medical school. (In this book the terms *doctor* and *physician* are used interchangeably.) Don't be confused by the fact that other professionals who have achieved advanced graduate degrees like Doctor of Philosophy (Ph.D.) or Doctor of Divinity (D.D.) can also be addressed as "Doctor." (It is a good idea, however, not to let either of the latter get a hold of your gallbladder.) Graduates of schools of osteopathy (D.O.) are also licensed to practice medicine and, except in a few states, represent the same specialties as medical doctors. They, too, are addressed as "Doctor."

To simplify a complex subject, I think of medical doctors as coming in three garden varieties. First are the family doctors (general practitioners), who cover most of the general field of medicine. They give what is called primary care and are logically enough engaged in "general" practice. Some general practitioners have completed specified training and passed a national certifying examination (board). They are called family practitioners. Second are doctors, called specialists, who have specialized in one particular area of medicine. For example, a pediatrician concentrates on children's health, covering the age span from birth through late adolescence. When physicians train further in a specific aspect of their field, they become what is called a subspecialist, for example, a pediatric cardiologist. Third, there are those physicians who operate on the body. They are called surgeons, and they, too, may specialize, for example, in pediatric surgery.

No matter what their specialty, doctors have different levels of responsibility in the hospital. The attending physician is the doctor ultimately responsible for a patient's care. Often your child's private doctor will fill this role; if not, the hospital will assign a member of its staff to supervise his hospitalization. Be sure to know the name of your child's "attending" and check with him regularly; he is the final authority on your child's situation.

Working under the supervision of the attending is the "house staff," consisting of fellows, residents, and interns, all doctors still in various stages of training. (A potential source of parents' irritation is that good medical training requires the frequent rotation of staff, which interrupts the continuity of patient–doctor relationships.) Also involved in your child's care may be consulting physicians, other senior physicians whom the attending calls in for expert advice.

If your child is admitted to a large teaching hospital, which should be aware of the most recent medical developments (one of the advantages of largeness), medical students may be involved in his care. The

students are the doctors of tomorrow, and they will be closely supervised by the attending and house staff.

Since all of these people may be part of your child's "ward team,"
they will regularly visit him to check on his progress (such visits are
called "rounds"). Sometimes when your child is disturbed, perhaps
from a deep sleep, by rounds or other hospital procedures, the whole
business may seem ridiculous, with overtones of a Gilbert and Sullivan
operetta. However, these routines are required for a specific purpose—
to see that your youngster receives the careful medical supervision he
requires. Be a patient parent. There is usually good reason for the latest
apparent outrage.

Finally, a relative newcomer to the medical field is the physician's
assistant, a health-care professional who often has had prior experience
in some form of medicine and graduated from an approved collegiate
program. He can perform certain medical practices under the supervision of a physician.

Nurses

Although physicians of all varieties can be critical to your child,
often the most important professional in his life will be his nurse.

Like doctors, nurses have different levels of training. A registered
nurse (RN) must have completed an approved program of nursing education and have passed a national examination. A licensed practical
nurse (LPN) must have graduated from an approved school for practical nursing and have passed a national examination. Nurse specialists
include registered nurses who have advanced training in various medical fields, such as a nurse anesthetist, nurse clinician, nurse midwife,
and nurse practitioner. The head nurse is in charge of all nursing services in a unit (for example, on the pediatric floor). The charge nurse is
in charge of nursing activities on a particular shift. Some hospitals have
a system called primary nursing, in which every entering patient is assigned one nurse, his primary nurse, who will be responsible for his
nursing during his entire stay.

Other Staff

SOCIAL WORKERS help you and your youngster in many ways: with
family problems, finances, and arrangements for after-hospital care.
The social worker can be your key nonmedical resource person—a lo-
cater of help and a provider of support, often acting as a liaison between you and community sources of assistance. (If you have trouble
locating him, ask your nurse.) Don't hesitate to contact him with any
problems, particularly those involving personal or financial matters. If
he doesn't have the answers, he can refer you to the person who does.

Although some social workers have received no formal degrees, many have earned a Bachelor of Social Work (BSW) or a Master of Social Work (MSW) degree. A doctorate of social work is given, but you are not apt to encounter persons with DSWs or Ph.D.s in your travels.

Here are some places where you might benefit from a social worker's help: schools for your child at all levels, hospitals, public and private organizations serving handicapped people, and community health and counseling agencies. Social workers provide assistance to parents and to their children and are often skilled in obtaining help in such areas as home care, homemaking support, family and individual counseling, financial assistance and planning, residential placement, diagnostic services, and support groups.

CHAPLAINS. Many hospital staffs include one or more chaplains on either a full- or a part-time basis. Besides being of spiritual support, they can be valuable counselors and community resource specialists.

PHYSICAL THERAPISTS. In general, the physical therapist (PT) works with the large muscles, such as those involved with ambulatory skills, i.e., walking, running, operating a wheelchair, and getting from the bed to a chair. A PT also "re-educates" some muscles to take the place of others that no longer function properly.

OCCUPATIONAL THERAPISTS. Although there is some overlap with the physical therapist in the jobs they perform, the occupational therapist (OT) concentrates more on the small (fine) motor skills, such as feeding, bathing, writing, telephoning, and self-care.

DIETITIANS AND NUTRITIONISTS are professionals who supervise food preparation and service, including any special diets. (Since Owen didn't use his teeth for chewing, everything he ate had to go through a blender. The dietitian hadn't ever seen anyone like him before.)

Another key professional is the PLAY or RECREATIONAL THERAPIST, often in charge of the pediatric playroom or recreation room, who is trained in child development and the therapeutic potential involved in children's play.[3] If your hospital has a pediatric floor but no place for the youngsters to play and let off steam, perhaps you can help establish one. Be sure it's well stocked with arts and crafts, video games, records, books, and play objects.

Another person critical to your child's well-being is the WARD SECRETARY or UNIT SECRETARY (or clerk). He can be a record keeper, appointment maker, wheelchair procurer, coordinator, pacifier, and general information disseminator. (Be nice to him. He works hard and often gets little credit.)

While I have not described them in detail, other people, such as

---

3. These rooms may also be supervised by a child life worker, some other staff member, or even a trained volunteer.

respiratory therapists, pharmacists, radiologic technologists, house-keeping aides, blood drawers (phlebotomists), and volunteers can all be key to making your child's hospitalization as comfortable and worth-while as possible. Treat them all with respect.

The Facilities

The community of medical experts it gathers together is the key ingredient in making the hospital an effective organization, and it is their skill that draws us there. These professionals would have a diffi-cult task, however, if they had to function without the buildings, equip-ment, and programs that support them. Thus another reason we seek out the modern hospital for our children and pay the high costs in-volved is to take advantage of the facilities and technology that it has to offer. Here follow brief descriptions of hospital services and "bricks and mortar" facilities. Becoming familiar with them may help you in the same way that it's useful to study a map of a city before you go there.

The hospital areas you should be familiar with are:

Admission and Discharge

The admissions office is usually located near the entrance where patients check in when they first arrive. It is often part of a larger book-keeping office, which also handles discharge arrangements when pa-tients leave. If your child is subject to unexpected hospitalizations, check to see how admissions are handled during nonbusiness hours.

The Pediatric Floor or Service

The pediatric floor is the area where children are treated. There may also be specialized facilities, particularly in the larger hospitals, to care for acutely ill children. These facilities have various names depend-ing upon local practice. Parents who enter these areas to visit or care for their children are often required to wear gowns and to scrub.

The Emergency Room (ER)

If an accident was the cause of your child's handicap, the ER may have been his first exposure to the hospital. In an emergency, it's impor-tant that you get your child to the hospital nearest you. After treatment, he can be moved to another, perhaps more appropriate, institution. Al-though patients can be admitted to a hospital through its Emergency Room, all the requirements of the usual admission process must be met. Some information, however, can be furnished at a later date. When you arrive, you will speak with a nurse, who will ask questions about your child's problem. If others are waiting, she will decide the priority of his case, i.e., how soon he will be treated; this process is called *triage* and she is called a triage nurse. Be sure to explain what has happened in as much detail as possible. She may also want to know your child's blood type, the date of his most recent tetanus shot, whether he is sensitive to any drugs, and if he has any allergies. Since the patient's personal physician will almost always be involved eventually, it is best to call him if time permits before going to the hospital.

The Operating Room (OR)

The operating room is where surgery and other specialized procedures are performed. More and more minor surgery is performed in clinics and doctors' offices on an outpatient basis. If general anesthesia is required, however, an operating room is almost always necessary, as is commonly the case for the insertion of a shunt or for involved dental work, particularly with some severely mentally retarded children whose behavior must be controlled.

The Recovery Room

The recovery room is a specially equipped room where such staff as anesthesiologists and specially trained nurses watch over patients immediately after operations. Nearly all patients are taken here for a period of up to several hours. Visitors are usually not admitted.

Living Spaces

Patients' rooms are usually designed for single, double, or multiple occupancy, but if the hospital is crowded, you will have to take what is available. Otherwise you can state your preference at admission time. (Do you want as much privacy as possible, or do you welcome company? Many multiple-occupancy rooms have curtains that can be drawn.) Of course, an important consideration will be cost. Private rooms can be extremely expensive. If you plan to stay overnight with your child, be sure to inquire, preferably before admission time, how this affects room selection.

The Cafeteria

The cafeteria is the area where staff, parents, and visitors eat— usually it is not locally renowned for its nouvelle cuisine or homey decoration. Food is important to morale, and parents should pay particular attention to seeing that their own meal hours are as heartening and regular as possible. Find out the cafeteria's location and hours, when and if it is possible to take your youngster there for a change of scene, and whether food can be taken from the cafeteria to your child's room. Many pediatric floors have a snack room with a refrigerator where special food may be kept, but find out the food rules and observe them, since patients' diets must often be carefully controlled. (Chapter 13 discusses nutrition for handicapped children in detail.)

Getting the News

The news referred to in the title above is news that is difficult to talk about because it's always bad news. There are many ways that parents can learn that their child has a serious handicap. A doctor may tell you of the ominous results of a prenatal test, or a state police officer may telephone you about your teenager's automobile accident, which can mean spinal cord injury. On the other hand, the news often is broken in the hospital, and while we are looking at this institution, it seems appropriate to examine the subject briefly.

Screening Tests

Sometimes disabilities are diagnosed through screening tests. Various tests are administered at birth or shortly thereafter ("newborn screening") to determine whether a newborn has, or may have, a potentially dangerous condition. The most common test screens for phenylketonuria (PKU), an enzyme deficiency that results, if untreated, in profound mental retardation. A special diet for the baby, if begun early, can reduce or eliminate the damage. (It's particularly important that a woman who has PKU notify her physician of this fact before becoming pregnant, as special diets are now prescribed for her during pregnancy.)

Many other screening tests may be done; some are required by individual state law, others are routinely administered in certain hospitals. Tests may be done for: tyrosinemia, galactosemia, maple syrup urine disease, hypothyroidism, homocystinuria, toxoplasmosis, and sickle-cell disease.[4] These tests are administered because they can trigger quick medical action that can eliminate the problem or reduce its severity.

The Initial Diagnosis

The initial diagnosis is the moment when many of us first receive "official" word that something may be wrong with our child. (The entire diagnostic cycle is discussed in Chapter 9.) As with our son, this experience can, of course, come not at birth but long after. Undoubtedly, this is a difficult period to get through, whether the unwelcome

4. If you have questions concerning any of these screening tests, consult your doctor. Your parents' group may wish to study your state's screening requirements. If in your collective judgment they are inadequate, your state legislators could be interested in your reaction.

news concerns your newborn child or comes as the result of the evaluation of a son or daughter who has been a family member for many months or years. The heavy responsibility of informing parents of problems at birth usually falls to the pediatrician; unfortunately, sometimes this job is not done well, and parents can be overwhelmed by the shock of the message. The burden can be made more tolerable if the news is broken in an unrushed, thoughtful fashion; you should remember this and try, despite your personal dismay, to be understanding when faced with the similar responsibility of informing your family and friends.

Breaking the news to family and close friends is difficult. There is no painless way, and the responsibility will not get easier if you procrastinate. However, remember that doctors can make diagnostic mistakes, and it is neither wise nor kind to concern those near you with worries that may be premature or medically unfounded. Once you are satisfied that the diagnosis is correct, however, and you understand it, you will probably want to speak personally with or write to the grandparents and close family members. Often a relative or intimate friend can help by making some contacts where appropriate.

No matter how distraught you are, be especially thoughtful when speaking to the grandparents. Remember that your former relationship to them (in which they were protective of *you*) may have to be reversed and you will now need to be considerate and protective of them. Grandparents may find it difficult to understand or to cope. Sometimes it is helpful to describe the situation as straightforwardly and specifically as possible, or it may help if the grandparents can speak directly to the doctor. Often it will help if they are able to do something constructive. Usually they want to feel involved, to share part of the sorrow with you, and to be needed as important family members. These are personal decisions. Mary and I decided not to tell her father, who was terminally ill with cancer, the bad news about his grandson. He died without ever knowing the truth. Obviously, we decided that honesty isn't necessarily always the best policy.

Usually no purpose is served by sharing the news with any but the closest of your personal friends and relatives. There will be time enough when you get home to worry about your neighbors and other friends. Consult with your doctor and think through exactly what is to be said. It is usually wise to be frank and specific. It may help to write down just what the facts are; that act in itself, separating fact from emotion, can sometimes make the information more understandable and help you begin to come to grips with reality.

Help from Someone Who Knows: The Support Group

During the first few days after the diagnosis, living with the knowledge of your child's handicap and attempting to put back together the unraveled threads of your family's life, you may find it helpful to talk things over with another parent who has faced similar problems. This sharing process is personal and shouldn't be hurried (perhaps later, when you have had an opportunity to sort things out, there will be a better time to consider seeking out others with similar experiences), but this contact can offer living testament that you're not as alone and isolated as you may have thought, and that there are others who understand and care. Many people gather together in groups, both large and small, local and national, for mutual support. Their name makes sense —they are called "support groups."

If you are interested in making contact with a group or with another parent who has gone through a similar experience, some hospital staff member—the play therapist, the social worker, the charge nurse, the doctor—should be able to offer suggestions. Actually, many hospitals themselves organize or act as hosts for such groups, who meet to hear speakers, to discuss mutual problems, to give one another emotional and practical support, and often to work with the hospital to improve practices and policies. The groups can consist of the families of handicapped or chronically ill children, or they can be for parents who have lost a child, but they all have a deep concern for their children and their aim is to help one another. Some parents find it helpful to locate another parent whose child has similar characteristics and who, as a veteran campaigner, can give advice on weathering the storm, particularly during the first few months. Such a relationship is, of course, a personal matter and not everybody's cup of tea, but Mary and I urge you not to overlook support groups. We did during the early years, although I'm not sure why. Possibly we thought we could and ought to battle it out alone. As it turned out, we were wrong; but then, we often were. (Support groups are discussed in detail in Chapter 12.)

Research

At some time or another after the initial diagnosis you may be asked for permission to include your child in a research project. This is not uncommon. I recommend that you give it serious thought. Most of us have benefited, often unknowingly, from the efforts of others who, through participation in research, have helped advance the fund of knowledge upon which we all depend.

Obviously, despite your willingness to help out, your primary concern will be for the interests of your child. Before becoming involved with a research project, understand all the facts and obligations involved. First, your *informed consent* must be obtained before your child can become involved. This means that those responsible must explain to you, in terms you can understand, what is involved for your child. (Another kind of informed consent is discussed when educational rights are examined in Chapter 16.) You will want to know if any of the research procedures will hurt, and whether there are medical, emotional, or psychological risks involved. Find out if the research program will take time away from your child's regular programs. If it is not conducted at his normal location, will transportation be provided? Will your child's identity be protected in photographs or written reports?

You should know what organization is conducting the research; check it out with your doctor. Don't feel any compulsion to "go along." It is unethical for a professional to hold your refusal against your child.

The potential benefits of research participation are numerous. It can offer specific rewards in terms of free services, as well as the general advantage of making possible expanded relationships with key professionals with whom you may have future contact. Finally, involvement may provide you with helpful information pertaining to your child's handicap and give you the warm feeling that comes from doing something for the good of other children like yours, and for society in general.

Now that we have discussed the bad news, let's explore how you can plan most effectively for your child's stay in the hospital.

5

Preparing for Admission

Your Plan

Make a list—not only does it reduce the chances that something important will be forgotten, but also sometimes just writing things down helps us organize our minds and prepare for action. Here are some things you may want to attend to before you leave home.

With the help of your doctor, get to know the medical details of your child's hospitalization. The medical necessity for the visit is often obvious, but if you aren't convinced, consider getting a second opinion and be sure that you satisfy yourself and know the answers to all the key questions (see the DOs and DON'Ts at the end of this section).

In Part One, I urged you to retain information for future reference in a looseleaf notebook (described in Appendix A). If you haven't begun to keep it, I suggest you do so at this time. Written reports of doctors' examinations and hospital stays are especially important. Be certain to include dates, locations, and the full names and titles of people present at meetings as well as a running diary—anecdotal records—of your child's progress as seen through your own eyes. Documentation can help both you and the doctor avoid misunderstanding and indicate over a period of time if a situation is becoming chronic. Include critical medical information for your child: allergies, dates and types of immunizations and booster shots received, height and weight at regular intervals, etc.

Prepare Admission Information

The hospital admissions process will require less time if you arrive with the required information in readily accessible form. Frequently the preadmission packet includes pertinent instructions. Admission people usually have a keen interest in such details as birth date, insurance policy number, doctor's name, next of kin, and Social Security number. Have your insurance and/or hospital card with you if you have one; if you carry no insurance, some hospitals require a deposit. You may be asked about any drugs or medicines that your child has been taking before entering the hospital. (Don't necessarily assume that all the information is passed on to your doctor.) Your doctor may request that certain drugs and medications that your child normally takes be discontinued during hospitalization. If you have brought them with you, they will be stored in a safe place and returned upon discharge.

The admission process can take as long as three hours, for, in addition to the paperwork, such routine medical procedures as an EKG, blood tests, and a chest X-ray may be required, but be of good cheer and show a happy face to your child; this business has to be taken care of and will go more quickly and effectively if you are cheerful, understanding, and prepared. In many hospitals, after your child is settled in his room, the nurse will check his pulse, respiration, and temperature, as well as height and weight, so that the appropriate quantity of medication, anesthesia, or intravenous fluids can be determined if their use becomes necessary.

The Consent Form

The question of who can legally speak for a minor when permission is required for a procedure is complicated (see Chapter 7). Although such requests are often routine, you would be wise to anticipate when they might be required and to know exactly what the release or consent form means before you sign it. The process can become legally complicated if parents are divorced or separated, or if the child is retarded but no longer a minor.

Probably somewhere in your child's hospital stay, often as part of the admission process, you will be asked to sign one or more consent forms. They can authorize the release of your child's confidential hospital records to a physician or to an insurance company or government agency concerned with payment of your bills, or to a social service organization involved with your child or family in such areas as placement, counseling, or advocacy. Consent forms can involve permission for your child to participate in a research project or for the hospital to take pictures of your youngster for use in scientific journal articles or for public relations purposes. (No one may take or use photographs of children without written consent from the parent or guardian.) Frequently, the request will be for authorization for a particular operation, or a general blanket consent required by a hospital to cover the kinds of procedures routinely undertaken by that institution.

It is rarely a good idea to search for trouble. Nonetheless, it is helpful to anticipate actions that you might need to take, such as the signing of release and consent forms. If you have thought things through beforehand, you won't freeze when action is necessary and people are standing around looking at their watches and waiting for you to sign. Just be sure you understand what is involved. The decisions that might be required are too numerous and diverse to discuss here, but, in your prehospital conference with your doctor, ask what decisions you might be required to make that can't wait. For example, in rare instances you may be asked whether a shunt should be installed or an operation performed on a baby with spina bifida. On the other hand, you may feel more comfortable waiting to face the problem only if you have to. This is a matter of temperament, but make the choice a conscious one. As with so many aspects of coping with your child's own special needs, being an *active* rather than *passive* parent not only helps your child but also makes you feel remarkably better about yourself and more in control of your entire family's destiny.

Communication

Since it may be crucial to act quickly and at odd hours, always maintain an up-to-date phone list, including doctors, pharmacies, ambulance services, and babysitters or people who will cover for you when you are at the hospital. At the same time, plan your method of communicating with home once you and your child are settled in at the hospital. (Remembering my long vigil at the phone waiting for news of my grandchild, I feel strongly about this subject.) Find out the extension number of the nursing station on the floor where you expect your child will be and keep track of nurses' names. Even with a telephone in your child's room it is probably a good idea to think through how and at what times you can most conveniently call home to see how things are going; conversely, decide when it's best for people at home to reach you.

Along with the communication network, you will want to prepare a list of people who should be notified of your child's hospitalization: close friends of your youngster or their parents, your minister or rabbi, and by all means your child's school, so that academic arrangements can be made. The school systems in many states provide tutors for students hospitalized over a certain number of days. If your child is in school, call the superintendent's office and find out what the school district's policy is. Teachers may wish to notify classmates so they can send cards or visit if appropriate. (The difficult problem of notifying those who need to know about a birth defect or handicapping condition was discussed in Chapter 4.)

Hospital jargon and medical terminology can be a nightmare for non–English-speaking parents. Your hospital may have on staff, or may be able to locate, a translator. It may take a little time, so inquire about it before admission. Don't be bashful! Other situations can also present problems. Your child may have special needs caused by blindness, deafness, or the inability to speak or to understand. He may be unable to walk or he may have difficulty with bowel or bladder control.

Let the hospital know of these conditions, particularly if this is a first admission.

What to Take to the Hospital

Plan in detail the things you will need for yourself and your child. Some patient handbooks provide helpful advice in this area. For instance, nightshirts (sometimes called "Johnnies") are often provided, but it is a good idea to bring along a comfortable robe. Check with the hospital, since children often can wear their own more familiar pajamas or street clothes. Include a favorite doll or toy, pictures of the family—anything that will make your youngster feel more at home— but keep things small, simple, and inanimate. The staff's welcome might be frosty if you arrive too late, too early, or with a band of raucous well-wishers, and pet toads are discouraged. With a chronically ill child it may save time and confusion if you organize, maybe even prepack, certain necessities in anticipation of emergency trips. Since few hospitals will be responsible for money or other valuables left in a patient's room, don't bring large amounts of cash, credit cards, or jewelry with you if you plan to stay in your child's room overnight. If you must take valuables, ask the admissions people to deposit them in the hospital safe.

Check Out a Distant Hospital

Sometimes it may be necessary for your child to travel to an out-of-town hospital. Medical arrangements will be made by your doctor (in consultation with you). Be sure you understand precisely what is involved and why the action is required. Additional planning will be necessary to provide for transportation and for parental living accommodations. Some large city hospitals have arrangements with nearby hotels, or you may be in luck and find a Ronald McDonald House nearby. The Ronald McDonald House is a low-cost, nonprofit housing facility, partially supported by the McDonald's restaurant chain, that provides lodging for the families of hospitalized handicapped and chronically ill children. Call or write the hospital admitting office. It will know about the local housing situation. As we have noted, many hospitals make provision for a parent to sleep in the room with a child. Pursue this possibility and take advantage of it if you can. It has many physical and psychological advantages, particularly when you are far from home.

Keep the Home Fires Burning

Whether your child is admitted to a local or a distant hospital, you must see that things are kept under control on the family front during your absence, particularly if you have other children at home. It is far more stressful to worry about your teenager who is at home and unsupervised if you are at the Massachusetts General Hospital with your baby and the teenager is in Caribou, Maine, than it is to worry about your teenager when you are both in Caribou.

It is natural and usually best to make arrangements with family and friends to take care of those left at home. However, if this is not possible, various organizations throughout the country provide such service. Some of these same contacts can help when you first return home from the hospital. As you would expect, urban areas offer more possibilities, but be patient, persistent, and thorough. Contact your doctor, clergy, hospital social worker, or discharge planner. Don't overlook the local reference librarian. Find out if there is a nearby information and referral (I&R) service or system. This service, often sponsored by such organizations as United Way or health and welfare councils, is in business to put you in touch with community resources. Go through the telephone routine discussed in Part One and check your phone book for such listings as "I and R," "Community Services," "Action" or "Hot Lines," and "Contact Help," or ask your local phone operator for help. Some of the following organizations may be able to help or offer suggestions:

- Meals-on-Wheels (home-delivered meals)
- Homemaker–Home Health Aide Services
- Visiting Nurse Association
- Family Service Agencies
- Catholic Charities, Jewish Family Services, or other religiously related agencies
- Local offices of the American Red Cross or United Way (sometimes called the United Fund or Community Chest)[1]

If your child has a specific handicap, such as cerebral palsy or spina bifida, a local branch of the national association for that disability may have suggestions for homemaker help, and your state or city Department of Human Services may have a division, sometimes called "patient services," that can assist you in locating help. Don't forget, as a

---

1. National Homecaring Council and Council of Better Business Bureaus, *All About Home Care: A Consumer's Guide* (1982), p. 9.

last resort, to cover all the bases, including the ones I have mentioned before: your town, county, or state officials, the mayor's office, the board of supervisors, your congressional representative, and departments of public health and mental hygiene. The State Department of Health can refer you to Medicare/Medicaid—certified home-health agencies.

Some of these suggestions may appear to be clutching at straws, but there were times during those years when Owen was home that straws didn't seem all that bad, and we clutched at anything. Bear in mind that it is a basic responsibility of public officials, bureaucrats, and agency employees to do their best to provide resource information to citizens who request it.

A Preadmission Visit to the Hospital

An exploratory, preadmission trip to the hospital will often pay dividends, and many hospitals welcome it. The excursion can make the actual stay less hectic for both parents and child and help reduce the fantasies and anxieties that children may have about hospitalization. Some hospitals even offer special preadmissions programs with a play session in the recreation room, a question-and-answer session with staff, and refreshments. Take advantage of them!

The preadmission trip, in addition to the obvious emotional advantages it offers, can help in little, unexpected, but practical ways. For example, it can make graphically obvious what arrangements must be made just to get to the hospital and back. Is there regular public transportation? What are its schedules? If you drive, what about parking? It should also become obvious that, in addition to the psychological advantage gained, it is highly desirable for practical reasons to have your spouse or another adult along. If your child is chronically ill and requires repeated or unplanned hospitalization, it may be worthwhile to contact a local volunteer ambulance service. If your child is not ambulatory, arrangements should be made to have a wheelchair available upon your arrival. A preadmission trip may be a pain in the neck, but it is the best way to get to know the layout of a rather complicated place before the pressure is on.

Most hospitals are pretty good about providing interior directional signs (some even furnish maps), and often an information-desk attendant will start you off in the right direction. However, to understand these directions and what the people are talking about when you get there, you should become familiar with a few of the more common technical expressions, listed here.

CATHETER   A tube that allows fluid to pass into or out of the body.

CAT SCAN (CT)   A very detailed internal picture of your entire body or a part of your body.

CBC   Complete blood count. A blood test to find out how many and what kind of blood cells a person has.

CENSUS   The number of inpatients in the hospital or on a specific ward. This figure indicates how many beds are available for new patients.

CHART   A patient's records—the complete history of the patient's illness, medicines, and tests from the time the person is admitted until he goes home. There can be inpatient and outpatient records.

EEG   Electroencephalogram—a study that may tell how the brain is functioning.

EKG (ECG)   Electrocardiogram—a study that tells how the heart is acting.

ER   Emergency Room. Sometimes called EW (Emergency Ward).

ICU   Intensive Care Unit.

INPATIENT   Patients staying in the hospital, as compared with outpatients, who come for part of the day only.

IV   Intravenous—a way of putting medicines, fluids, or nourishment directly into a vein.

LOA   Leave of absence. Allowing the patient to leave the hospital for a brief period of time.

NPO   Nothing by mouth. The patient may neither eat nor drink.

NURSING STATION   The centralized location on the ward at which nurses carry out their professional duties (think of Captain Kirk's desk).

ON CALL   Health professionals who are on duty (either in the hospital or available if needed).

OPD   Outpatient Department.

OR   Operating Room.

RADIOLOGY   The X-ray department.

SCRUB   To wash carefully so as to remove all harmful bacteria.

STAT   Immediately.

TEAM   All people involved in a patient's care.

VITAL SIGNS   Temperature, pulse, respiration, blood pressure.

You can make a game out of learning this new language and, using flash cards, see how many expressions your child can learn before admission. The nurses will probably be delighted to give him positive reinforcement when he demonstrates his knowledge of "their" language. He will already be an insider, and you will learn something, too.

Emotional Preparation

Most children share common questions and fears about a hospital visit. They ask why they must go, if hospitalization is a punishment for something they have done wrong at home or at school, how long they will have to stay, and if they will ever come home. They probably will also be concerned about where Mom and Dad will be, whether the operation will hurt, or even the possibility of death. Teenagers, particularly, may wonder if they will look different afterward. Underlying these questions in part is the fear of the unknown. Since reducing anxiety may even improve medical results, are there ways you can help? For many of the concepts that follow concerning children's hospitalization, I have drawn from the Association for the Care of Children's Health (ACCH) pamphlets *Preparing Your Child for Repeated or Extended Hospitalizations* and *A Child Goes to the Hospital.*

Be Truthful but Be Supportive, Too

Whatever your child's age, facing the future honestly and openly is the best approach. Select a quiet moment to talk with your youngster about the upcoming hospital visit. Try to find out what particular things are on his mind. If your child is four or younger it may be best to talk things over only a few days before admission, since young children have a different sense of the passage of time from adults and, if given too much warning, may begin to worry and fantasize about what could happen to them at the hospital. As the child grows older, he usually requires more time to become accustomed to new circumstances and to think things over. You, the parent, will have a sense of the timing most appropriate for your own child.

It's important to be well prepared for your discussion with clear, simple, and correct explanations of anticipated concerns, contacting your doctor, if necessary, for clarification. Your child depends upon you, and the information you give him—even if it is painful—should be correct. If you tell your child a needle won't hurt and it does, your child learns a lesson more lasting than the needle's sting. Be careful not to undermine your child's confidence in his doctors or nurses by making promises they can't keep. Don't tell him, "The doctor isn't going to hurt you" or "The nurse won't take any more blood" if they might have to. Wishful thinking can be a dangerous indulgence.

You can help your child by responding to his natural need for information. This is true of all kids, but it's even more important for a handicapped child. His sense of isolation and differentness is bound to be even greater and more difficult to face than that of the normal sick youngster. His questions, those he asks and those he doesn't, shouldn't be ignored. The need to communicate, the need for the parent to try to understand and to help is very important. Neither excessive sympathy, which incapacitates, nor an unreasonable toughness, which discourages, is the answer. Professionals are particularly aware of the importance of open, sensitive, two-way communication between parents and child.

> Always listen to your child's comments and be sensitive to hidden fears. Some common misconceptions of the school-age child are: during a blood test all the child's blood may be drained away; after the application of a leg cast, the leg is no longer there; or the child's throat is "slit" during a tonsillectomy. Also, don't dismiss fantasy stories. Find out what they mean. Remember, these [fantasies] are very real to your child . . . their source could be TV programs, tales from friends, or bits and pieces of conversations heard from you or other family members. Talk these fears out, explaining and showing calmly what will really happen.[2]

Like an adult, a child when worried and afraid may respond in ways not typical of his normal behavior. He may become more irritable, aggressive, and active, or may withdraw into himself. Don't be surprised or overreact. Maintain normal home routines and behavior expectations as you prepare for the hospital stay.

Help Him Allay His Fears

Many children feel that the hospital and everything involved with it, even the illness, are somehow a punishment for something they have done wrong. A simple explanation to the youngster of the reason for the hospital visit, emphasizing that he hasn't in any way been naughty, should help. Your words should satisfy his curiosity about why he must go: "This is the best place to fix what's wrong." The answer to the question, "When can I come home?" can be more difficult, especially since you yourself often won't know. To say, "We can go whenever the doctor says you are well enough" may seem like a cop-out, but in many instances it's the truth of the matter. And it doesn't hurt to admit that you don't know. One of the major worries in your child's mind is the possibility that he will be cut off from you, possibly forever. This fear of

2. Association for the Care of Children's Health, *A Child Goes to the Hospital* (1984).

separation from parents is particularly evident in children age six or younger. The assurance that this will not happen and the manner in which you handle the necessary periods of separation are extremely important and are discussed later in this section.

Fears are sometimes reflected in questions. Be alert and sensitive to them. As children grow older the nature of their anxieties tends to change. They become more concerned about the body and what will happen to the part where something has gone wrong. Will he lose forever something other kids have? Will there be a scar? Will it show? Why must it hurt before it gets better? Your doctor, if you have chosen wisely, should be able to help explain, in terms your child can understand, what will happen. Some do a first-rate job of understanding and being understood and in the process gain your child's confidence and relieve and divert his mind. One pediatrician I know has delightful comic book figures painted on the back of his white coat, wears a large bow tie, and always seems to be trailed by two or three small patients as he makes his rounds.

If your child suffers from a chronic condition, frequent hospitalizations are double-edged experiences. A few advantages are that the faces, places, and routines eventually become familiar and less disquieting. On the other hand, previous treatment that in your child's eyes failed to cure can form a basis for anger, disappointment, and resentment. He can be understandably afraid of repeating a painful experience (Chapter 6 deals more generally with the hospital experience of the chronically ill child). From an emotional point of view, it is imperative that you learn from experience to safeguard and to improve not only your child's but also your own mental health. You can take specific actions that will relieve boredom and anxiety as well as quiet your child's anxieties and make him feel better about himself and his treatment. Use your imagination: involve his food, his room and roommate, visits from friends, school relations, and daytime activities. (See Chapter 6 for more ideas.)

Siblings

During a period of stress it is easy to forget your other children. They, too, are under pressure and will have their own questions and fears. Try from the beginning to be sensitive to their needs, even when you are probably having difficulty keeping yourself emotionally afloat. (Ongoing sibling problems are discussed in Part Three.) Circumstances vary so much from family to family that generalization is difficult, but we found two principles helpful in dealing with our children, no matter what their age: It is your responsibility to provide leadership and to see to it that the interests of the entire family are considered as sensitively and realistically as possible. And, for the most part, the interests of all are best served when your youngsters are well informed.

Visits to the hospital may help. Under certain circumstances a family conference with the doctor (perhaps without your sick child) may help everyone. Once again, a sensitive physician can be extremely effective in helping a family stay on an even keel. He should be concerned for the family as a whole, since family harmony and support are bound to affect the sick child positively. Brothers' and sisters' teachers also need to be advised of the situation at home, since siblings' academic performance and behavior can be affected.

If There Is No Formal Language

Our son's almost complete lack of an ability to communicate has always been the one characteristic of his many disabilities most difficult for us to bear. Through the years we never really knew what went on in his mind, whether he was smiling and yodeling on the beach or standing alone in a dark room staring at the wall. "I wonder what Owen is thinking" has become a familiar family litany.

But no matter how severely handicapped and apparently isolated from the world around him your child may be, no matter how little or how much you think you know about what goes on in his mind, don't assume that he is not subject to the same emotional forces that affect us all. No matter how disabled, he is a human being and not an inanimate object. Never forget this! His disabilities may make him even more sensitive to disruption of his routine and to unfamiliar places and faces.

Your own emotions will be very much under pressure during this period. You can help yourself most if you have a doctor in whom you have confidence (if you don't, think about a change); you and your spouse (in fact the entire family) work as a team, sharing responsibilities, disappointments, and triumphs; you become as well informed as possible about everything that is involved in your child's illness; you seek out and accept the help that is available; and you consciously try not to overdo. Some nurses with whom I have spoken mention this last recommendation as a high priority, suggesting that often the best thing an exhausted parent can do for a child is occasionally to go home and get a good night's sleep. The nurses suggest that sometimes parents exaggerate the effect that an occasional separation will have on their child, especially if the child has settled into the hospital routine, the separation is anticipated, and the child is properly prepared for it.

6

The Hospital Stay

If you have diligently taken care of all your preadmission chores, the actual admission process and settling yourselves and your child into the hospital should be considerably easier than it would be had you arrived at the hospital with no money for the taxi, a suitcase that keeps flopping open, and a sinking feeling that you may be one day early. There is enough necessary confusion eddying about the corridors of a hospital without adding to it.

Humanize Your Child's Hospital Room and Get Acquainted

As soon as you complete the admission process and locate your child's room, make it as happy and as homey a place as your ingenuity and hospital rules allow. Put up pictures, posters, cards. (First find out what adhesives are permitted; hospitals can be touchy about the condition of their walls.) As much as possible, see that your child's room is a haven, free from unpleasant and painful experiences, and that regular home routines are maintained. His room and the playroom should be places where he can feel safe, where he can rest and be secure. Get to know the names of the staff members and what they do. Write things down so you will remember them. See to it that your child gets acquainted with the people instrumental to his care and that his primary nurse, in particular, knows his nickname, his likes and dislikes, favorite foods, and so on.

Take a walking tour of the floor. (Your preadmission visit should have left you already fairly familiar with the maze of corridors, swinging doors, desks, rolling carts, and such key places as the playroom and the pantry.) In particular, find out the playroom's hours, its rules, and where they keep such invaluable staples as modeling clay, video games, and Barbie dolls. Meet the play therapist if there is one on the staff and find out if there are any foster grandparents, whose laps and hugs can help induce a healing chemistry that modern medicine sometimes overlooks. When things have quieted down, get to know the social worker (discussed in Chapter 4). He can be a real help in your attempts to cope with the outside world, particularly in the running of your home while you are away and in posthospital planning.

Be Good Hospital Citizens

Observe the rules of your floor, and be sensitive to the rights and responsibilities of the institution, of the doctors, and of your child as a patient. Most hospitals have written policies that cover these important relationships and often have assigned one person to respond to patients' questions and complaints (sometimes called an ombudsman). If you didn't receive a pamphlet setting forth these policies in your preadmission packet, ask for one and read it carefully. It's a kind of Patient's Bill of Rights, but it considers the rights of the doctors and the hospital as well. Here is how a typical hospital might view the relationship.[1]

What Are the Hospital's Responsibilities?

Your child has the right to competent and compassionate care that responds reasonably and with courtesy to his needs, irrespective of your ability to pay. Any rudeness or apparent incompetence should be reported. Ask the head nurse how to lodge a complaint. Some hospitals have a patient advocate (ombudsman) or what is sometimes called a patient care committee to represent the patient if he is dissatisfied. You have the right to discuss complaints with professional staff, but for your part, be courteous, too, and not unnecessarily demanding. You may be harried and worried about your child; the staff may be harried and worried, too—but also frantically busy. You have the right to expect that all matters concerning your child's care are treated as confidential. This right to privacy applies to *all* professional relationships. The patient also has the right to be informed of the hospital's rules and regulations (he may have to ask for them); the right to be told the name of the physician responsible for his care; and the right to examine his bill and to be given a full explanation of its charges. The last hospital responsibility is the obligation to make all medical information pertaining to a patient available to him, his parents, or his legal guardian, although most information of this nature will have to be interpreted by a physician to make it understandable.

What Are the Physician's Responsibilities?

The physician has the responsibility to keep you always informed (in ways you can reasonably be expected to understand) about several

1. Some concepts drawn from the pamphlet *Rights and Responsibilities of Patients, Physicians, and Maine Medical Center*, adopted by the Staff and Trustees of Maine Medical Center, November 1974.

important areas affecting your child; for example, the diagnosis, treatment, and prognosis for his condition; the medical consequences if you refuse proposed treatment for your child; the reasons for transferring your child to another institution (and alternatives to such transfer). The physician has the responsibility to tell you if he is involved in a research project affecting your child (you can refuse such participation); to recommend consultation with other doctors or specialists, either when you ask, or when he feels it's appropriate; and to give you all the information necessary so you are able to give thoughtful approval before a treatment is begun. Unless there is an emergency, he should give you a description of the treatment, its risks, its benefits, and an evaluation of alternatives. Finally, the physician has an obligation to discuss any complaints you may have concerning your child's care and the responsibility to arrange for appropriate continuation of care after your child leaves the hospital.

What Are the Patient's Responsibilities?

As your child's representative you have the responsibility to see that he is on time for appointments or to let the hospital or his doctor know if he will be late or must cancel his date. Inconsiderateness on your part will inconvenience both the staff and other patients. You should make every effort to understand your child's health-care instructions and to let the doctor or hospital know if you are confused on any point, or if your child is unable to follow instructions. You can't expect clear, concise language, free of jargon, unless you make it clear that you don't understand what is being said. Don't just sit there smiling and nodding.

You have the obligation to provide the doctor with all important information about your youngster's former illnesses, hospitalizations, medications, and such other pertinent facts as allergies and unusual reactions to drugs. Your notebook can come in handy here. You also have the responsibility to see that you, your child, and the entire family are good neighbors and are considerate in matters involving noise, TV use, and smoking. Finally, it is your job to make available all necessary information to help the hospital work with you in making financial arrangements for payment. Hospitals can't be responsive to your financial needs and at the same time lower health-care costs unless they have this information.

Hospitals have responsibilities to the community, but the community, as well, should support its hospital if it is to expect first-rate health care. This support can range from individual financial contributions when fund-raising efforts are necessary (for not-for-profit hospitals) to the efforts of individual volunteers, who perform the many nonprofessional jobs necessary for the hospital to operate efficiently and humanely.

Balancing Your Life

The days that you and your child spend away from home, under the best of conditions, are unnatural for the entire family. If your child is multiply handicapped or chronically ill, you may sometimes find yourself logging more hours at the hospital than at home. To get maximal coverage and to reduce individual loads, it is usually desirable to split things up between father and mother, and it is important that both parents be a continuing supportive force. Often mothers carry almost the entire responsibility, with the father either absent or arriving for a visit fifteen minutes before bedtime. The ideal arrangement is a balance in which the floor nurses, the mother, the father, and the child all have contributions to make. Nurses can become partners in the behavioral as well as the medical management of your child. For example, in your absence they must respond to what's called "inappropriate behavior" in your youngster. Check with the nurses to see how things go when you aren't around and together work out a consistent approach to discipline.

Always Say "So Long"

Naturally, it's difficult for you to leave your child, even if only for a few hours. I have seen parents wait until their child becomes distracted by a game or another playmate before trying to steal away. Sometimes while working in the playroom I have been asked by parents to play with a youngster so that they could leave unobserved. Parents often rationalize this behavior by thinking that it's easier on the child. It isn't. It's easier only on the parent, as they would know if they could see how their youngster reacts when he suddenly realizes that his mother and father have disappeared—gone for good, for all the child knows, and without even saying goodbye. Basically, it's a dirty trick—perhaps unintentionally, but still a dirty trick. When you have to leave, always explain why you're going and make clear when you will come back. Stick to your word! If you are delayed, and this will happen, get a message to your child so that he won't be left waiting by the door. You can expect that your child will act up when you leave, but if he knows you will return, and when, his tears ordinarily will be short-lived; anyway, hospital staff are very good at drying them. It's normal and healthy for a young child to cry when separated from his parents. Indeed, quiet acceptance of separation on his part may be a cause for concern.

Difficult as it will be, part of your own adult growth and development in becoming an effective parent of a handicapped child is a necessary toughening-up process. To a certain extent it is a natural evolution-
ary process, so make no excuses to yourself. If you are to hang in there
and provide the most effective support to your child, you have to be
understanding, warm, and flexible when the occasion warrants, and
inflexible and demanding, too, when such an approach is called for. As
you grow and become a real partner with your child in his struggles,
you will learn the difference. Growing tough will also allow you to be
helpful during painful procedures. Your influence can be of real help to
the medical staff, particularly during a long, chronic illness, but you
have to *develop* the inner fortitude that will enable you to step in and be
helpful when your child is in pain.

Prolonged Hospitalization

Families who must adjust to protracted periods at the hospital, either with a chronically ill child or with a brand-new baby, face special
problems. Although they have suffered through the same initial period
of shock and adjustment as those involved in a one-time visit, the family
of a chronically ill child must adapt to a prolonged ordeal in which the
duration of the treatment may be unknown and the chance of a positive
outcome is sometimes slim. The families who wage this struggle put
into perspective problems that other, luckier, parents complain about.
Quick, spur-of-the-moment courage is admirable, but it pales in comparison to what is required of those who must stay the course over long
periods. On the brighter side, parents of a child who faces prolonged
hospitalization can take actions that lighten their load. Although some
of the suggestions that follow apply to any child on any hospital visit,
most are particularly applicable to chronically ill children involved in a
long hospitalization. How you can help your child depends on the nature of his disability and his age.

The New Baby

All infants need stimulation during their early months of life. If
they are to progress normally and develop a sound relationship with
their parents (a process called bonding), they should be held, sung to,
played with, cuddled, and caressed. An infant who, after birth, must
remain hospitalized for long periods of time needs this sensory interaction even more, particularly if he is preterm or has been isolated (in
neonatal intensive care, for instance). Although the importance of early
infant stimulation and bonding is discussed in detail in Part Three, I
make a few suggestions here.

Many barriers may stand between you and your small baby in the Neonatal Intensive Care Unit. There he lies in his isolette, almost an inanimate object, 90 percent tubes, catheters, valves, and apparatus and 10 percent diaper and baby. Don't be intimidated by all the equipment surrounding or attached to him; ask the nurse to explain its operation. It may be difficult for you to participate in many aspects of his care at this early stage, but do what you can. Try to develop a hospital routine that matches as much as possible the one you follow at home. At the very least, both father and mother should get involved with his feeding and changing. Rocking chairs are sometimes available where you can hold your new child, rock him, and get acquainted. Chances are the hospital will welcome and encourage you. When parents aren't available, some institutions enlist volunteer "huggers" to be surrogate parents and to fill this need temporarily.

Since the stimulation of all senses is important, find out if you can bring in some of your own things from home—a music box, a mobile, a colorful poster, a family picture, or brightly contrasting fabric to hang on his crib. Many neonatal intensive care units provide mobiles especially designed to stimulate infants. Ask what the hospital has available. Drawing a colorful picture may provide your older children with an opportunity to participate. Choose crib decorations that are attractive, effective, and safe, and position them so your baby can observe them. Remember, they're there for him, not you, to look at. Finally, seek advice from a nurse about what kind of stimulation is good for your baby. Too much or the wrong kind can do more harm than good, and what is appropriate will vary with the developmental age of your baby. Researchers in infant development are learning what babies can see at what age and what colors and patterns they prefer.

Probably the most important contribution you can make during this period is just to be there and to make yourself a physical reality to your child, providing all the demonstrations of love that mean so much to his development.

The Toddler/Preschooler

As we have seen, preschoolers tend to fear abandonment, pain, and damage to or loss of body parts. In a prolonged hospitalization involving many medical tests and treatments and increasingly frequent separations, it is particularly important to talk with the medical staff to enlist their advice and support in minimizing these fears. If you work as a team and are sensitive to your child's vulnerabilities, time and the repetition of even unpleasant experiences may bring acceptance. It is possible to transform painful experiences into normal routines, but that isn't likely to happen spontaneously.

In general, it's good to be on hand when particularly scary or painful procedures take place. With younger children, however, who see their parents as "protectors," sometimes it's best not to be directly involved but to return immediately afterward. Often staff will prefer this approach, since children may resist more strenuously if their parents are within sight. Talk it over with the staff involved. Find out if you can be with your child before an operation when he receives the anesthetic and later in the recovery room. If you can't be on hand, explain who will be looking after him. Tell him exactly where you will be and when you will return. Plan so that no new procedure is begun when you aren't with him, or if that's impossible, see that he understands what's going to happen and why. I have found that nurses are likely to be particularly responsive to a child's needs, sometimes more so than doctors. Often nurses will spontaneously take pains to reassure your child. Ask them for help and advice. They're a wonderful resource.

Inquire if difficult procedures can be done by a staff member whom your child knows, likes, and trusts. Do what you can to avoid unpleasant surprises and strange faces. If your child's illness requires taking many blood samples, or if he is particularly upset by needles (many kids are), talk with the nurse and see if the procedure can be performed by the same person. Another way to reduce the impact of frequent unpleasant experiences on both you and your child is to gradually take over as much of the routine hospital care, treatment, and medication as permitted. You may be able to help with such things as special feeding, changing surgical dressings, bathing, and physical therapy. Participation allows you to practice the toughening-up process, and it helps get the "bugs" out of procedures while doctors and nurses are available to give advice. Remember, later, at home, you will need to be able to perform these jobs alone.

Sometimes you yourself can reduce your youngster's pain and discomfort. For example, learn how to handle a portable IV so as to make your child's movement as comfortable as possible; be sure to know what to do when the IV alarm goes off and the red button lights up. If your child is in traction, in a wheelchair, or bedridden, learn from the nurse about ways to give him more flexibility. Ask for specially designed writing and coloring tables or rigs so that your child can read, write, or watch TV no matter what his position. Your ingenuity sometimes can compensate for lack of medical know-how. Be tenacious and find out what you can do in a practical way, but never underestimate the power of tender, loving care. We all know that when Mom or Dad kisses a hurt finger "to make it better" it does feel better, never mind why. Hugs and kisses are generally pretty good medicine, and it's one area in which you probably have at least as much experience as your doctor.

Parents often worry about their children being spoiled during the hospital stay. This is a complex and personal matter that you can discuss with the staff. Do be alert that in some instances overindulgence can harm a chronically ill child, particularly in the area of nutrition (see Chapter 13).

RELIEF OF FRUSTRATION. No matter how well things are going, hospitalization, particularly a long one, is likely to generate frustrations. Conversations with your child, play, and reading sessions all can help, but don't overlook purely physical outlets. Depending upon your child's age and physical condition, provide appropriate games and materials through which he can vent some of his pent-up indignation. Modeling clay, bean bags, safe punching bags, and hammering benches may be noisy or messy but they can be beneficial.

Seize every opportunity to divert your child's attention. If he is well enough, the play or recreation room can do wonders for his frame of mind. Young children learn and develop through play. They also need its activity to work things out in a new environment. Encourage this. Many hospitals have toys available, some of which are specially designed to simulate hospital activities. Get involved yourself and join in. Your child will love it. I have spent hours being examined by five-year-old neonatologists with their doctor's kits or playing Nurse Brown with hand puppets. It often helps a child if he can make up games and act out hospital experiences both in the hospital and at home. Get your child his own play doctor's kit; it helps him to become familiar with the tools of the trade and to become less fearful of the real instruments.

Some effective games can be improvised. Here's one that works well for me. You and your child can construct a building out of dominoes, each adding one domino at a time. Whoever places the domino that finally topples the structure loses, but even if he loses, your child receives the benefit of a wonderful noise and general confusion as the building tumbles. (You receive wonderful exercise picking up after each game.) It's great for frustrations and can give your child a rare opportunity to beat an adult at something, and even to make a mess legitimately. (This domino game is especially attractive to youngsters age six to twelve.) See if the playroom has a large easel with newsprint and water-based paint. Brush and finger painting also offer creative escape and release, but be sure to use a mat, a smock, and water-based paint, and close supervision is recommended. Finally, be sure you have permission from the charge nurse or the person responsible for the playroom before you launch into any of these enterprises. The unsupervised results of creative painting can be extraordinary!

THE PLAYROOM. In many ways the recreation room or playroom can be the center of activity for the entire pediatric floor. Play is a child's work, and through it he will grow, mature, and develop in both mental and physical areas. Often children feel overpowered in a hospital, with little control over their lives, and ordinarily they are right. Play offers them the opportunity to gain some control and to make choices and decisions. Even if a child is bedridden, see to it that he has many things available around his bed to play with. Better still, see if he can't be wheeled down to the playroom to watch other children and to share in that stimulation.

Normally the toddler or preschool child is involved in learning various skills naturally. Your child's skill level will depend upon the nature of his handicap. Don't be discouraged if the progress he was making at home comes to a standstill or even reverses itself while he's in the hospital. The setback is most likely temporary. On the other hand, he may be eager to continue and even to develop new skills while he's in the hospital. If this is the case, encourage him and give him all the help you can. Learning new skills will keep his mind from dwelling on the medical problems at hand.

School-aged Youngsters

For children for whom school is a possibility, concerns tend to branch out beyond the immediate family group to include more of the outside world. A long hospital stay can trigger fears of falling behind in school, of being forgotten by friends, or perhaps, even worse, of being laughed at when back among their peers. Call or visit your child's homeroom or Sunday School teacher and discuss ways in which contact can be maintained with the class and schoolwork can be kept up to date. If the hospitalization is planned, assignments often can be done beforehand. Some hospitals provide special educational programs coordinated with the school curriculum. If elective surgery is involved, schedule it so that important events in your child's life are not missed. Many hospitals offer a "leave pass" (LOA), which allows a child to leave the hospital to take part in special activities at home or school. Television, sometimes an effective tranquilizer in itself, is available in most hospitals and can offer distraction from discomfort, continuity of home routines, and sometimes even educationally oriented programs.

Teenagers

As every parent of an adolescent knows, the teenage years can be turbulent times under the best of circumstances. Adolescence is a developmental period when acceptance by one's friends is painfully important, and being in any way different can be crushing. To be either a handicapped person or a teenager is not easy; being both is at least doubly challenging, and parental patience and understanding are required.

At a time that your child's natural development makes him seek more independence, circumstances may actually dictate less independence and require more reliance upon you, his parents, and upon professional caregivers. This can be a bitter pill. You can help him by involving him in as many decisions affecting his care as possible. (Remember that at age eighteen your child is no longer a minor and may become legally responsible for making his own decisions.) Encourage him to be independent and to speak directly to the doctors and nurses, rather than always working through you. Consult with the health professionals involved and enlist their cooperation. Don't underestimate their sensitivity. They deal with these problems every day and should understand. A telephone, the importance of which transcends adult understanding, can be an alter ego for a teenager. See that he has one in his room if it's at all possible. If not, there should be a pay phone nearby. Find out where change can be obtained. When your child's mobility is limited, a phone can be one of his few links with the friends who are so important.

I have found that in many instances, particularly in the late teen years, teenagers can feel awkward on the pediatric floor, where support services are often oriented toward the younger patients who make up the majority of the population. Teenagers may view most playroom activities as "kid stuff" and stand aloof. Making available appropriate magazines, such as *Seventeen* and *Sports Illustrated,* can help. Some hospitals have video games available. Find out if radios or tape players brought from home are allowed, but caution your son or daughter to be sensitive to the needs of roommates or neighboring patients, who may find noise objectionable. (Put name labels on all personal items so they won't be lost.) Sometimes hospital staff can find worthwhile nontechnical chores that young-adult patients can perform to fight what can be the debilitating boredom of long hospitalization. This boredom can manifest itself in rebellion, apparent indifference, or such symptoms as "forgetting" medical appointments and medication or overlooking hospital rules and regulations. The hospital volunteer coordinator can be helpful in finding ways to make life more livable for your older child. (Sometimes older patients are encouraged to act as big brothers or sisters to the younger children.)

Sometimes teenage volunteers from local high schools work regularly at the hospital and are able to relate to young patients in a way impossible for adults to achieve. In many instances this ability to relate will follow unorthodox but lively channels. One day, from my vantage point in the playroom, I noticed unusual activity centered outside one young patient's room as interns and doctors on rounds crowded to get a look inside. Afraid that the patient, a special friend of mine, might have taken a turn for the worse, I investigated. To my amusement I found him to be in high spirits: he was displaying a gift that one of the young volunteer assistants, the captain of the local high school soccer team, had brought him. It was a large poster of a buxom blonde whose bathing suit wasn't up to the job at hand. To the consternation of many, the administrators decided that the poster had to go, but my young friend's day had been made.

Be Sensitive

You or your child's teacher can arrange an exchange of tape recordings by which the class sends its greetings and school news, and your youngster sends back word about how he is doing in his new environment. This can be an enjoyable and stimulating activity. Encourage visits from classmates during appropriate hours—if the doctor approves and your child is up to it. First, find out what the rules are. At some hospitals, visitors under a certain age are not admitted. If your child's appearance has changed, the teacher can prepare the class in a thoughtful way. Photographs can be of help, but this is a sensitive area, particularly in the teenage years. Talk the problem over with the teacher or guidance counselor. In all your attempts to arrange things for your child, you walk a tightrope between doing too little, thereby missing opportunities to help, and doing too much, thereby embarrassing him and making him appear babyish in his friends' eyes. There is no absolute rule stating how much help is too much, but open, frank conversation with your child can establish general guidelines. For example, you might say, "I'll be seeing your teacher today about your homework; the class will be anxious to know how you are. She'll probably want to know how the class can keep in touch. Do you have any ideas?"

Keeping busy and in touch with friends is an important consideration in maintaining good mental health, but there will be times when your child wants to be left alone, particularly when he's feeling bum physically. Unfortunately, privacy is a rare commodity in what is basically a public place. Do your best to see that your child can be alone when he needs to be. Don't let your efforts to encourage contacts with school friends and family intrude upon this need. On rare occasions, a private room may be desirable, but not realistic in terms of cost or availability. Most hospital rooms are equipped with curtains that provide at least visual privacy. Don't hesitate to use them.

Roommates can be great sources of mutual entertainment and support, but they can intrude during difficult moments when privacy is desirable. If your child and his roommate don't get along, particularly if your youngster is very sick and needs quiet, speak with the nurse about the possibility of switching rooms. When I have discussed possible roommate conflict with nurses, their response has been that generally the kids get along fine; it's the parents who are apt to cause the trouble. (There's a lesson to be learned here.) However, nurses are almost always good about seeing that children, whenever possible, get rooms that are most appropriate to meet their needs and where possible will make switches if it seems in the patient's best interests. Your child may find privacy in some quiet corner of the hospital. Ask the staff for suggestions, but be sure your child lets both you and the nurses know where he will be.

Routine is important, but special breaks in routine can give your child something to look forward to and shorten the long hours. The play therapist may make arrangements for such nonmedical activities as holiday and birthday parties, movies, and puppet shows. (You might volunteer to give a hand if it seems appropriate.) Food treats offer another kind of pleasant break in routine. Snacks approved by the doctor can offer relief from the monotony of institutional food. If brought from home or your child's favorite store, they offer another tie with the nonhospital world. (For more on dietary concerns, see Chapter 13.)

In the teenager's world of conformity an unusual appearance presents a real problem, since often little can be done to improve the obvious physical effects of some conditions and treatments. Be sensitive, use ingenuity, and help any way you can. If hair is falling out as the result of chemotherapy, locate an appropriate cap (baseball caps are usually popular) or even a wig. Wearing a wig or a hat can and does help; it is a case of what alternatives are possible. The oncologist (cancer specialist) may know a local store where wigs are available. A parent's reaction to a child's change in appearance can go far in shaping a child's view of his disability. For that reason, try to keep things in perspective, to focus on the positive, and to be as upbeat as possible; this approach focuses more on what practical things can be done than on becoming bogged down by what cannot be changed. Again, you have to be tough and realistic for your child's sake. Focus on the child, not the handicap!

Repeated Visits

Some of the tedious administrative procedures required in normal hospital routine can occasionally be simplified when frequent visits are necessary. Admission and discharge routines may be streamlined, and all the lengthy recitation of medical history to a constant flow of health professionals can be shortened. Discuss with your doctor or the admitting office what, if anything, can be done. It may help if your child can be placed back on the same floor, with familiar nurses and technicians. Such an arrangement may not be possible, but if it's medically appropriate, it's worth a try.

Finally, in all your efforts to be helpful at the hospital, it's important not to be a pushy parent. That usually is counterproductive. Try, instead, to act as a thoughtful and informed advocate for your child in a courteous and positive fashion, being aware not only of your own problems but also of the pressures and frustrations of those around you.

7

Hospital Discharge and Some Further Questions to Think About

Normally your child will look forward to his return to home or school, but it may present difficulties. This is particularly true when his absence has been prolonged or if his appearance or ability to function has changed; casts, colostomy bags, special medications, and scars all present challenges. The health professionals involved will have had experience in handling these challenges, and the school nurse, too, should be advised and consulted. If your child must have special assistance or transportation arrangements, be sure to notify school officials well in advance of his return. (Part Four discusses the school's responsibility to make its buildings accessible to handicapped students.) Sometimes, depending upon the circumstances and personality of the child, a festive occasion can be made of the homecoming. A cast can be painted and autographed, a wheelchair decorated—but take your lead from your child. A welcome-home party can be embarrassing to a youngster who wishes to slip in as quietly as possible.

One way to pave the way for re-entry is to prepare gradually beforehand. The problems involved in moving back into the normal world differ from child to child and depend upon circumstances. The child with a disability can't help worrying about how he will be viewed by the healthy population. Encourage special friends to visit either the hospital or your home the last few days before the big event. The attitudes of nondisabled people often contribute to the social uneasiness of handicapped folks, and helping the "normal" of all ages understand is a big assignment. Many good programs available for school use are designed to improve understanding on the part of the nonhandicapped population, but timing is important, and any presentation at school should be scheduled so as not to embarrass your child.

Preparation for Posthospital Treatment

The planning required for the return home will depend upon your child's age and illness and the availability of services in your geographic area. Although there may be some similarities, there may be almost as many variations in posthospital treatment as there are different children, because good educational/medical plans must be individualized to be effective. For the first few months at home, the primary consideration is that the medical treatment begun in the hospital be continued without interruption. Fortunately, resources should be available. Your challenge is to locate and coordinate them. The entire hospital medical team involved with your child should give you specific direction, through the leadership of your doctor, who has a responsibility to provide reasonable continuity of care and to inform you about any continuing health-care needs after discharge.

The nursing staff will instruct you about posthospital care. They will also help arrange whatever drugs or equipment your child may need. Also, sit down with your doctor to discuss all aspects of your child's posthospital care. Be sure you understand the technicalities. Get critical instructions in writing, including exact descriptions of his medications and the names and addresses of health professionals involved in his care, particularly the medical team coordinator if he is not your regular pediatrician. Enter them in your notebook. If you will be continuing some procedure started in the hospital, insist that you be allowed to begin to take over its performance well before you leave. Arrange for all equipment necessary for the first few weeks at home through your pediatrician or the visiting nurse before leaving the hospital. Some independent organizations also supply home medical equipment and supplies (see Resources: Suppliers). You may have to master changing a gastrostomy tube, the sterile techniques used with a Hickman catheter, feeding a baby who can't suck well, handling a child with abnormal muscle tone, catheterization, and so on. You will never have a better opportunity to learn than in the hospital.

Don't be afraid to find out whom to call when you need help. Often, the floor nurses, who are available by phone twenty-four hours a day, will be willing to answer questions that may panic a parent in the first few weeks at home. Finally, ask for an overview of what you can expect in the weeks ahead. This will save the doctor some phone calls and you unnecessary anxiety. Sometimes you will be unable to provide care at home without assistance. Often the social worker, together with your doctors and nurses, will be able to help you develop a plan that provides necessary support. With their help, see what kinds of services are provided in your community. If your child is seriously affected, a visiting nurse may be able to meet with you and your pediatrician before you leave the hospital. This could be extremely helpful. (Part Three deals with various kinds of professional home services available, both public and private.) Arrangements often can be made to provide whatever personal help you may require and to ensure that necessary medical supplies and equipment are in place in your home when you arrive from the hospital. Sometimes it is desirable to move a youngster from the hospital to some other care facility. Many of the problems involved are likely to be similar to those you encounter if you are forced to consider institutionalization of your youngster. (See Chapter 23.)

First things first. Make plans for your transportation home and arrange for the help necessary to make it a smooth transition. If possible, both parents should be there when the child comes home. The hospital social worker may be able to help you understand and anticipate the stresses, both physical and emotional, you are bound to encounter upon your return home. He may be able to suggest supportive community counseling resources and possible sources of financial assistance for expenses encountered as you start up your new life. The business office at the hospital could be another source of financial information.

The Discharge Process

Before you leave, the hospital will usually require that:

- Your doctor write a discharge order, which indicates that it is appropriate for your child to be released from the hospital.
- You visit the business office to take care of your child's bill. When this has been done by cash payment, insurance coverage, Title IX (government assistance) payment, or other individual arrangement with the business office, you will receive a discharge slip.
- You give the discharge slip to the floor nurse.

You are now ready to go home.

Paying the Bill

Many hospitals refer to financial plans in the same way that funeral directors mention "final arrangements." Whatever arrangements they are, they should be planned before admission, although the exact amount of the bill will be unknown at that time.

Meeting hospital and doctors' bills can be a worrisome financial obligation, but be of stout heart. (For sources of financial assistance, see Chapter 15.) If you are covered by a good health-insurance policy, with major medical protection, you should be in pretty good shape. Some hospitals operate a so-called open door policy, which means that in emergencies and if they have available beds, the hospital accepts any patient irrespective of his ability to pay. The patient is expected, however, to make every reasonable effort to meet his financial obligations. Some not-for-profit hospitals state in their philosophy that even though they expect full payment—and some require deposits when there is no insurance—they will cooperate with the patient or family to work out financial arrangements. This policy can mean that the hospital will point out sources of public or private assistance or that it will accept some sort of long-term or even partial payment plan.

If you require financial assistance, the hospital will undoubtedly ask for financial information, the nature of which will differ from state to state. It is important to be prepared to answer such questions as:

- Do you have hospital insurance that covers your child and does it include major medical coverage?
- If yes, what is the name of the insurance company and your policy number?
- Does your youngster receive Medical Assistance, and if he does, what is the card number and expiration date?
- What are the names, occupations, and places of employment of all wage earners in the home?
- What is your estimate of total family income, monthly rent or payments on your home, and the total of other sizeable monthly debts, medical bills in particular?
- Is there any other organization, such as Crippled Children's Services, for which you are eligible and from which you would accept help?[1]

Many hospitals have, through the years, received grants and bequests to be used for special purposes, or even for people from certain geographic locations. The hospital business office or social worker should be your best source of information about them. Remember, federal law requires every state to have a crippled children's agency, funded by both state and federal monies, which, in addition to providing no-cost diagnostic services for children under twenty-one with disabling conditions, may help parents with financial planning and locating medical resources. In certain limited instances, depending upon the family's ability to pay, this agency may assume part or all of the cost of care. Since the crippled children's agency goes by different names in different states, ask your local health department or the hospital social worker for information about your state's agency.

An important point should be remembered about public financial aid. Parents who receive such help should in no way feel that it is charity (or that the resulting medical care will be second class). Most citizens receive help directly or indirectly from the government in their jobs, businesses, or private lives: there are price supports for farmers, import quotas for automobile manufacturers, unemployment benefits for peo-

---

1. Loosely drawn from a financial form used by the John F. Kennedy Institute for Handicapped Children in Baltimore, Maryland.

ple out of work, and mortgage interest deductions for homeowners. Much of this assistance is paid for by the taxes you pay, so relax and accept financial aid when you can find it.

A Checklist of Predischarge Questions

Here are some posthospital questions you need to have answered:

- Who is responsible for helping to organize posthospital medical care? (It may be a pediatrician, neonatologist, social worker, or discharge planner, depending on your hospital's organization.)
- Have you been thoroughly instructed in the home care of your child? Do you feel confident that you can perform the tasks required?
- Do you have a manual that describes appropriate new home-care responsibilities? (For example, *Handling the Young Cerebral Palsied Child at Home,* by Nancie Finnie (Dutton, 1975) or *Home Care for the Chronically Ill or Disabled Child,* by Monica Loose Jones (Harper and Row, 1981).
- Will the necessary equipment, medical supplies, and material be on hand when you get home? Do you know how to replenish supplies?
- If your child requires involved home care and you feel uneasy, have arrangements been made for a visiting nurse or therapist to help you on a regular basis, and will he visit you at least once in the hospital to get acquainted and to plan his schedule? (This applies to any professional who will be involved with home care.)
- Do you know whom to call, at all hours, if you have medical questions to ask?
- Have specific plans been made to provide necessary orthotic supportive devices (braces, special shoes, casts, etc.) and do you know the locations and telephone numbers of those who will provide and maintain them?
- Who is responsible for helping you plan for your nonmedical posthospital concerns? (This is usually a social worker or a discharge planner.)
- Has someone counseled you concerning expenses involved and possible methods of payment?
- Has your home been prepared, physically, to accommodate your child?
- If you need a breather, who can give you information on respite care?
- If your home tasks, combined with the new medical duties, get too

heavy and you feel you need an extra hand or emotional help, where might assistance be found?

- If you want to contact other people who have children with similar problems (a support group), do you have their names and addresses?

Many of these questions are discussed at length in Section III; don't leave the hospital without satisfactory answers.

Moral Questions

As discussed in Part One, ethical problems can be raised during genetic counseling and prenatal diagnosis. Here we consider the ethical dilemmas that arise once the child has been born.

When prenatal diagnosis has identified the problem before the child's birth, parents have the opportunity to prepare themselves both practically and emotionally. The situation, difficult at best, is made more anguishing when the birth defect is unexpected. In either case, life-or-death decisions sometimes need to be made quickly and at a difficult, emotional time. Should the child immediately be placed in specialized foster or adoptive care if the handicap is so severe that the family feels unable to cope? (Rarely do conditions require institutionalization.) Should corrective surgery be performed to address a life-threatening problem, even if the child will probably suffer paralysis and severe retardation all his life?

Recently, the right of parents to decide to withhold critical medical treatment from disabled infants with life-threatening conditions has been challenged by the Department of Health and Human Services (Child Abuse and Neglect Prevention and Treatment Program) as the result of a court decision in the so-called Baby Doe case. States receiving federal support are required to establish "programs and/or procedures within the State's child protective service system to respond to reports of medical neglect,"[2] but appeals have been filed, and it may be years before the issue is settled. However, even under the regulations as they now stand, exceptions can be made and treatment withheld under certain complex circumstances. If you need to know the current guidelines, consult your doctor or lawyer.

Parents with profoundly disabled infants can face exquisitely complex problems. So much depends upon the individual family's circumstances and perspectives, the quality of life predicted for the child, and

2. *Federal Register,* vol. 50, no. 72, Monday, April 15, 1985, Rules and Regulations, p. 14878.

how one views the rights of the newborn with a handicap in relation to those of the parents and society. The questions posed are too involved and too personal to be answered in a book, particularly because of the unresolved legal questions, but three general suggestions might be helpful if you are involved in such a decision:

- Except when medical necessity makes immediate action imperative, do not let yourself be rushed into making a decision.
- Be sure to get as much specific information as possible about such critical areas as finances, the institutional and foster home and adoption options in your state, the possible effect on your family of caring for the child at home, and the predicted quality of life for the child.
- Get advice from more than one person. Possible sources (besides your doctor) are clergy, a representative from your state's department of human or social services, your attorney, a respected family friend, other family members, and other parents who have faced a similar problem.

Take nothing for granted. For example, before you launch yourself on a counterproductive guilt trip because you assume adoption is either out of the question or a heartless action that will place your child in an unfeeling home, you should know you're mistaken. One adoption agency I know of, the Down Syndrome Exchange (56 Midchester Ave., White Plains, NY 10606; phone 914-428-1236), specializes in placing special youngsters and has a waiting list of parents who seek just such children to include in their family. You could be doing both the prospective parents and the child a kindness.

Lawyers and the Law

Although legal services may be necessary even before your child is born or an older child is hospitalized for diagnosis or treatment, such counsel generally becomes particularly important later, as you plan for your child's educational, social, and financial future. On the other hand, during your hospital stay, legal consultation with a *local* attorney familiar with disability issues may be desirable to help answer some questions, since the law's position on certain issues can vary from state to state (see Resources: Law). Here are some questions that can be critical:

- Who has the legal right to act for a child or mentally retarded adult?
- What rights does a child have, regardless of his mental competency?

- Under what conditions must a hospital provide services for an individual?
- What financial obligation does a parent have if he is unable to meet hospital bills?
- Under what circumstances can life-support systems be initially withheld or later removed? What obligation does a parent have to authorize lifesaving surgery for a severely/profoundly handicapped child?
- What can a parent do if he believes the professionals engaged in his child's care have not operated in a responsible fashion?

One word of caution concerning irreversible legal obligations: If you have become concerned about your child's financial future and are considering establishing a trust fund, I urge you to go slowly. What may seem a prudent move can, if mishandled, eventually work to your youngster's disadvantage (see Chapter 15).

Malpractice

The subject of malpractice carries numerous negative connotations. To ignore its existence, however, would be to overlook a fact of life. In your role as your child's advocate, you face the problem of what to do if it becomes apparent that a professional has acted in an irresponsible or unprofessional fashion that adversely affected your child's welfare. The person involved could be a doctor, an educator, an institutional staff member, an administrator, or any professional who, as a part of his duties, comes in contact with your child. (In some states the courts have specifically precluded educational malpractice suits.) Of course, physicians, nurses, and others directly involved in health care have figured most prominently in malpractice suits, for obvious reasons. Heavy malpractice judgments have helped contribute to ever-increasing health-care costs, since the expenses of high malpractice insurance premiums are eventually passed on to the patient. (However, do not fool yourself. Even if a negligent doctor is involved, there is absolutely no assurance that any money will ever be received by the parents.) Unfortunately, another outcome of the preoccupation with this aspect of medicine is that it can erode the physician–patient relationship and transform it from a team effort, where all work together, into an adversarial contest. Still, if malpractice has occurred, you may owe it to your child to seek legal redress.

Is there anything you as a parent can do to lessen the chance of malpractice? You can make every effort to select the best medical team available. You can become, wherever possible, a knowledgeable, participating member of your child's health-care team. You can make certain that your communications with the professional are always frank and direct. Mutual confidence must be the starting point if your child is to prosper in his treatment. With few exceptions, our country's medical system is well regulated and the personnel superbly trained. Many medical practitioners have spent more than ten years after college learning their specialty. Unfortunately, the news media are more apt to report the rare mistakes than the everyday successes. Doctors are neither saints nor sinners; in general, they are conscientious people, deeply interested in your child's welfare.

In the rare exceptions, mistakes have been and will continue to be made. (Admittedly, it is easier to discuss this area dispassionately when it's not your own child who is involved.) A professional has a real and tangible responsibility to his patient to perform his services in accordance with acknowledged standards. This is part of what being a professional means, and if he fails to do so and as a result of his error the patient suffers harm, the practitioner should be held responsible. A reputable lawyer can give parents helpful counsel. He will be able to suggest whether you should take legal action, and, if so, how it should be done. Resorting to legal action is a drastic step, one that should be taken only after careful consideration. Remember that even when unsuccessful, a lawsuit can affect a doctor's reputation. (A far less drastic step, albeit one that does not offer the possibility of financial remuneration, is to complain to the state commission on medical discipline or another professional body having jurisdiction over a particular profession.)

Dos and Don'ts
for Your Hospital Stay

1. *Choose your doctor according to the professional qualities that are important to you.* Consider affability (Do you have confidence in and get along with him?), availability (Can you reach him when you want him?), ability (Is he professionally competent?), and affordability (Will his bills fit into your budget?).

2. *Know the details of your child's impending hospitalization.* Get clear and complete answers to critical questions, such as: Why does he need to go? What will be done? What is hoped to be accomplished? What will it cost? Are there alternatives?

3. *In hospital selection, give your newborn every advantage that modern medicine provides, particularly if he is at risk.*

4. *Plan what things can be done before entering the hospital; draw up a checklist of chores and then take care of them.*
   - Obtain and become familiar with all preadmission material available from the hospital and make a get-acquainted visit.
   - Arrange for your family's needs while you are away, and arrange for your lodging if the hospital is far away.
   - Make transportation arrangements, including emergency provisions if unexpected hospitalizations are likely. (If it is practical, have a bag packed and ready to go at all times.)
   - Notify those who should know about your visit and establish a plan for hospital–home communication.
   - Prepare your child emotionally for the visit and, in consultation with your doctor, think through decisions you may be required to make.

5. *Seek help with difficult moral questions.* When difficult decisions must be made, be sure that you have the benefit of a wide range of advice and that you take enough time to make your decision. If you are upset, and it is possible to do so, postpone your decision making until later, when you're calmer.

6. *When the diagnosis is definite, decide who needs to know about your child's condition, and when, how, and by whom the notification will be made.*

7. *Both father and mother should be with their child as much as possible and involved in his care.* In addition, the child's progress will be helped if his entire family understands the situation, doesn't feel left out, and is encouraged to work as a team.

8. *Learn how you can make your child more comfortable physically and emotionally.* Work on the assumption that you can do something practical to help your youngster.

9. *Plan your posthospital life while you have experienced advisors readily available.*
- Consult with the doctor who will coordinate your child's post-hospital programs. Become familiar with all aspects of your child's home care.
- If it's appropriate, make arrangements for a visiting nurse to help out when you get home and meet with her while your child is still in the hospital.
- Be sure you have available all necessary medical supplies and equipment and that your home is physically arranged to accommodate your child's needs.
- Identify and make preliminary contact with sources of advice and emergency assistance that can help you once you have left the hospital.
- Continue to keep an accurate, organized, current account of all pertinent facts about your child in your notebook.

10. *Complain—and compliment.* Offer positive criticism, with suggestions for improvement, but compliment staff, too, when a job is well done.

11. *Anticipate discharge requirements.*

PART THREE

Now this is not the end. It is not even
the beginning of the end. But it is, perhaps,
the end of the beginning.

SIR WINSTON CHURCHILL

It's a New World: Coping with the First Few Years at Home

Prologue

The early years with Owen were difficult. But memories of living with this "crazy kid" bind our family together in ways outsiders would never understand: the sound in the night as he swayed back and forth in his crib banging his head; Mary rocking him in her arms when he was unhappy, humming into his ear and making the only sound of comfort he could understand; Owen sitting for hours, leaning back on his haunches in that characteristic way of his, watching in rapt attention as tiny dust particles danced in the rays of the afternoon light.

He was an embarrassment to all of us—except to Mary—and as the years passed he grew "curiouser and curiouser." Stimulated by shifting visual patterns—waves rolling onto a beach, clouds moving across the sun—he would rock back and forth, flap his hands in the air, and yodel. (He wasn't a very good yodeler.) This was unusual behavior no matter how you looked at it and tended to draw a crowd, particularly of young children, who watched his every action with rapt attention. His brothers and sisters, sitting with him at Little League games, would edge away, afraid of what their friends would think and what Owen would do, because you never could tell for sure, except you knew it would be interesting.

Gradually, we toughened up, and Mary never gave up in her efforts to breach the communication barrier that so completely isolated Owen. She worked on it even at the very end of the long day after he had kissed everyone good night—sometimes two or three times—brushed his teeth, and was finally ready for bed. Dental hygiene was not one of his strong points, and if I was slow in my supervisory responsibilities at brushing time and hesitated even for a second, he'd dash into the bathroom ahead of me. Looking over his shoulder to see what I was up to, he would squeeze out some toothpaste, gulp it down, wave absentmindedly at his teeth, and scoot back out into the living room before you could say "Jack Robinson."

After the predictable bathroom encounter, Mary would lead him through the routine that eventually became a family tradition. We all knew what was coming, and conversation quieted as the two of them slowly climbed the stairs and we heard Owen clumping around over-head. Soon would come the familiar words: "My name is Owen. You are Mommy. I love you. Good night." To this day I have never learned whether these short phrases have any meaning for him at all, and it's a shame not to know. Certainly, his almost unintelligible grunts haven't changed much down through the years.

Physically, he's a grown man now, a far cry from the kid in pajamas with toothpaste on the front, but some things haven't changed at all. Mary and I know that when Owen comes home from school "on vaca-tion" and his brothers and sisters gather from wherever they are— home for the holidays—we will hear again his evening litany. It's one thing we can count on. As a matter of fact, now that I think about it, maybe his yodeling has improved.

8

The Transition from Hospital to Home

No matter how self-assured you are and with what infinite care you made plans while at the hospital, the first few weeks at home with your new baby will probably be bedlam. But be of good cheer; you will make it! Most parents are sure the period they're in is the worst they'll ever face. They're right! Today's decisions are critical. Often there doesn't seem to be enough time or emotional energy to worry about tomorrow. And yesterday? "Well, you wouldn't believe yesterday." However, despite the importance of other moments in a lifetime of critical moments, the span from birth to five years is often the most crucial of all, and the insensitivity of many professionals to the pressures families face can mark the beginnings of an adversarial climate between the doctor and parents that is difficult, once begun, to reverse. The early years are a time of transition when the family needs all the support it can muster. Sometimes too much is expected too soon. It was of us, and yet we managed to muddle through.

For some of you, this period marks the first time you have had to worry seriously about anyone else. Or even if you have had other family responsibilities, you felt you could handle them. Now, suddenly, circumstances seem to be getting out of control; it's easy to feel you're no longer the master of your own destiny no matter how independent you may have been in the past. Because when you return from the hospital with your baby in your arms and the door of your house closes behind you, you know your universe will never again be the same. Your handicapped child becomes a factor in everything you do. Even your decision-making process changes, and the quality of your family life will be determined by the manner in which you're able to cooperate both with one another and with the professionals who will play an increasingly important role in your future.

This section deals with six broad responsibilities you will have to shoulder. You must:

1. Acquire the skills necessary to weather the first months at home. Your experience during this period will set a pattern for the future. It's a time to trim ship, not to abandon it.

2. Have your child thoroughly examined in every area—physical, social, emotional, and mental. The terms you will encounter—*diagnosis, assessment, evaluation,* and *prognosis* (all defined in Chapter 9)—are confusing, since they often overlap and are sometimes misused.

3. Make sure that a program is developed for your youngster that utilizes all available resources inside and outside your home, to put into action the recommendations of the professionals.

4. Educate yourself and your family to be effective participants in your child's daily management.

5. Ensure that your entire family, including yourself, live healthy, well-balanced lives in spite of your changed circumstances.

6. Plan and act early to prepare your child for the formal school years and maximal eventual independence.

Establishing an Initial Medical Safety Net

Even if you strictly follow my preparing-to-go-home suggestions, problems will arise. Try to reduce these inevitable surprises by taking first things first. Establish your own medical safety net. To get a sense of what constitutes a real medical emergency, ask your pediatrician what symptoms and secondary problems might develop and how to respond to them. For example, a child with a cleft palate can be susceptible to infections of the eustachian tube, with resulting middle-ear problems and possible hearing loss. Youngsters who have spina bifida are vulnerable to kidney damage, if unattended, since they frequently are unable to sense a full bladder. Kids with Down syndrome can be vulnerable to upper respiratory problems.

As a child, Owen was susceptible to chest colds, and Mary and I would take turns holding him in our arms under a steaming shower trying to relieve the congestion. Each breath seemed to be his last. We became an effective team, shuffling back and forth under the shower curtain in the wee hours of the morning (when being a good team member isn't all it's cracked up to be). The hot water never seemed to bother Owen. Not until later did we realize he was almost completely insensitive to pain and would, if unsupervised, stand motionless in a scalding shower until his back became raw and blistered (a more complete physical might have detected this condition earlier). This absence of the safety alarm that pain normally provides caused continuing problems, particularly after Owen was institutionalized.

An important part of any safety net, after learning what kinds of problems constitute an emergency, is knowing how to get medical assistance in an emergency. As you become experienced, you learn which alarms you can handle yourself and which ones require outside help "stat" (in a hurry). In the early days it's natural to call your doctor about matters that won't faze you later, but it's better to be conservative than to risk delaying too long.

Some of the signs of serious trouble for which you need immediate medical consultation are: unusual difficulty in breathing (the skin sometimes turns blue), indication of severe or persistent pain, sudden or extreme alteration in your child's usual behavior pattern (lethargy, excessive sleeping, marked change in temperament, disorientation, etc.), loss of consciousness, ingestion of possibly toxic substance, convulsions (body may get rigid, eyes become fixed and turned to one side, arms and legs twitch), vomiting that has a green color or that dramatically spurts from the mouth (projectile vomiting), a significant change in the frequency of urination or color of urine, blood in the bowel (stool will look black), extreme diarrhea, dehydration, excessive bleeding, or a body temperature that you and your physician have agreed beforehand is a cause for concern.

Before you call the doctor, get organized: Have a pad and pencil handy to write down instructions and have at hand the name and phone number of your pharmacist in case the doctor wants to call in a prescription. In a real emergency, inform the person who answers your call, "This is Mrs. Jones. I have an emergency," so that you won't be put on hold. Also know which emergency room to call if your doctor is unavailable. If your child has swallowed a possibly toxic substance, have the container available so that you can read its contents from the label. Prepare yourself for the doctor's natural questions: How long has the problem been going on? What is the child's temperature? In the event of severe congestion, what does the mucus look like? (Is it yellow or green?) How many sessions of diarrhea has he had? Is the baby's skin moist or dry, hot or cool?

Make sure you can reach important people at all times. Post key nighttime and daytime telephone numbers for your medical "team" (particularly the coordinator and visiting nurse), the suppliers of medical equipment and supplies, the poison control center, the hospital emergency room (some triage nurses will give you general advice over the phone about the seriousness of the problem, although they may not be supposed to), the druggist, and the local ambulance service. Before leaving the hospital, you should have established who is in overall charge of your child's treatment. As time passes, this responsibility may change, but see to it that you, and all the individuals involved with your child's care, know who is in charge and how to reach him. Most parents well know the frustration of being "bounced" from one professional to another. Being told by Dr. Jones that "You'll have to check with Dr.

Smith" can be the last straw, particularly when just getting past Dr. Jones's secretary and finally running him to ground has already represented a full morning's work.

Medication or Drugs

If your child requires special medication, be sure you understand everything that's involved. It's the doctor's and the pharmacist's job to see that you're thoroughly briefed. It's your job to see that you understand their instructions. Ask questions! If an error is made and your child suffers, it won't matter who made the mistake. Medication can do wonders, but, improperly used, it can be dangerous. (One study has suggested that half of the prescription drugs dispensed are used incorrectly.) Here are suggestions to help you avoid mistakes:

- Ask the doctor the purpose of the medication or drug.
- Find out what side effects, if any, the drug could have and if aspirin or other nonprescription drugs should be avoided while the medication is being taken. Side effects vary; some are very mild, others are serious. (For example, if a drug can cause drowsiness or upset stomach, the time the medication is taken is important. Knowing what to expect will allow you to report unexpected effects to your doctor, which he may be able to reduce or eliminate by reducing the dosage.) Ask the prescribing physician or the pharmacist for a list of possible side effects of your child's medication and be sure to include a drug side-effect chart in your notebook.[1]
- Give the doctor all pertinent information. Does your child have any allergies? Has he had a reaction to other medications? Is he currently taking other drugs or medicines? Don't assume the doctor knows or remembers these details. Review them carefully each time a drug is prescribed.
- Be sure you understand how often, precisely when, and in what dosage the medication is to be given. Should it be given before or after meals or near bedtime? Is it desirable to take the medication in conjunction with a glass of milk? Should certain foods or beverages be avoided? Must the entire course of the prescription be taken to achieve optimal results? It's natural to want to stop the medication as soon as symptomatic relief is obtained, but resist

---

1. A handy "Drug Chart," including side effects, as well as seven side effects of chemotherapy, is included in the excellent publication *Young People with Cancer: A Handbook for Parents*, produced by the Office of Cancer Communications, National Cancer Institute and National Candlelighter Foundation, NIH Publication no. 83-2378 (March 1983).

this temptation and never discontinue medication without your doctor's approval. Don't alter the amount of your child's dosage without first consulting your physician and don't share medication prescribed for one person with another. Finally, be sure to destroy unused medication when it is discontinued (this is one time when it doesn't pay to be frugal).

- Decide with your spouse who is responsible for dispensing the medication and work out a system so that you neither double-up nor omit a scheduled dose. Some pharmacies sell medication dispensers that help eliminate errors.

- Drugs can be expensive, although the cost may qualify as an income tax deduction. Generic medications are usually less expensive; ask your doctor to prescribe them if possible. If your child requires medication over an extended period, and if you belong to a national association, the organization may offer an inexpensive group purchasing plan. A growing number currently do.

- Keep medications in a safe place, and never leave them lying around the house. Find out if they must be refrigerated, and always have a sufficient supply so as not to run short at night or over the weekend.

- Enter all the details in your notebook, including dose frequency, date prescribed, form (injection, liquid, pill), and your own observations of the results, particularly if your child requires frequent medication.[2]

Learning How to Be Effective

To become skilled nurturers of both their special child and their family, parents must become students of the world they all are entering. They must learn their new "trade" by reading, by asking questions, and by doing. Much valuable information is available on videotapes and filmstrips and in books, pamphlets, and magazines. Books are the most plentiful resource and range from personal accounts of real-life experiences (usually written by parents) to technical works by professionals (usually written in language often difficult for the layperson to understand). Many specific manuals offer guidance on living, working, and playing with handicapped persons.

A word of advice: since research findings are constantly revised and expanded, get the most recent information available (medical texts

2. Some of these ideas were drawn from the article "Are You Ready to Take Your Medicine?" by Robin Frames, included in the National Multiple Sclerosis Society publication *Inside* 4, no. 4 (1986): 24–26.

are said to be out of date in five years) and don't be surprised if experts sometimes disagree; despite what you may think, medicine is not always an exact science. When you receive conflicting opinions and must make a decision, review the current literature on the subject (if you have time) and make up your own mind. Many parents complain they aren't able to locate satisfactory information about their child's disability, but today in many cases the information is available; it's up to the parent to locate it.

Getting Organized: Aids to Basic Competency (ABC)

Some parents prefer to face challenges on a day-to-day basis and find checklists vaguely distressing. Others, like myself, need external structure to organize their thinking and support their shaky memories. To the former I offer my envious admiration. For the latter I have constructed a two-part system that, combined with the notebook already described, offers a fledgling parent two advantages: first, a structure to keep track of key human resources (people and organizations), and, second, suggestions for a home reference library of basic books and materials designed to establish a foundation of general information. I call it Aids to Basic Competency (ABC), having invented the title because it's easily abbreviated and sounds reassuring.

The first part, dealing with the support network, uses a form (included in The Notebook, Appendix A) that is filled in by the parents (perhaps with the help of a social worker) as they progressively record basic information about people who are, have been, or probably will be key to the family's efforts in such areas as education, church, the library, recreation, law, advocacy, housing, medicine, politics, the bureaucracy, finance, employment, and respite care—all in the sequence in which they might ordinarily be needed.

The second part contains the basic home library, which can be expensive, although a number of documents suggested are free. Some books will serve you a lifetime, while others may have to be updated or replaced periodically. Inspect books before you buy them by borrowing them or looking them over in your library's reference section. If funds are short, you can try to borrow key material when the need arises, but the books may not be available when you need them. Appendix B contains the description of the material to include in your basic library.

Of course, neither the ABC nor any other plan in itself can meet all needs. However, if you are able to keep both your notebook and the first part of your Aids to Basic Competency up to date and eventually to acquire the home library, you should have adequate, general reference resources from which to work.

Information about Specific Problems

Your health professional should be the best source of up-to-date information about specific management problems, such as the gastrostomy tube, the ostomies, catheters, and feeding tubes; however, medical assistance is only one form of help you will need. Some national organizations concentrate on certain special areas—for example, the HEATH Resource Center (see Resources: Clearinghouses), a first-rate clearinghouse, specializes in postsecondary education for handicapped individuals, but it also offers much of general interest. Here are some informational sources to help you expand your knowledge as time goes on and your child grows older:

1. The National Information Center for Children and Youth with Handicaps (NICHCY; see Resources: Clearinghouses) will furnish a wide range of free information dealing with handicapping conditions, including information specifically geared to parents. Their extremely valuable "State Resource Sheets" list addresses and pertinent information about organizations serving handicapped persons in each state in the union. Send for yours. Although the organization charged with the responsibility of compiling this information may change, the overall responsibility to provide citizens such service has been assumed in recent years by the U.S. Department of Education, Office of Special Education and Rehabilitative Services, in Washington, D.C. (see Resources: Federal Agencies). Check with them if NICHCY no longer provides the service.

2. ERIC Clearinghouse on Handicapped and Gifted Children. ERIC (Educational Resources Information Center; see Resources: Clearinghouses) is a federally funded system that collects literature in all areas of education. The ERIC clearinghouse dealing with the exceptional child is operated by the Council for Exceptional Children (CEC; see Resources: Clearinghouses). Either write them directly or ask your librarian for information on how to utilize their services. Databases, such as ERIC and NARIC, are wonderful resources. Talk to your nearest reference librarian for help locating, understanding, and using them.

3. NARIC (National Rehabilitation Information Center) is another federal service, funded by the U.S. Department of Education. NARIC (see Resources: Clearinghouses) furnishes specific information about rehabilitation. Although this organization should be of greater help to parents of the older child, it can be a useful resource for others as well. Since both ERIC and NARIC also serve professionals, some material will be specialized and technical.

4. Several national organizations, such as the National Easter Seal Society, the March of Dimes Birth Defects Foundation, the Muscular Dystrophy Association, and the Association for Retarded Citizens of the United States (ARC) (see Resources: Associations), are remarkably good resources, particularly—although not exclusively—in the area of their primary interest.

5. The American Council on Rural Special Education (ACRES) of the National Rural Development Institute (see Resources: Associations) is a resource for the parents of handicapped children living in rural areas. Efforts to provide adequate services for these children are often complicated because of the distances separating them from large urban areas and the facilities concentrated there. ACRES works to improve this situation. Although ACRES offers its members several services, including a resource book, I have found its materials, to date, of limited value in areas of interest to the handicapped population.

6. The United States Government Printing Office (Washington, DC 20402) will send free current bibliographies on such subject areas as "The Handicapped" and "Children and Youth" (which deals with both handicapped and nonhandicapped children). Write the Superintendent of Documents. Some representative titles included in these categories are *Sex and the Spinal Cord Injured, Pocket Guide to Babysitting,* and *Young Children and Accidents in the Home.* A fee is charged for some documents. Many of their telephones utilize a series of recordings which defy logic and give me acid indigestion.

7. *Exceptional Parent* (see Resources: Periodicals), which is discussed below, offers an excellent way to keep up to date. Its annual "Education Issue," which includes a directory of organizations, is particularly helpful.

When searching for information it saves time if you have composed one form letter that can be sent to many organizations. Type the letter on 8½″ × 11″ white paper (see fig. 1).

If your child's diagnosis is indefinite, describe his handicap as specifically as you can. For example, in our case we might have said, "Owen is a two-year-old boy who, for unknown reasons, is developmentally delayed. As yet, although he crawls, he neither talks nor understands language. He will not eat solid foods and is slow in all his motor development." Enclose a stamped, self-addressed envelope; it will speed up their reply. Make a copy of the letter for your notebook.

The Public Library

Although materials from associations or public agencies are often either free or inexpensive, commercially published books can be costly.

Date

Dear _____ :

I am the parent of a handicapped child. [Fill
in the details of your child's age, sex, and
handicap.] I am seeking information bearing
on my child's disability or related areas and
would appreciate it if you would send me a
list of available materials, including information on document cost, procedures for
ordering them, and a description of your
organization.

Sincerely,

[Your name and address]

Fig. 1

Don't forget your neighborhood public library and its reference librarian. Librarians are a superb, but often neglected, resource. Ask them
how to solve your information problems. You won't be disappointed!

If you know the title of the book you need, look it up in the card
catalog. If you're not familiar with library procedures, ask for assistance. Don't give up if your book is out of print or not included in
your local library; it should be available through the interlibrary loan
system, a nationwide computerized network that has been helpful to
me time and again. Locating a book that is not on the shelves is part of a
librarian's job, but you have to ask for help.

Many local libraries have access to state and university collections,
which may contain titles of interest, particularly if special education
courses are offered at the institution. (When a librarian uses the word
title, she means the entire printed work, and not only books but also

any written material—pamphlet, government document, periodical, etc.) The reference librarian or the interlibrary loan librarian can help you track down a particular book and she may suggest other sources of related information.

To locate a book through the interlibrary loan service, give the librarian its author's name and its title (date of publication and publisher are helpful but are usually unnecessary). If you don't know the exact title, the librarian can probably locate a list of the author's published works. Current and back-issue magazine articles can also be obtained through the same network. You need the article's title, its author(s), and the publication date of the periodical or some other identification (such as volume or issue); the page numbers of the article are helpful but usually are not necessary. If the librarian finds a library that has what you are looking for, it will usually send you a limited number of photocopies free of charge. One helpful pamphlet deals specifically with locating hard-to-find material: *How to Find Information about Your Subject: A Guide to Reference Materials in Local Libraries*, by Merete Gerli (see Resources: Bibliographies).

To look for additional material—especially if you don't know exactly what it is you want—it helps if you can communicate in terms understood by an automated system that deals only in symbols. (Many libraries make use of various computerized systems.) Having to describe your child and his condition in this fashion—putting him in a cubbyhole or category and labeling him—can seem insensitive and raise your blood pressure, but be realistic. When dealing with computers it's unavoidable.

Be as specific as possible in your search for information, but don't necessarily restrict yourself to one area. It pays to be creative; do not expect that everything that could be of interest to you will be collected under one category. Say, for example, your child is eighteen years old and mentally retarded. "Mental retardation" is obviously one category to search under, but many other areas may be of interest: "affirmative action programs," "independent living," "occupational programs," "sex and the mentally retarded," and "Supplemental Security Income" are examples. Your librarian, doctor, or special education teacher can help by suggesting topics (labels) to use in your search, particularly if your youngster's disability does not fall neatly into one of the recognized categories.

Periodicals

Magazines are a more up-to-date resource than books because they are published frequently. *Exceptional Parent,* a magazine published six times yearly, is "exceptionally" good for keeping parents current in many areas. One of the magazine's helpful features, "Readers' Search," provides parents who have similar needs a way to contact one another and exchange information. For example, one reader wrote, "I am interested in corresponding or finding information about our daughter's condition, partial trisomy." The magazine is required reading for parents and should be perused from cover to cover. Don't just select appealing articles from the index; articles that appear to have little relevance can turn out to be invaluable.

Often in the search for pertinent magazine articles it's hard to know where to begin. The *Reader's Guide to Periodical Literature*, which can be found in most libraries' reference sections, is a valuable resource, since it lists past years' articles, by subject matter, from a large number of magazines. The *Education Index* can also be helpful. The "search" (locating particular information) can be made into a constructive project for siblings that offers two advantages in addition to information gathering: siblings can contribute to the family and feel good about themselves while at the same time developing valuable library skills.

Another way to keep up to date is to get on the mailing list of a publisher who specializes in matters affecting handicapped people (see Resources: Publishers). Some publishers allow customers a number of days to inspect books during which time they can be returned without cost. Finally, your librarian, local school system, or church may have, or be able to locate, pertinent audiovisual materials and the equipment to show them. By inviting interested teachers and parent groups to join you in a viewing session, you can get acquainted with people who share your interests.

The National Library Service for the Blind and Physically Handicapped (NLS/BPH)

The NLS/BPH (see Resources: Clearinghouses) is an underused and often misunderstood organization that can be a valuable resource for both you and your child, even if he is not visually impaired. (I wish we had known of it earlier.) The service publishes "books and magazines in Braille and in recorded form on discs and cassettes for readers who cannot hold, handle, or see well enough to read conventional print because of a visual or physical handicap." If your child qualifies, more than 50 regional and more than 100 local libraries across the nation will lend materials free of charge and often can provide special reading equipment, such as amplifiers, page turners, talking-book machines, headphones, pillow phones, and remote control units. There is a special music library for handicapped musicians, music students, and those who simply enjoy music. Ask your librarian how to contact the library that serves your area and get an "Application for Free Library Service—Individuals." To qualify, "Persons must be certified by a doctor, nurse or other professional as unable to read ordinary print, or to hold a book or turn pages." You can also request information and an application form directly from the Reference Section of the NLS/BPH.

More and more material is being recorded, by both nonprofit and commercial organizations, and can be valuable even if your child is not visually impaired. You can use recordings to divert his attention or entertain him in the hospital, on long trips, or at home when you have run out of energy and can't read one more story. And if you can afford it, buy a Walkman—for your youngster this machine can be a status symbol as well as a tie-in with the nonhandicapped world.

In addition to reading materials, other services of the NLS/BPH include a bimonthly publication and a Reference Section, mentioned above, which I find particularly valuable even though some of its activities are directed toward the professional. The NLS/BPH explains that its Reference Section will answer individual "questions on a wide range of subjects to handicapped persons, their families, and professionals who work with them. For questions that do not fall within the scope of the NLS/BPH reference collection, e.g., medical and legal questions, alternative information sources are suggested." This information-gathering service covers many areas of interest: "commercial sources of spoken-word and large-type publications, special aids and equipment designed for use by handicapped persons, . . . national organizations and federal agencies with programs benefitting the handicapped population, [and] research and technology having application to training, employment and independent living for handicapped persons and major social issues directly affecting the handicapped population." Furthermore, it accepts inquiries either by telephone or by correspondence.

The Reference Section also publishes much free material, including such reference circulars as *Becoming a Volunteer: Resources for Individuals, Libraries, and Organizations* (1981), and *Parents' Guide to the Development of Preschool Handicapped Children: Resources and Services* (1984). The latter circular is first-rate: it offers concise annotated listings of a variety of things, including suppliers of recordings of stories, songs, and learning activities, and of educational games, toys, and play equipment; national organizations concerned with handicapped children; and magazines of interest to parents (ten listed) and children (four listed). Over all, NLS/BPH is a particularly valuable resource, and I am optimistic that its references will be updated on an ongoing basis.

Recording for the Blind

A service of particular interest to disabled students and professionals is Recording for the Blind, Inc. (RFB). Write them for details (see Resources: Suppliers for their address). RFB is an independent, nonprofit organization that lends free recorded textbooks and other educational materials to the qualifying blind, perceptually handicapped, or learning disabled person. A student or professional can apply to RFB to have them record a book that he needs in a work-related area.

For all disabled people, whatever their handicap, vast quantities of information are available, much of it free. If you are unable to provide material for yourself or your child, chances are you just haven't looked in the right place.

Home Management

If you were actively engaged in your child's care at the hospital, the first days at home will be more comfortable, but even with this preparation and the written directions you should have received from your doctor, you may still be ill at ease when the responsibility is all yours. Help from a visiting nurse or a physical therapist is wonderful, but try to become self-reliant as quickly as possible. Self-reliance includes knowing what to do and whom to call if equipment fails or malfunctions as well as knowing how to tell when equipment is performing properly. Any unfamiliar apparatus (a portable IV, for example) can be intimidating until you learn its idiosyncrasies. Remember, hundreds of parents have successfully performed the same tasks you face. Furthermore, many equipment-rental companies offer technical assistance to customers on a 24-hour basis, and some maintain libraries dealing with illness-related equipment. Nurses with whom I have spoken praise the average parents' ability to cope with their child's equipment after instruction and a little hands-on training, and they insist that generally all the parents need "is a pat on the back and assurance that they're doing O.K." Most nurses, however, make a point of adding the reassurance that if any problems come up when the parents get home, "We're always here near a phone to bail them out."

The nature of the skills required will depend upon your own situation, but most parents of young handicapped children need to know such basic techniques as feeding, bathing, dressing, diaper care, and toilet training. In addition, you must handle your child's specialized medical requirements. Sometimes the work involved in their child's care exceeds the physical and emotional resources of the parents and fosters a "siege mentality." As many family members as possible should become competent in the techniques required, and responsibilities should be divided among family members. Siblings should help out, but don't expect too much—they have their own needs and developmental tasks. Fathers, on the other hand, often tend to stay too much in the background. They should learn the skills so that they gain confidence and become involved in their child's care; a bonus is how easily they also establish a positive relationship with their handicapped child.

Outside Help

Without question, you will need professional assistance and supervision during that period at home before your child's first assessment is completed and a care plan can become a reality. (The time required to develop the plan and the difficulties encountered will vary widely, especially depending on your location. Do your best to get things going—Chapter 10 describes specific things you can do.) If possible, make arrangements for a visiting nurse to meet you upon your return from the hospital. The nurse can act as a liaison between you and your doctor, keeping him informed of your child's progress. Another goal of the visiting nurse is to provide information regarding your child's health and to help you find needed resources. She is a coordinator, so take advantage of her knowledge of local resources. In some states, visiting nurses can also provide actual medical assistance. At various critical moments in our own early years we hired a former registered nurse to give Mary a hand with Owen. Looking back now, we seem to have been unbelievably naive; we didn't even know visiting nurses existed.

In recent years many national and local companies have entered the home-health-care market and offer comprehensive 24-hour services, including respite care (see Resources: Suppliers). I am referring here to private, independent concerns that charge for their services. These companies can often provide registered nurses, licensed practical/vocational nurses, home health aides, and home managers, as well as companions and live-ins—a wider range of home assistance than is generally available through public agencies. They frequently have help who are qualified to assist with monitoring devices, tube feedings, chemotherapy, dialysis, intravenous antibiotic therapy, fluid replacement therapy, and tracheostomy care, as well as such other services as locating ambulance transportation and arranging for home-care equipment and medical supplies. You should also explore whether the organization that helped you cover your home responsibilities while you were at the hospital offers other support services and can continue to be of assistance after your return home. (The financial considerations involved in home health care are discussed in Chapter 15.) For information on local home-health-care companies, contact your pediatrician or hospital social worker, or look in the Yellow Pages under "Home Health Services."

In your search for help don't forget or downgrade that wonderful American institution, the babysitter. Like everybody else, babysitters are becoming professionals, with advanced degrees. The American Red Cross operates a nationwide instructional program, and occasionally parents' organizations and local branches of national organizations, such as the Council for Exceptional Children, offer babysitting registers. In some locations United Cerebral Palsy affiliates provide both basic and specialized training for sitters (often called "cerebral palsy monitors"), and local agencies give additional training to graduates of the Red Cross program in preparation for work with children with special needs. If you live near a university or large teaching hospital, find out if they have special education or nursing students interested in such duty. Be creative, but be prudent. Discuss the question of reliable supervision with your health professional. Perhaps with his guidance, you can train two or three responsible neighborhood kids as babysitters. Draw up a written checklist with specific instructions for them. Whether a local sitter pool is a realistic possibility and at what point it might be appropriate will depend upon your child's age and the nature of his handicap. (Chapter 14 discusses babysitter safety and includes checklist information and Appendix A contains a profile form to be used in describing your child to a sitter.)

Another outside resource is the parents' support group. Establish a relationship with such a group early on. They may be able to provide an experienced parent willing to shepherd you through your learning period on a one-on-one basis if you'd like. Parent training in home-management techniques, education, and health care is currently a priority of two federally supported parent-centered programs: Collaboration Among Parents and (Health) Professionals (CAPP) and Technical Assistance for Parent Programs (TAPP). (See Resources: Support Groups.) These programs are discussed in Chapter 12.

To be efficient as well as comfortable in your new life, rearrange your home as much as is practical to save steps and reduce anxiety. Appropriate physical alterations can lower the stress on you by reducing worries about fire or concern that you will be unable to hear your child's cry or labored breathing; however, during your first months at home, probably only an improvised arrangement will be possible. Do what you can! The best place to locate your youngster's bed will depend upon many factors, but often a spot in or near your own bedroom and close to a bathroom is desirable. A location on the first floor can be important for safety reasons. Just be flexible and creative. (During one period, Owen wouldn't sleep in a bed—or crib, for that matter—so Mary bought him a warm rug that he could curl up on. After he fell asleep on the rug, we would swoop him up and sneak him back into his bed.)

There are many ways to adapt your home to make it more liveable, particularly for the older child. Ramps, an elevator, a bathtub lift, and a roll-in shower are all possibilities. Your visiting nurse, physical therapist, or occupational therapist can give you practical advice on other little things you can do around the house, and they can sometimes recommend companies that offer equipment that will help you "make do" until a more professional—and costly—job is possible. (For more information, see Resources: Adaptive Housing.)

Informing Neighbors

Once you return home from the hospital, you will have to tell your acquaintances and neighbors about your child's condition. Don't postpone this. The word will spread quickly, no matter what you do. This is a painful task, but it's better to get on with it and see that the picture of your child's condition is as free of distortion as possible. If you don't, you'll only have to set things right later, over and over again. Some parents will find that describing their child's condition in objective, matter-of-fact language is easier and takes less time than becoming involved in emotional discussions about the future and what might have been. If some neighbors or friends have trouble handling your news, recognize that it's their problem, not yours.

Finally, during the first few weeks at home, keep in mind that these difficult early days, too, shall pass. Remember, all of us experience tears and sleepless nights, and be kind to yourself. Try not to be overwhelmed by the seemingly impossible problems, and don't assume that this is the way it's going to be forever, because it's not. It's normal for you to be a bit shell-shocked, but better days are coming, and your attitude will help shape them. Although Mary and I complained about our heavy workload, I'm convinced that being so busy we had little time to worry about ourselves was probably our salvation. Like us, you may have to cut back drastically on nonessential activities for the time being. People will understand. Now is the time to get hopping and stop worrying.

9

The Diagnostic Cycle and the Person Who Helps You: The Care Provider

Defining the Problem

At the beginning, when your child's diagnosis is indefinite, trying to find out exactly what's wrong with your youngster can surely test your inner resources. This is a particularly harrowing time, since often you will harbor the hidden hope that you're all wrong and that your child will eventually be found to be absolutely "normal" (whatever that is). On the other hand, even when the defect (and diagnosis) is obvious at birth, getting specific and understandable information about it still can be difficult. The bewildering language used in the search for answers doesn't help matters. For example, you'll find that the various professionals with whom you deal will, for no apparent reason—except (you think) to confound you—assign different names to fundamentally similar activities. What a physician may describe as a complete diagnosis, an educator might call an evaluation, and a social worker, an assessment. To bring some clarity to this confusion, a few of the more commonly used terms are defined here. However, you also should ask your professional to explain, specifically and simply, what he means and what the implications are for you when he uses an expression you don't understand. (Please excuse me if I use some jargon, myself. In this area it's hard to avoid it.)

- *Diagnosis* (ordinarily a medical term): The doctor's judgment as to what is wrong with the patient and the cause of the problem. Sometimes the term is broadly used to refer to the entire process, including a prediction of future effects and what steps can be taken to improve the situation.
- *Screening:* The process that identifies individuals who are functioning below levels appropriate for their age or those who may have a particular condition or be at higher than average risk to develop it. Beware of the term "at risk." It does not reflect a firm diagnosis, nor does it indicate that the person described is, in fact, affected. It merely suggests that the person may be vulnerable and that more extensive testing or continuing observation is prudent. It should never be used to label children nor should it act as the basis

for corrective action (remediation). Screening tests are, as a rule, short, superficial, and inexpensive. Common screening tests are the Apgar test for newborns, routine vision and hearing tests, testing for scoliosis, the Brazelton Neonatal Behavior Scale, and the Denver Developmental Screening Test (DDST). (See Resources: Testing.) (In educational circles, for reasons that escape me, tests are often called "instruments.")

- *Evaluation:* A testing program, which can be started in many ways, including as the result of a request from you as a concerned parent, on the recommendation of your family doctor, as a result of a screening test, or on the recommendation of a public school's special education committee. The tests prescribed can be given in the specialist's offices, at school, or in the hospital. The tests are sometimes designed to provide information about only one area of a child's functioning (for example, an occupational therapist interested in your child's perceptual-motor integration [his physical coordination] might give the Berry-Buktenica Test of Articulation). Parents should always be told why and how a certain test is being given, and recommendations for treatment should ordinarily accompany test results. Often this information will be transmitted through the medical "coordinator." In educational usage, "evaluation" has a very different meaning, particularly under the provisions of P.L. 94-142 (see Chapter 17).

- *Assessment* (or *Developmental Assessment*): The ongoing overall process by which specialists from various fields (a multidisciplinary team) attempt to discover the nature of the handicap and recommend what generally must be done to improve the situation. Occasionally an effort is made to find the cause of the problem, although often a diagnosis will already have been made. In many instances one professional conducts the assessment, particularly when the problem is relatively straightforward and there is little need for input from other specialists. An assessment team might include a pediatrician, physical or occupational therapist, social worker, nutritionist, speech pathologist, public health nurse, and hearing specialist. The assessment should always relate to both the screening that has gone before and the program that evolves from it, and should include such areas as the child's social and medical history—including behavior observed during the interview, his gross and fine motor development (generally speaking, the coordinated use of large and small muscles), his ability to handle activities of daily living, including communication, and his learning skills and ability to understand more complex ideas.

- *Prognosis:* A medical term referring to a prediction of the consequences of a disease or condition and an estimate of the chances of, and nature of, recovery.

- *Program:* The specific plan meant to eliminate a handicap or to reduce its impact, drawn up on the basis of the assessment or educational evaluation team's recommendations. To be effective it should cover all areas affecting the child (medical, educational, social, emotional, and home environment), and it should reflect not only a child's limitations but also his strengths and potential to grow and enjoy life. This is an opportunity for parents to shine; in your dealings with the professionals, particularly in program planning, accentuate the positive. It's easy for people—even professionals—to become preoccupied with defects and overlook potentials. To be most effective, be positive yourself. All plans should be based upon goals and objectives and should include procedures to review and evaluate program effectiveness on a regular basis.

A Search for Answers

How to Begin

There are many ways a family can enter the diagnostic cycle. It's difficult to generalize. Too many youngsters, too many families, and too many problems are involved for anything to be typical. (Except the pain; maybe the pain is typical.) One way the process can begin is for the mother and father to start the ball rolling and to make the referral themselves (ask that their child be tested). This isn't an easy route, nor does it happen overnight, for just reaching the point at which parents can ask the question "Is my child really all right?" can take a long time. Our family's story is, in many ways, similar to the experiences of others who, like us, didn't know at first that there was a problem and had to wait it out—wait with a child who gradually, almost imperceptibly, grew more and more different. Uncertainty is difficult to live with; it can launch a family on an odyssey in search of answers, answers that may not be there to find.

The first year of Owen's life was uneventful. Actually he appeared to be that ideal baby we had heard about but never seen: he seemed happy and content, and never fussed. He hardly ever got into things and was a joy to have around. All our other kids got into things all day long. I don't remember when I first began to feel concerned. There was just a growing, almost imperceptible uneasiness in the back of my mind that something wasn't right. As the months passed, my concern increased and became more specific. I found myself watching Owen more closely, not really knowing why or what it was I looked for. Yet I couldn't bring myself to talk with Mary about it. I didn't know what to say, what words to use. Maybe I hoped if I ignored "it," "it" would go away. Surprisingly, Mary was slower than I to realize that our fifth child was different in a fundamental and important way. Perhaps, for her, the thought was unthinkable. Maybe she was too busy or too happy just having a child who didn't fuss, but the day came when there was no question that he lagged far behind the developmental pattern we had become accustomed to with our other children.

Later, we learned that this reluctance to face the possibility your child might be "retarded" is a common phenomenon in which both father and mother hide their concern, afraid of transforming a bearable unknown into an unbearable reality. During this period it's possible to lose the power of effective action, to become immobilized by desire to protect your partner, and yet to be concerned that by waiting things out you will lose irreplaceable time. Of course, now I wish I had talked things over earlier. Down through the years I have had lots of time to worry and wonder. Was that time, in fact, irreplaceable? When we finally got going, was it already too late?

Our search for answers began with a trip to the Johns Hopkins Hospital in Baltimore, Maryland, to consult with Miriam and William Hardy, experts in the field of audiology. It was obvious that Owen had a hearing problem, but since he couldn't communicate at all, testing was difficult. Eventually our family moved to the city of Baltimore with its large medical center, but we chose it more for personal than for medical reasons (Mary's mother lived in Maryland, and we wanted to be near her). Within a year—we were hardly unpacked—our family was again uprooted by the move to Baltimore County to qualify for a program the doctors thought would be more appropriate than the one offered in the city. Our private odyssey was under way.

Owen at various times in our odyssey was diagnosed as massively retarded, deaf, autistic, receptive aphasic, and—of all things—normal. Eventually, the experts threw in the towel and gave up. (They never said so, but that's what they did.) In effect they admitted that they didn't have the foggiest idea what was wrong, using that wonderful euphemism: "Owen's diagnosis is not clinically comprehensible."

Normal Development

Despite the fact that Mary and I came to grips with our problem only as a result of comparing our son with the norm—with other children of the same age—we're still not completely comfortable with the concept of normalcy that the comparison suggests. Nor should you be. Are the adjectives "normal" and "average" any different from other labels, which are really only convenient generalizations, misleading and potentially mischievous when misused? Labels tend to concentrate on the negative, describing a youngster's limitations, ignoring his strengths and potentials, and implying that the condition described is both correctly diagnosed and irreversible. The concept of "normal" development, on the other hand, is actually nothing more than a rough gauge indicating the growth that is generally anticipated at various ages. If a child is relatively slow in reaching certain generally accepted milestones, such as rolling over by himself, sitting without support, or beginning to use words with meaning like "Mama" or "Dada," it doesn't mean that he has a serious problem or that he won't eventually catch up and develop into a happy and healthy adult. Of course, there is no question that knowledge of growth patterns is important to you, for unusually slow development can be a sign that something is happening that needs closer examination. Parents, at the point at which they are trying to decide whether or not to seek professional advice, should become familiar with this generally accepted frame of reference. Ask your doctor, nurse, or librarian for a current human growth and development chart. Many good ones are available; get one that goes into some depth and isn't over-simplified.

The Colorado Department of Education had a creative idea when it published a combination baby book and developmental chart (*My Baby's Book*, in Spanish and in English), which you, with some ingenuity, should be able to adapt and include in your notebook. Each 10″ × 12″ page represents a certain age. On one side the page displays colorful pictures of babies performing a variety of tasks, illustrating the development expected at that age. For example, babies are shown "raising their heads" and "turning to a loud noise" at four months, and "reaching for a piece of banana" and "bearing most of their own weight" at six months. Each facing page is titled "My Baby's Pictures," with blank space provided for snapshots of your own child taken at a corresponding age. Also included is a schedule of recommended immunizations and doctor visits. If you are concerned about your child, keep a running written and pictorial record of the ages when he performs these "milestone" actions. An added benefit of this routine is that it will force you to keep records and take photos that someday you will be glad you've got.

Beginning the Actual Diagnostic Cycle

Getting Diagnostic Information

In some locations it is possible to ask for very general diagnostic help over the telephone, and some organizations occasionally will send a staff member to a parent's home to make a preliminary assessment, but usually it's not that easy. You can begin to gather information and enter the diagnostic cycle in a number of ways. Some processes can be initiated by you and others will result from the action of others.

1. Many programs (at the state or local hospital level) have been developed for possible at-risk newborns, to check these babies' progress after they leave the hospital. The North Carolina High-Priority Infant Tracking Program is an example. In this voluntary program, each child meeting certain conditions at birth (called a "high-priority" infant) is carefully checked on a regular basis (monitored) during the first year to see they receive the best of care. When the baby leaves the hospital, the family's local health department is alerted and given certain information, including the conditions that caused the baby to be so identified and the name of the doctor or organization responsible for medical supervision once the infant is home.

At regular intervals—four, seven, and thirteen months—representatives from the local health department contact the "responsible" doctor or agency to see how the baby is progressing. At the end of the first year, the baby's development is checked, and a public health nurse keeps in close touch with the situation, offering help whenever the family has difficulty obtaining adequate care. If you are interested in this kind of program, ask your doctor if there is anything similar to the North Carolina program near you and, if so, whether he feels your child could benefit from participation.

2. You as a parent can begin the cycle by sharing your concern with your family doctor, who may already be familiar with the situation. If his response doesn't satisfy you and serious questions remain, ask him to arrange for a complete diagnostic work-up, which may involve referral to an appropriate specialist or clinic. Referral is the process in which a professional makes arrangements for a patient to see another professional (often a specialist) for consultation. Parents themselves can sometimes refer their own child directly, although some organizations prefer or even require referral by a physician. A representative of your local department of human services or department of health, a visiting nurse, or a social worker should also be able to tell you where local diagnostic services are available.

Every state has an agency, ordinarily called Crippled Children's Services, which provides funding for diagnostic and health-related programs for handicapped children (the term *crippled* is misleading, since the disabilities covered can be mental as well as physical). While programs funded vary from state to state and can include research projects and/or direct services, in some instances the agency will help with financial planning and, if parents meet financial guidelines, may pay for all or a portion of the services involved. Contact the responsible state agency to see what services are provided; your local health department will have their address, or it will be listed in your own state's Resource Sheet available from the National Information Center for Children and Youth with Handicaps. For example, if you live in Alaska, Crippled Children's Services are administered in the Family Health Section of the State Department of Health in Juneau. The Alaska Resource Sheet also sets forth "agencies . . . [that] can help you find the services your child needs." One of these resources, for families who qualify for Medicaid, is the Early and Periodic Screening, Diagnosis and Treatment Program (EPSDT), a national program. If you think you qualify, contact the agency listed in your state's sheet to see if they can be of help.

Currently there is little interstate uniformity in what state agency, if any, is assigned the responsibility of giving parents a hand in arranging for and monitoring the diagnostic cycle, although help is in sight. Fortunately, there is some federally mandated national responsibility. Public Law 94-142 stipulates that every local school system *must* identify each child from birth through school age with a physical, emotional, or intellectual handicap that could interfere with his education. Although this program goes by such names as "child find" or "project search" in the various states, "child find" is how the program is identified by federal law, and it is the term you are most likely to hear (see Part Four for more discussion of the law).

To satisfy their obligations under this legislation, many local school systems cooperate with other agencies in testing and follow-up, and your special education director should be able to give you information on locally available diagnostic services. Another promising source of help, Public Law 99-457 (discussed in Chapter 10), is currently in the second year of a five-year cycle. Although its emphasis is on assisting states in establishing early intervention networks for children from birth to three years old—from birth to age five where no state program is currently in place—it also provides participating states with support in organizing the planning and eventual provision of "early identification, screening, and assessment services." This legislation should place even more emphasis on the child-find provisions of P.L. 94-142 and eventually ensure that *every* child with a problem—physical, emotional, or cognitive—is identified. Contact your local school system if you have questions about your preschooler's development or to obtain up-to-date information, and contact your local state representative if your state doesn't appear to be participating in the new program.

A common complaint of many parents is that their pediatrician was slow to alert them to possible trouble—and was resistant, later, to their requests for testing. "The doctor said, 'Don't worry; he'll grow out of it'" is a refrain I have heard time and again from parents whose children never did grow out of it. Pediatricians deal with hundreds of patients, and statistically they are correct; most children do eventually grow out of their problems. Parents, admittedly, are apt to take a more personal, and perhaps skewed, view of statistics. My advice is to trust your instincts. If they warn you that something is wrong, don't over-react and lose your cool, but don't worry quietly by yourself either, hoping that everything will turn out all right. Share your concerns with your spouse and ask your professional for further study. You have ulti-mate responsibility for, and must eventually answer to—and for—your child.

3. You may be referred or, in some instances, may refer yourself to a local child development clinic. Every state has such organizations, al-though their names vary locally. They provide complete diagnostic and evaluation services (sometimes called D & E) either free of charge or for fees based upon a parent's ability to pay. Every state also offers services for the evaluation of particular problems, such as eye and dental clinics, language and speech centers. In your own geographic area, services probably exist of which you are unaware. Take advantage of what is available.

4. Another kind of center offering comprehensive D & E services that is becoming increasingly common is sometimes called a "one-stop" clinic. Often located in teaching hospitals and universities, the one-stop clinic gathers specialists from many disciplines and is sup-ported by the most sophisticated equipment. Although the clinic is called "one-stop," several appointments are frequently required: one for medical-neurological (nervous system) examination, another for psychological-educational testing, and others for specialized evalua-tions, such as hearing and speech and physical therapy. In some in-stances the institution's social worker meets with the family. One rea-son parents should not procrastinate once they have decided to seek diagnostic information is that there may be considerable delay before an appointment can be scheduled—six months is not uncommon. Na-tional organizations, such as the Muscular Dystrophy Association, March of Dimes, and United Cerebral Palsy, sometimes also offer diag-nostic and follow-up care at their affiliated clinics, which naturally tend to specialize in one handicapping condition; contact their area affiliates for information.

In your search for answers, be sure that your child receives a thor-ough physical examination (a complete medical and neurological as-sessment) even though his problems may appear to spring from an emo-tional or cognitive origin. Sometimes apparently unrelated physical causes can lie at the root of mental problems. Hearing and vision must be checked, for hearing loss or language difficulty can be mistaken for mental retardation. As you pass through the diagnostic labyrinth, keep the test results in perspective. Owen, you will recall, has a serious hearing problem—at least we think so. But for reasons that defy explanation, his auditory test results sometimes fluctuate wildly, and every once in a while, nestled in between readings that indicate continued severe loss, one test will reflect perfectly normal hearing. (Sometimes at home this "deaf" child will practically jump into the air when someone inadvertently crinkles paper behind his back.) This inconsistency troubles us all, but we learned an important lesson from this baffling and unnerving testing pattern: never view test results as infallible indicators or accept their results without question, particularly when they appear to contradict your own insights gained through years of personal observation. Remember, the purpose of diagnostic testing is to provide a basis for treatment; even the most reliable test indicates conditions present only at a particular moment. Since the human body is never static, a test result even a few years old may have little relevance today. Still, a comprehensive testing program can be invaluable; often it's the only objective information we have to go on.

Preparing for the Appointment

Much can be done to make the visit to the doctor's office or the clinic a positive experience. However, you have to work at it. Preparations will vary depending upon your child's age and condition, but here are some things to think about. If you have any choice at all in scheduling your appointment, some times may be preferable: the middle of the week and first thing in the morning or right after lunch are times that staff are fresher and that require less waiting. (Mondays may be crowded with weekend overflow. Fridays? Well, you know how Fridays are!) Be on time and go equipped with something to occupy your child. Preferably, take books and toys from home (not small things that other children might swallow or roller-type devices that could send other, unsuspecting adults on their ears; you have enough trouble as it is).

Take along snacks that are easily handled and not gooey or drippy: a small box of raisins, an apple, or cheese. Fruit juices can be purchased in small plastic containers, or you may have a little thermos you can use for milk or some other beverage. And speaking of milk, don't be hesitant to nurse your child while you're waiting—and bring an extra diaper. If your spouse is along, or even an older sibling, one or the other can play with your child outside the office while you wait your turn or if the physician wishes to speak to you alone for some reason. With an older child, ask the staff beforehand about ways to amuse and prepare him emotionally. Try to avoid surprises for either you or your child by asking questions. If you know, in detail, what procedures will be necessary, you can talk them over with your youngster (if he can communicate).

Finally, do not hesitate to seek help for financial concerns. Find out what diagnostic services seem most appropriate for your child first, and then ask how payment can be worked out. Alternatives are often available: a sliding scale based on family income, insurance coverage, or some kind of public medical assistance.

Working with the Professional

As you begin reaching outside your own family for help, you will become increasingly involved with "service or care providers"—people whose job it is to assist you and your child when you need it. Whether you like it or not, your effectiveness will depend upon your ability to work with them. Here are some suggestions that may help.

Of prime importance is the initial selection process in which you decide with whom you will work. The professional's time is valuable (so is yours) and therefore it's critical that you get maximal benefit from every meeting you attend with him. The suggestions just made for dealing with a doctor's appointment as well as those made in Chapter 2 concerning preparation for a conference with a genetic counselor are equally pertinent here.

In all your relationships with professionals, ask that communications, written and oral, be carried on in lay English. Misunderstandings can be frustrating and dangerous. Whenever Mary and I were confused, which we often were, we never hesitated to ask questions like, "What exactly do you mean by that, Doctor? We don't understand." Over the years we persisted, no matter how long it took, till the point became clear, and although sometimes we felt foolish, we did manage to learn. Sometimes it wasn't a doctor with whom we spoke, but a teacher, or a bureaucrat, or an institutional director, and occasionally it became evident that the professional, himself, didn't understand what it was he was saying. On the other hand, speak up and say what's on your mind in a clear and organized fashion. It's equally vital that he understands you, too. Always be courteous and considerate.

Whether you are in a group meeting or an individual conference, you will be asked certain questions time and again. There can be no escape, but you can anticipate and prepare for them. When you call the secretary for an appointment, ask what you should bring with you and what information the doctor will require. Here are some of the kinds of questions he might ask, depending upon the nature of the situation:

- "When did you first notice the problem?"
- "Can you give specific examples of the symptoms?"

- "How old was he when that happened?"
- "Do you have any idea what could be causing the condition?"
- "What have you done to try to correct it?"
- "Have you given your child any medication?"
- "Have any of your blood relatives experienced similar conditions?"
- "Has the situation affected your family life?" And those old standbys you should always be prepared for: "Does your child have any allergies?" and "Is he up to date on his immunizations?" Have your answers down pat. It's thoughtless not to be prepared.

Use your notebook to record the information you know you will need to have at your fingertips in the future, and take it with you to appointments and meetings. If you don't record things when they happen, you may lose them forever, and they may be important. It took us years and a number of hard knocks before we got this lesson through our heads. Record test results, reports, and your own observations of your child—sometimes called "anecdotal" records. It's vital that you be knowledgeable about testing procedures. In your meetings with diagnosticians, who could represent any number of specialties, don't sell yourself short. You know your child better than anyone else and have information that is available only through you. (As is discussed in later chapters, many federal and state laws stress the importance of parental participation in decision-making or information-gathering meetings.) You should ask to be included from the beginning wherever it's appropriate. Record-keeping responsibilities should be shared, like all other duties, by mother and father on the basis of interest, ability, and availability. In our family it is Mary who keeps neat, dated records, and always has. I stuff things in shoe boxes. Mary is tranquil and organized and finds things she's filed. I am given to periodic fits of housecleaning and can never find anything. It didn't take us long to decide that Mary should keep our notebook.

A Second Opinion

In a parent's sometimes love-hate relationship with the medical profession, the period when the initial diagnosis of handicap is arrived at can be difficult. The parent, for many reasons, may question the doctor's conclusions and want another opinion. This is a very reasonable request. Today, many insurance companies require a second opinion before certain surgical practices are performed. Be frank with your doctor; there is no need to feel embarrassed. If you are polite and he acts offended, perhaps you have the wrong doctor. This is a moment when you must be as thorough as possible in a matter involving decisions of critical importance to your family. Make clear that your decision is in no way a criticism of the doctor's professional ability (unless it is). He should be glad to suggest at least two competent doctors from whom you may make a selection and he should make all your child's medical records, test results, X-rays, etc., available to the consulting professional. Unless there is particular reason to do otherwise, I suggest using your own doctor's suggestions, but you can, of course, locate a physician on your own if you wish. Just be assertive—but in a reasonable, polite, and understanding fashion. With rare exceptions you can rest assured the professionals you encounter are doing everything they can for your child's best interests.

How the Doctor Passes on a Diagnosis Is Important

Because doctors are usually extremely busy, occasionally they communicate sensitive information in a hurried, even impromptu fashion. I believe that such action, no matter how necessary it may seem, should be avoided at all cost and that parents have the right—as consumers, if for no other reason—to be given such news in a humane fashion. They deserve to be told in an environment that offers them privacy during that truly awful moment. They need the opportunity to get a grip on themselves and to ask the questions and to discuss the fears that often flood immediately into their minds.

Some psychologists suggest that even if the report is bad, the elimination of uncertainty can bring relief after months of worry. The mind is complex and often unfathomable, but if there was any relief for Mary and me when we heard the news, we were unaware of it. The doctor told us that we had a massively retarded son in much the same way that a telephone operator might report, "I'm sorry, but the number you have dialed is out of order and the lines are down." The doctor's insensitivity was compounded by the fact that his diagnosis proved to be incorrect. We were furious with the doctor and have never really forgiven him. Our lives appeared to have been irreparably damaged—a remarkable reaction as we look back on it now with the perspective time gives us, since we then had four other kids who were normal to a fault and were giving us fits because they were so healthy. But a mind numbed by grief often loses perspective. Also, it's an interesting commentary on our family's own particular coping style that Mary fought back her tears till we had left the doctor's office and then, in the privacy of our car, broke down. I remained outwardly stoic until I was alone so that even she wouldn't see me in my "weakness." It was the first time in my adult life that I had been moved to real unrestrained tears. I'm still not sure for whom I wept.

Obviously, parents have limited control, if any, over the way the professionals break the news. If in their judgment their experience was needlessly clumsy or cruel, any action they take to improve the situation will obviously be too late for any benefit to themselves, but if later they become active in a support group or gain influence in an advocacy position, their criticisms and suggestions can be brought to the attention of the professional community. However, no matter how you receive the mind-chilling news, it is only the beginning. More than any other attribute, success in this first stage of information gathering requires perseverance—the kind of tenacity that characterized Mary's insistence that our son could and would learn to speak. It's the kind of tenacity (some might call it stubbornness) that continues despite setbacks, despite inconvenience, despite disappointment.

10

After the Diagnosis

This chapter considers resources, ways you can help relieve your child's disability and make the most of his capabilities. Once the waiting is over and you know there is a problem, your inclination will be to roll up your sleeves and to get going. That's as it should be. The plan generated by the multidisciplinary team, the most important result of the work done by the assessment team, is designed to give specific direction to the remedial action that should be taken. It will probably involve two basic and interrelated concepts that you should understand: "early intervention" and "infant stimulation."

Early Intervention

To develop normally, every newborn, handicapped or not, needs to exercise all his senses—sight, smell, hearing, touch, and taste—as well as every part of his body. Most infants will do this naturally. Spend an hour watching a month-old baby in his crib and write down everything he does—everything. If you're a careful observer and are quick, you will develop a whopper of a list. Later, at eighteen months, observe him again and follow along as he careens around the room, crawling, jumping, picking things up, checking them out. He'll rub toys over his mouth, throw them down, rap a toy drum, listen, frown, laugh. Nothing escapes his inspection. Nothing in the house is safe! You will be exhausted and your list will probably lie crumpled in the corner. What you have witnessed is nature's way of seeing that the whole body is exercised (stimulated) so it will grow and develop properly. When such spontaneous activity is limited, as it can be by slow development, a handicapping condition, or prolonged isolation, growth can be ad-

A number of the concepts in this chapter are drawn from *One Step at a Time* (1981), a U.S. Department of Education booklet by Barbara Scheiber. The publisher, Closer Look, is no longer in existence. Carol Tingey discusses this subject in "Early Intervention, Learning What Works," in the November 1986 issue of *Exceptional Parent*, as do Rosalyn Benjamin Darling and Jon Darling in their chapter, "Helping Techniques II: Intervention," in *Children Who Are Different* (St. Louis: C. V. Mosby Co., 1982).

versely affected. The attempt to supply additional, compensating stimulation to the child who may be deprived of it is called "infant stimulation." Such special stimulation is also a form of early intervention, since *to intervene* means to take some action you hope will improve an undesirable situation that you fear is developing. In this case intervention supplies stimulation that is lacking. Wresting what's left of a box of chocolates from the sticky hands of a two-year-old before he finishes it off and gets sick is an example of practical early intervention with which every parent is familiar.

Although it's desirable to ensure that a child receives compensatory stimulation for any normal stimulation that he may have been deprived of, it's also important to realize that not all stimulation is beneficial. Bright, flashing lights and loud, unexpected noises can be definitely undesirable. It's not a question of the more stimulation the better, so consult your doctor before attempting any "home therapy." It's important that the advice you get in this sensitive area is the best available. More is discovered every day about the effect that stimulation—the total experience we receive through our senses, which researchers call the "sensory diet"—has on a young child during the first years of life and its impact on later development. Much has been written on the subject, and I recommend that you familiarize yourself with some of the concepts (see Resources: Early Childhood).

There is tremendous value in the spontaneous stimulation that takes place as the natural result of parents' love for their children. It's critical that your child not be deprived of these natural physical demonstrations of affection, even if you are convinced he's not aware of or benefiting from your actions (you could be wrong). Talk to your baby, no matter how unresponsive he may be. Such stimulation can be even more central to his language development than it is for the nonhandicapped child, since your child may be isolated from many of the cues upon which language development normally depends. Pick him up. Sing to him. Rock him and kiss him as you would any "normal" child. This natural "therapy" doesn't require a doctor's prescription! No one in the world is able to do it as well as you. Perhaps no one else will do it at all.

Owen's early stimulation was drastically reduced. His inability to derive meaning from sound, his poor gross motor control, and his reduced sensitivity to tactile sensation all contributed to his lack of stimulation and his resulting loss of contact with the world around him. This deprivation, I am convinced, added to his handicapping condition, despite all of his mother's natural affection. He loved to have Mary hold him tight in her arms and hum tunes into his ear. Of course, we knew nothing about sensory deprivation then, and it was only later that we realized it was the stimulation of the vibration and not the lullaby that delighted him—who knows, he might even have liked modern atonal music.

At one time Owen was diagnosed as autistic, in part, I believe, because of his bizarre "fits" of hand flapping and his mannerized bowing and bobbing, in which he would roll and pitch like a ship at sea. These interludes always occurred when he was exposed to a flood of visual or auditory stimulation. Perhaps only extreme sounds or sights were strong enough to break through to him and register on his starved system. If we had known then what we know now—and if we had had the information available to parents today—perhaps we could have provided additional sensory stimulation specially designed to penetrate the barriers that surrounded him. But neither we nor the medical profession knew enough to be of help.

Much Is Still to Be Learned about Early Intervention

Intervention can take place anytime in a special child's life when it's needed, but because of the rapid development that should take place between birth and age five, action during this period can be particularly effective. Some researchers suggest that an even earlier period—birth to age two—is most critical of all, and they urge that a planned program begin as soon as possible after birth. However, some professionals have reservations about aspects of the early intervention approach, and, admittedly, the research currently available is limited, inconclusive, and conflicting. Even such questions as to what degree parents should be involved, what the long-term effects are, which programs are most effective, and how early intervention should begin have not been adequately investigated. One result of this lack of scientific verification is to place even more emphasis upon the parents' judgment about what kind of early programing is best for their child, so don't hesitate to speak up and give your doctor the benefit of your ideas.

It's not helpful for our purposes to discuss why the research is inadequate, except to point out that questions raised have, in general, not suggested that a professionally planned and controlled program will be harmful, but that there is a lack of evidence proving that early intervention will accomplish any permanent gains that would not have been realized later by the child as a result of his own natural growth and development. (Do recognize, however, that this ambiguity does not apply to desirable medical or surgical action taken early to correct a physical defect.) Despite this lack of substantiating data, and based only on my experience as a parent, I suggest several reasons why early action under the direction of a competent professional is ordinarily preferable to waiting things out. However, remember that one of the most effective interventions of all in your child's life is living in a happy, supportive, and loving family. Don't get so stressed out about arranging intervention that you distort and depersonalize the natural family environment upon which he depends for natural nurturing.

First, many parents feel better about themselves and function more effectively when they are actively engaged and believe they are doing everything possible to help their child. Waiting and doing nothing can be debilitating. Next, if a youngster progresses faster after receiving early intervention than he would without it, the period of personal failure and frustration he endures is shortened and the negative effect on his self-esteem is reduced. Thus, acceleration of development has value in itself even if the child never exceeds the ability level he would eventually have reached without intervention. Furthermore, just the process of developing a plan for your child requires activities that, in themselves, are useful: setting up small, incremental developmental goals, keeping records of your child's progress, and making an analysis of his strengths and weaknesses. Finally, if your child is able to learn basic living skills earlier than he otherwise would and thereby functions more independently, your family will be more quickly relieved of some custodial chores, which can sap energy and destroy morale. However, before you undertake any formal program, you should realize that even ardent supporters of the early intervention concept do not suggest that success can be achieved without hard work or that it will be realized overnight.

To be a contributing partner with the professionals in implementing the assessment program, you should have thought through your own informed reactions to such questions as: When should the program begin? Who, with you, will provide the necessary coordination? What will be the nature of the program? (What will be its syllabus? Where and by whom will it be conducted?) What must be done to monitor the program's effectiveness? How can expenses be covered? In other words, think things through.

When Should the Program Get Under Way?

Ordinarily, the sooner the better. There will be enough unavoidable delay without your contributing to it, so don't sit back and expect that progress is going to be made automatically. Many parents feel inadequate because of their lack of training and experience in an area that seems to require knowledge and skills completely beyond their capabilities. That attitude can lead to self-defeat. Most parents have the potential to do what must be done, so have confidence in yourself. Over the long run a host of care providers will play vital roles in your family's life and will share responsibilities with you. However, it is the nature of things that professionals come and go, and when each successive phase is over and the professionals move on, you will remain the only consistent influence shaping your child's future. Prepare for this leadership role. Seek out the most capable specialists to share the burden. Welcome them and cooperate with them to the fullest, but never abdicate your ultimate responsibility.

Coordination

Who will be responsible with you for organizing the program and providing the services required? Ideally, the assessment team will make specific recommendations and help with all the important details. However, that does not relieve you of the responsibility for getting to know the territory—what must be done—and for seeing to it that the program doesn't get bogged down. The nature of local resources will, or course, influence your options. If your child has a specific disease, such as cerebral palsy, muscular dystrophy, or epilepsy, a national association may offer clinical services. For example, some area associations for retarded citizens provide infant stimulation and treatment programs beginning as early as the fourth week of life, and the Shriners support many hospitals in the United States, Canada, and Mexico for children who have orthopedic problems (see Resources: Facilities, Schools, Clinics).

Often the center or clinic that conducted the original assessment or identified your child as being at risk can provide many of the services called for in the intervention plan. Although some clinics may be sponsored entirely or partly by state or local governmental organizations (the department of health or board of education), some may still function, to a degree, independently and operate under their own locally incorporated names (i.e., "Project Search," "Project Co-Step," or "The Infant Stimulation Program"). So don't be confused when they are listed separately in the phone book. Whatever the name or funding source, the agency providing services should be responsible for overall coordination. If you are to stay on top of things, you must receive, read, and understand regular progress reports as well as reassessments of your child made as conditions change or in response to a reasonable request by you. Ask your doctor how you can make this request and when you should receive the reports.

Part Four discusses the rights of parents under P.L. 94-142 to free special education and evaluation for their children. Some of these rights may also apply in the preschool years, although there is significant variation from state to state in the age at which children become eligible for these services. The tendency has been for federal legislation to gradually lower the mandatory age. For example, in 1986, P.L. 99-457 updating P.L. 94-142 stipulated that by 1990–91 states not offering services to children three through five years old become ineligible for federal funds. (This act is sometimes *informally* referred to as the Handicapped Infants and Toddlers Act, although such designation, technically, identifies only Title I, Part H, of the act.) The same legislation encourages states to provide many services set forth in the bill to children from birth through two (as is mentioned in the previous chapter, diagnostic services are included). Thus, one by one, the loopholes are being closed up.

In addition to supporting state-level research, experimental, demonstration, and outreach programs, the new law includes provision that each handicapped infant or toddler in participating states have an Individualized Family Service Plan (which in many ways is similar to the individualized education plan described in Part Four). The plan is to be a "multidisciplinary assessment of unique needs and the identification of services appropriate to meet such needs . . . developed by a multidisciplinary team, including the parent or guardian" (Sec. 677. [a]). In other words, the plan must describe what early intervention is needed and what resources are needed to provide it. Grants are also available to "plan, develop, and implement a statewide, comprehensive, multidisciplinary, coordinated program of early intervention services," which should be invaluable in states where there is currently little or no coordination. Remember that this law is not currently mandatory, and since programs are complex, change from time to time, and are influenced by individual state law, keep yourself informed about what is currently available and take advantage of any resource that meets your child's needs. Note, also, as you begin to think of your child's possible admission to federally supported programs for handicapped youngsters, that eligibility is not limited to the physical or emotional handicaps, but includes intellectual/cognitive impairment as well.

Parents are, of course, free to begin their child's intervention program at whatever age they feel is appropriate and to secure professional services at their own initiative and expense, but, irrespective of the funding source, public or private, parents should ask to participate in their child's assessment and in any decision-making group involved with his future. You'll find that most programs will welcome and encourage your participation. This comment from a program in Maryland is typical: "The [program's] philosophy is that the parent is the child's primary teacher. Staff members can assist—but never replace—parents in the difficult job of raising a handicapped child."[1] In many states, organizations overlap one another in the functions they perform. Such duplication can cause problems, particularly when many professionals are involved, and makes it even more necessary that you insist that you have only one coordinator (sometimes called a case manager) with whom to work. Fortunately, many states assign responsibility for the coordination of all special preschool services to one particular agency or to a coordinating agency to improve efficiency. Your local education department or the department of health and human services should be able to tell you whom to contact in your area.

Types of Programs

The Home-based Program and What Goes On in the Home

Services for the newborn to five-year-old child are generally offered either in the child's home or in a central location (such as an unused public school classroom, a health clinic, or a room in the YMCA). An intervention program in which professionals regularly visit the home to provide direct treatment or to offer advice and training to parents is called a "home-based" or "home management" program. Often families can accomplish wonders on their own with only a minimal amount of consultation and monitoring from the outside. However, a home-based service program requires professionals who are located nearby and are willing to make house calls and an assessment team familiar enough with local resources to be able to locate these professionals, or a center that will organize such a program and that has a staff prepared to work on an itinerant basis.

Generally it's considered preferable for the young child (up to about the age of two) to receive his primary treatment in the nurturing environment of the home. If during this period his home life is interrupted by outside distractions, he may be less able to establish the close relationships with his mother and father—and to a degree with the rest of the family—that will reinforce future healthy development. During this age span the child is most vulnerable to disconcerting and possibly harmful outside forces.

The advantages a period of initial stability offers to a newborn are obvious and commonly acknowledged. Less obvious is the parents' need to accept and to identify with their child and, in a way, to bond with him. It's frequently difficult for parents to recognize and to accept what is normal and human in their handicapped child and to love him for all the things he is, rather than despair about what he is not. It's easy to be overwhelmed by the magnitude of the disability and to lose your

---

1. "A New Commitment: The Infant Stimulation Program" (Brochure, school year, 1979), sponsored by Anne Arundel County Public Schools and Anne Arundel County Department of Health, Anne Arundel County, Maryland.

perspective. Only a very few, lucky parents seem to escape this period entirely. (It took us a long time to work our way through, and I'm not sure that I ever have.) Acceptance evolves more quickly when parents participate in their youngster's program and work hard at it.

Under normal conditions the home-based program, with its ability to provide on-the-spot advice and support, is ideally suited for the period of settling in and getting to know one another. An added advantage is that transportation problems are reduced or eliminated. For those in rural areas life can be particularly complicated by the distances involved and the frequent scarcity of services, although more and more urban-based educational and medical centers are reaching out into rural districts with "outreach programs." Delivery of services in rural areas is often still unsatisfactory, but progress is being made. ACRES (American Council on Rural Special Education) may be helpful to rurally located families (see Resources: Associations).

Maximize the home environment. No matter how well organized the home-based program is, you and the influence you exert will be the key ingredients. Make the home environment as stable, warm, and upbeat as you can. If possible, provide a comfortable, "sheltered" work space for the visiting professionals, and encourage family members to cooperate with and to welcome them as though they were guests in your home. Provide healthy stimulation by showing your youngster, in all your actions, what an exciting world he lives in (his formal plan should include specific ways to help you do this). Encourage your child to explore—to grow comfortable with the world and with you and to utilize as many of his senses as possible in the process. Although it's important that you receive positive feedback from your child, you may have to be patient. This satisfaction may come at unexpected times in unexpected ways. Don't be discouraged or feel cheated if your baby doesn't respond to you in ways you think he should—smile in response to your smile, grasp your finger, or giggle in delight when you toss him into the air. This lack of response is one of the most difficult things some parents have to face, but the worst thing you can do is let yourself subconsciously seek revenge on your child. By withdrawing, by smiling less, by laughing less with him, you reduce the stimulation he needs so much. Where else will he learn to smile? My own relationship with Owen was sometimes clouded by anger, lodged somewhere at the back of my mind; I seemed to say, "If he's not going to play the game with me, I won't play it with him."

You, as his parents, make up the animate (human) environment for your child, but don't forget the inanimate environmental forces around him that constantly, although sometimes imperceptibly, exert their influence. Fortunately, they frequently can be controlled, and you can help. Ask your care provider or discover through your own research what specific colors, shapes, movements, and designs are most appropriate for your child's walls, furniture, and mobiles. Even the nature of the sound coming from record players, radios, and tapes can have an influence. (Owen loves to ride in my car with the radio blasting. A grin spreads across his face and sometimes he vibrates so much I'm afraid he'll hop right out of the car; it's worth it just to see him react directly to something I have done, but don't take your baby for a car ride like this.) Needs vary from child to child, and since what is appropriate stimulation for your child when he is very young will change as he grows older, be flexible and adapt your actions and his environment to changing conditions.

Keep in mind that play can be the best and most natural stimulation available and the home is where it should begin. The platitude "Play is a child's work" doesn't go far enough. Play is one of the primary ways that children develop in all areas, and it fills their need for stimulation. The give-and-take of play offers obvious advantages for physical development, and emotional development also depends significantly upon play. It provides the framework for the social interaction through which children learn to live with and trust others, to find ways to control their impulses, to cope with conflicts, and, if the environment is sympathetic, to gain the satisfaction of successfully completing a task. Since a disabled child is unable to play normally, his parent's natural role as his playmate assumes an expanded significance. In some instances you will be your child's only playmate, although you hope siblings will fall into this natural brother-sister role. If his handicap is severe, as was Owen's, or if the handicapped youngster is an only child, the patience required can put the entire family to the test.

For example, I remember how Owen once hung Burdock, the family's irascible cat, from the clothes hook on the back of the bathroom door. Our daughters doted on the cat with a devotion that defied reason. When we found him, swinging suspended in a sling Owen had improvised from an elastic female garment, Burdock was out of breath and about as exasperated as a cat can be who is accustomed to the finer things in life. (Fortunately, the story ended happily, and Burdock escaped intact, with only his dignity impaired.) Similar episodes, which are bound to happen in even the best-regulated families, can be healthy experiences for your other children and become oft-quoted lessons in understanding for years to come. It's interesting that so many of the Owens of the world seem to possess a rare talent, an unusual aptitude for just plain and simple raising Cain, and it's reasonable for siblings to be provoked. In fact, letting your handicapped child get away with murder isn't fair to anybody, especially not to him, since it encourages an unrealistic picture of the outside world's reactions.

Although the parent plays a vital role as a partner in his youngster's play, he should not take control. Play should be as spontaneous as circumstances allow, and if play isn't fun, it isn't play. Bear this in mind if your youngster must endure long physical therapy every day. He deserves a break, and relaxation can be as important as the therapy. Parents should also remember that a handicapped child can tire easily, and a few relatively short sessions of romping together are better than single long periods of relatively high-intensity activity. It's a question of quality. ("Let's Play to Grow," a national program that incorporates structured play into family life, is described in Chapter 26.)

> The value of adult-directed play lies in the ability of the adult to provide the child with the opportunities, equipment, experiences, and encouragement appropriate to his abilities and interests, but without imposing adult standards upon him. . . . But above all, play belongs to the child! It gives him pleasure, satisfaction, and the opportunity to develop into a vital, motivated, creative human being. Through an understanding of the developmental nature and changing levels of play during the first 3 years of life, the infant's caregiver can provide the optimum space, materials, situations, and interaction for the fullest benefit to baby and family.[2]

Another approach utilizes play as a way of advancing a child's lagging development in an organized manner. In this approach, the parent makes games out of specific therapeutic exercises in the hope of accelerating both physical and mental development. This is really nothing new; for years mothers and fathers, trying to make often tedious home therapeutic exercises less a chore, have invented their own games out of daily home routines. Federal Handicapped Children Early Education Program (HCEEP) grants have encouraged the development of playground equipment and household furniture that is therapeutically stimulating to help children develop motor functions. Eventually, the equipment should be available for sale to the general consumer. Consider building some things yourself (for example, a chair designed for a child with poor muscle tone). Some parents organize "lending libraries" so that toys designed to meet the specific needs of handicapped children can be shared. Such an undertaking not only circulates the often expensive playthings in the community but also makes the supervising par-

2. From *Program Guide for Infants and Toddlers with Neuromotor and Other Developmental Disabilities*, edited by Frances P. Connor, G. Gordon Williamson, and John M. Siepp, Ch. 1, p. 36 (New York: Teachers College Press, 1978). (The main contributor to this chapter is Frances P. Connor.)

ents more effective with their own children, since they must be able to explain and demonstrate the materials before they can be circulated (see Resources: Play, Toys; Early Childhood).

Furthermore, some programs, such as the Montessori, Portage, and Lekotek methods, use play and specially designed toys in their approach to early childhood development for the handicapped child. You may want to read about these techniques and programs and then ask your professional about them if you have any interest.

As soon as you are able to get beyond the "one day at a time" period—unless an overwhelming disability makes inevitable institutionalization obvious—begin to set your sights on the goal of eventual maximal independence for your child, no matter how far in the future it may seem. The time will come when his ability to function in society, even at a minimal level, will control his destiny and yours. Many parents don't face this day of reckoning until they are forced to. It may happen when their child's age exceeds the ceiling mandated by the state for educational coverage. If the child still can't perform the minimal tasks required for independent living at that magic date, the alternatives will be limited to institutionalization or continuing and perhaps perpetual home custodial care. Or the moment of truth may come later, when suddenly you realize that your "child" is no longer a child and that you—who would never grow old—have indeed grown old. It will become obvious that you can no longer postpone preparing for the day when your child must live in the world without you, and you will hope it's not too late.

Perhaps your child will never reach the point at which any degree of independent living is possible. Whatever his ultimate placement, however, you will regret it if you have not made every effort to prepare him or have failed to offer him the benefit of every doubt. Think about the skills necessary for independent living early in the game and include them in your long-range goal. At times it's necessary to live one day at a time to maintain sanity, but to fail to plan for the future is to invite disaster. Do nothing for your child that he can—with your help—do for himself, although it may seem cruel to watch him struggle. It's often temptingly easier to do it yourself in the short run, but in the long run your continual help can severely limit his future. It's better to teach him to crawl or to turn over (forcing him to strengthen weak muscles) than it is to turn him over yourself or to always carry him. Your service provider can give expert advice on how to help without getting in the child's way, and many manuals deal with the subject. (For specific help in this and in many areas, I particularly recommend *Home Care for the Chronically Ill or Disabled Child*, by Monica Loose Jones—see Resources: Guides.) As your child grows older, concentrate on the self-help skills without which eventual independence will be impossible—e.g., toilet training, personal care, safety, and hygiene. In later years, when you can, involve your child in routine household chores that teach necessary manual skills and sharpen motor coordination, such as vacuuming, sweeping, window washing (be sure they're ground-floor windows!). There are probably far more things to do around the house that have inherent instructional value than you ever realized.

The Center-based Program

As your child grows older, moving him out into the community and exposing him to the additional social stimulation of the larger environment should be advantageous for both child and parents. The youngster has an opportunity to mature in a more normal fashion, while his absence from the home for significant periods provides the family time to themselves. One of the responsibilities of any good development center and its programs should be a concern for the health of the entire family. (Today the increasing number of households with two working parents makes special day-care facilities particularly important, since some handicapped children move to a community setting earlier. When this is the case, the day-care setting is the "home" as far as early intervention is concerned, and close communication between parents, day-care workers, and early intervention providers is vital.)

Center-based programs operate from sites where a variety of specialists and specialized equipment can serve the handicapped children of the surrounding area. In many instances the center serves as a focal point for parent activities as well. The center may be called an "infant development center," "early intervention center," "infant treatment center," or even "rehabilitation center" if it includes clients of all ages. Here is how one center with a combined home and center-based program, the Infant Development Center in Portland, Maine, describes itself in its brochure (I have entered my comments in brackets). As you read, note how many important services are offered by this organization. If similar offerings aren't available in your area, they should be, and you could serve your community by working with staff to obtain them.

INFANT DEVELOPMENT CENTER [Portland, Maine]
Purposes 1. To provide early intervention services for infants and preschool children who have been identified as developmentally impaired or at risk for potential developmental problems. 2. To provide parents help, support, information, and involvement in the provision of services

to their child. . . . [Irrespective of what support is offered, the parent still has a responsibility to take some initiative. If you expect to be "spoon fed," you may lose out.]

Methodology 1. On referral to the Center, a staff member will visit the home, make an initial assessment, and arrange for a developmental screening either at the home or the Center. Following the screening, staff will meet and assign a primary person to coordinate whatever program is indicated. If a more comprehensive program evaluation is needed, that will be scheduled with one or all of the following: physical therapist, occupational therapist, educator, psychologist, speech and hearing therapist. A program will then be designed and with the parent's approval will be implemented. [In this center the parents participate in the assessment and meet again with the team within three weeks to go over the report and resulting program. As you move into the educational maze, be sure that all programs proposed for your child are individualized, and not "packaged" or prepared for a heterogeneous class of children with different abilities and/or problems.] 2. Depending on the needs of the infant/child and family, either one or both of the following types of programs will be used: a. Home management programs: Periodic visits by Staff to the home to help the family manage the child's program. b. Developmental classes at the Center for socialization and pre-school skill development. 3. Full re-evaluation of the child will be done whenever necessary. Additional services offered: a. Preparation of child for pre-school and school program and assistance to the teacher during the adjustment period. [Communication between the classroom teacher and the medical representative or special education teacher will remain a vital consideration throughout your child's development. Never let these two critical staff members get out of touch.] b. Consultation with other agencies, day care centers, etc. c. Baby sitting services from 10:00 AM to 4:00 PM, Monday through Friday, at the Infant Development Center. [This has recently been eliminated; however, other services, including a kind of respite-care clearinghouse, have been instituted.] d. Participation in a parent group, if desired. [These are the services I have in mind when I speak of concern for the entire family.]

The specialists whom you encounter during this early period will depend upon the nature of your child's disability. A pediatrician or an orthopedist is often a regular member of the team. Other specialists— an ophthalmologist, a dietitian, or a neurologist, for instance—may also be included when their expertise is needed. The specialists needed should be described in the assessment document, since they are the people upon whose shoulders the success of the plan will rest. Become familiar with them, with their training, and with the tasks they perform. The center should have written "job descriptions." Staff selection should be of concern to you. Never feel you necessarily have to take what you get or accept performance with which you are dissatisfied. A director of a development center once said to me, "A great deal is said about the importance of selecting a doctor in whom you have confidence and with whom you feel comfortable. But, often, other staff specialists can be just as important to your kid's future and are either overlooked or their skills underestimated. Their selection and performance should be a top priority item to you."

Evaluating a program's effectiveness is rarely easy, particularly during the early years, when both diagnosis and prognosis may be unclear and when goal setting—a vital part of the process—is difficult. Later, when your youngster reaches school age, formal goal setting and subsequent efforts to evaluate the program's success in reaching those goals will be easier. A good development center should lead the way and set patterns for the future by encouraging an attitude toward your child that focuses on the things he will be able to do—with their help and yours. Your active participation in the goal-setting process and your review of progress with staff on a regular basis should give you an overview of how your child is developing in relation to his potential. Learn as much as you can about your child's disability and cooperate actively with the professionals. Don't be just an observer or, even worse, a chronic complainer, or else the center's staff may eventually discount your comments and discourage your participation.

11

Emotions and Stress

Once when I was trying to help a parent who was going through a particularly bad period, he stopped me short by saying, "Look, you mean well, but I don't need your sympathy or a lot of bull about interpersonal relationships or sibling rivalry, whatever they are. I need concrete ideas that are going to get me through the next couple of days." His irritation was understandable. I've felt the same way, myself, and have often wondered if it really makes sense to be concerned with such nebulous concepts as emotions and psychological factors when the immediate priority is getting through tomorrow. It took a while, but I've finally answered that question for myself in the affirmative and am now convinced that all of us—researchers, care providers, professional schools, and certainly parents—pay too little attention to the influence emotions have upon a family's ability to function.

For better or for worse, the mental health of a family will affect how a disabled child sees himself and, as a consequence, how well he will progress. It will influence the parents' ability to cope with their new responsibilities and hence their effectiveness in managing affairs for and responding to the needs of other family members. Finally, it will affect the parents' control over their own personal lives, now complicated by the pressures of trying to hold their family together. Marital problems, drug and alcohol abuse, and deteriorating job performance all can result if emotional pressures are not understood and attended to. Of one thing I am convinced: those who believe that living with a handicapped child will create a family somehow stronger and more cohesive through some spontaneous process—distinct from careful planning and practical action—are badly in error.

I don't suggest our family's experience is typical, if indeed any can be. Unquestionably, Mary and I were more fortunate than most during the early, difficult years, because although four other young children competed for our attention at the time, we lived in pleasant surroundings, had room to get away from one another when necessary, and were economically well enough off so that Mary didn't have to work outside the home. In addition, active grandparents living nearby provided real support. But in many critical ways, our experiences echo those of many parents, for in the years since Owen we have run a battery of emotional hurdles that have left us a little bit sadder and a great deal wiser. Through our friends we learned there are many threads of experience common to all parents of handicapped kids, despite the fact that families have different life styles, economic resources, and emotional characteristics. The consequences of ignoring emotional problems make up a whole bundle of these common threads.

"We don't know what to do. We're being driven to the breaking point." This is a complaint I've heard so often that I'm convinced it's a rare parent who doesn't have vivid memories of the time when he, too, wondered just how much more his family could take. Most can remember the exact moment. With us it happened when Owen's school was abruptly closed by the state, and he was back in the family, not for vacation or a weekend, but, as far as we knew, forever. All day he trailed either Mary or me around the house, even to the bathroom, restless and discontented unless he could actually touch one of us—a hand on the back, head, or thigh, an arm around the shoulder. When I went to my desk to work, he came too, sitting on a stool opposite me, gazing at me for hours, unblinking, without moving, as though waiting for some sign. The other kids were in school, and the room would be quiet except for the scratching of my pencil and Owen's characteristically heavy breathing, which, as time passed, seemed to grow louder and louder.

Eventually we entered a "furious period," when everyone became furious with everyone else over the most insignificant things. Finally one evening at supper I admitted that although I had previously said, "We Callanans can take care of our own, and Owen is our own," perhaps I had been hasty, and it wouldn't hurt if we looked into respite care. This was the moment our family hit rock bottom. Fortunately, it was also the time we began our climb back up to the surface. Respite care saved our sanity by demonstrating that willingness to accept help is a skill as important to survival as any a parent can acquire. So, although our family isn't typical in all things, we are typical in many. After all, we paid our dues, sharing that singular culminating experience with many others: we reached the breaking point and survived.

The Causes of Stress

Stress occurs when outside pressure makes us feel tense. It's a condition experienced by everyone in varying degrees and, if improperly handled, may impair our ability to function. However, its effect is not necessarily bad, since it is nature's way of preparing us to cope with emergencies. Stress can be caused by such things as changes in a person's life style, job pressures, financial problems, family changes, or personal injury or loss. This chapter considers stress and the emotions from the particular perspective of the special family and suggests ways to avoid or cope with some of the common pitfalls. In general, we found difficulties sprang from four sources of conflict:

- The family's efforts to adjust to the child's handicap, particularly during the early years—and the resulting change in the nature of individual family members' expectations for the child and for themselves.
- Frictions that develop between family members, particularly father and mother, as the result of conflicting opinions about child-rearing approaches and the extent of each family member's individual responsibilities.
- Conflicts caused by interaction with the outside world, particularly the professional community.
- Needless frustration resulting from parents' "doing things the hard way." Lack of information about the nature of the handicap and resources available to combat it, unwillingness or inability to organize adequately for today and to plan for the future (when the future may be as close as tomorrow), lack of attention to the many little details of living that will eliminate or reduce the severity of problems that generate stress in the first place, and unwillingness to accept help from the outside all contribute to this frustration.

The Nature of Stress

The First Stage: It Can Be Like a Death in the Family

When a family learns that one of its members is handicapped, everyone is affected. Some are stunned, some are concerned only with their own private misfortune, and others retreat, isolated and stricken, into their own private cell—at a time when they most need support. Mary and I learned that one of a parent's most difficult chores is to control his own emotions while being sensitive to the pressures on other family members. Even when relationships are close and communication is open, the search for emotional stability can be an up-and-down affair in which spirits fluctuate from day to day, perhaps from one blood count to the next. As the years passed we learned that although we could take certain actions to strengthen our coping ability, there was no such thing as an inviolate state of mind that, once attained, would forever ensure emotional tranquility. Ongoing adjustments must be made as circumstances change, and as all of us grow older.

When we first learned that Owen was "massively retarded," we felt alone, bewildered, and betrayed. I don't remember feeling anger or despair or guilt then—only a numbness and a shock that dampened all sensation. Mary and I didn't say much. There didn't seem to be anything worth saying. Now, looking back over our long journey (writers always seem to call emotional experiences "journeys") and reliving the violent exhilarations and crashing disappointments, I'm sure it would have helped us had we known more about our minds and what happens to them under the impact of a crushing shock. I think we would have felt better about the way we were behaving had we realized that a person's emotional state, like his body, can be strained, thrown out of kilter, and even temporarily dislocated, and had we known there was nothing to be ashamed of if we behaved in ways unusual for us. Some professionals who study the mind suggest that this kind of upheaval ordinarily follows patterns.[1] For instance, they say that in grief, people pass through emotional stages before they can heal and adjust to new circumstances. Not everyone will necessarily react in the same way at the same time, but people are apt to follow similar patterns. However, and this is a big "however," stages do not necessarily consistently follow one another, and individuals may either entirely skip one or revert back to an earlier stage. For me, an apparently minor event will trigger something in my mind, and I will go back to a moment fifteen or twenty years earlier and relive the anger or despair I felt then. It doesn't take much—an unexpected call from Owie's institution, the birth of a grandson, the sight of another handicapped youngster walking through a crowded terminal; it doesn't take much.

The deep-sea diver, if he is to survive, must return to the surface in slow and regular stages after his body has been exposed to the pressures of the deep. Similarly, the parent must allow himself time to adjust to the reality of living with a handicapped child. In retrospect, I'm convinced that it would have helped, when we were in a despair from which we feared we might never recover, to know of the experience of others who had come back to the surface. We didn't know then that we had lots of famous company, that President Kennedy's sister was severely handicapped and that Pearl Buck, the author, wrote about her own disabled child in *The Child Who Never Grew* (see Resources: Personal Narratives). This is a sensitive gem of a book about how one mother came to terms with the issues many of us face: interaction with the out-

1. In this section I have drawn upon concepts suggested by Elizabeth Kübler-Ross in *On Death and Dying* (New York: Macmillan, 1969) and "You Are Not Alone: For Parents When They Learn That Their Child Has a Handicap" by Patty McGill Smith, in the 1984 newsletter of the National Information Center for Handicapped Children and Youth (now National Information Center for Children and Youth with Handicaps).

side world, the pain of institutionalization, the unsuccessful search for a diagnosis, and planning for a child's life after one's own life is over. In some ways it is a description of Pearl Buck's "journey" through the grieving process.

When parents first hear the disastrous news, they are said to grieve in much the same way they would had their child died. One awful moment came for me in the early hours of a winter's morning when I lay, sleepless, in bed and the thought crossed my mind, for the first time, that perhaps it might have been better for everyone if Owen had died at birth. It's not a happy memory, and I doubt if caregivers could ever understand just what this means. I've often wondered how many parents are haunted by the same memory. Parents of a severely handicapped child are said to mourn for the normal child they had planned for and dreamed of, who now is "dead." I, for instance, had hoped for a son to take fishing.

The first reaction is often numbness, disbelief, and denial. Parents sometimes won't believe the diagnosis and shop around for a second and even a third opinion, like a cancer victim searching for a diagnosis he wants to hear. For us, even before we first consulted a doctor, stress had begun to build, as we fretted and stewed and worried. Sometimes when the period of uncertainty is prolonged, parents feel relieved that they finally have an answer, even if it's one they didn't want to hear, preferring a known problem to the continuation of the awful waiting period. Parents who are ashamed of what they see as an "inhuman" reaction on their part can take solace from knowing they're not monsters but are only reacting in a very human way.

The first few weeks after leaving the hospital can be stressful for another reason. It's now thought that as many as 30 percent of all new mothers, whether their children are handicapped or not, experience what is called "postpartum depression," which is characterized by difficulty in adjusting to the new demands of motherhood. Some doctors suggest that this condition can be detected sooner and attended to earlier if the mother does not terminate the relationship with her obstetrician at birth, as is often the case, but schedules at least one more appointment a few weeks after delivery. This advice is particularly applicable to the mother of a handicapped infant, since her adjustment problems are considerably more complex.

The Next Stages: "If Only" and "Why Us?"

In time, the initial numbness fades, at least to a level at which parents can function, and mother and father begin to come to grips with the realities of their new life. But parents, being rational people in a generally rational world, find blind acceptance difficult and naturally seek explanations. They wonder what they did wrong and often experience feelings of guilt. "If only we had acted earlier"; "If only I hadn't smoked during pregnancy, the baby might be O.K."; "If only," "If only." Our family's history is filled with similar recriminations: If only we had isolated our daughter Martha when she had German measles. If only we had read more, learned more, talked to more people. *Then* things would have been different.

Inevitably another thought creeps into your mind that is as old as the story of Job: "Why me?" It's a pernicious question that saps both time and energy and has no answer. Such questioning accomplishes little more than encouraging a search for someone to blame: the doctor, a spouse, the hospital, even God. Sometimes even the infant can be made the scapegoat, which is doubly destructive, since directing anger at the child increases parents' guilt and decreases their ability to function as the child's advocate. It's a vicious circle that can lead to a state of paralysis in which the more you blame yourself, the less effective you become, and the less effective you are, the more need there is to assign blame. We found it became difficult to understand and retain information or to make thoughtful and responsible decisions. At this moment it's wise, whenever possible, to postpone critical decisions until you have had time to get yourself organized and together. Take time to read *When Bad Things Happen to Good People*, by Harold S. Kushner (see Resources: Counseling).

I never met a parent who, when speaking of emotional problems, didn't mention feeling angry and isolated from society. For some the anger and isolation are temporary and gradually disappear as they become hardened and as society's attitudes slowly change. Although my own anger has diminished with time, it has never completely left me, remaining long after feelings of grief and guilt have disappeared. Perhaps my inability to face the mainstream of society when my son is with me is attributable to Owen's mannerisms, which have remained so flamboyant that, even today, every excursion into the world can embarrass and anger me. The anger is hard to bear, since I begin by being angry with Owen and end up by being disgusted with myself for being angry.

Sometimes I know I exaggerate the stir we create when Owie and I walk arm-in-arm through an airport terminal or into a crowded restaurant, arms linked so Owen won't pace like a benign appendage behind me. Every eye seems to be on us. We are suddenly the source of uneasy attention. I have developed a game that helps. When I notice adults following Owen's every movement with unblinking attention, I try to catch their eye, nod my head, and wink as if they and I shared a personal and quietly amusing secret. It's fun to watch their faces. Their reactions vary widely: some obviously think they must know us from somewhere else, but aren't sure; others seem worried about just what the wink might mean; and there are always some who look back and forth from Owen to me as though trying to determine which one of us is the "crazy one." In our family, the word *crazy* is used, not cruelly but as a term of endearment as far as Owie is concerned, but we wouldn't want others to use it who didn't understand. In the same way, when we meet a group of retarded individuals on a field trip or at a concert, we speak of them, in the family, as "Owie's crowd." (I suppose the experts would call this part of our "coping mechanism.")

As we gradually worked our way out of the depression that characterized our early years, we found a sense of humor to be a wonderful tonic and an indispensable survival tool, one of the few we had to combat emotional fatigue and maintain perspective. Some may find it offensive or callous to laugh or apparently make light of situations that from other perspectives are tragic. (Abe Lincoln said that he laughed because he didn't dare to cry.) You may have thought some of the passages in this book to be in poor taste. Just keep in mind that tears and long faces rarely solve problems, but a merry heart and a laugh can keep people functioning. In our family we have learned to poke gentle fun at ourselves and our special child, and often find something to smile at in even the most unlikely situations. There is a bright side. Life for handicapped folks has improved, and continues to improve, as society's attitudes mellow and some stereotypes are discarded, primarily as the result of the deinstitutionalization movement, which has allowed more disabled people to escape their prisons and mingle with the outside world. But back to our journey.

The "Bargaining" Stage

As if things aren't bad enough already, most of us pass through yet another stage on the road to final acceptance. It's sometimes called the "bargaining" stage, although I think of it as the "wait till" stage. It typically begins with the parent's refusal to accept the reality of the situation, hoping that once some particular action is taken, things will suddenly turn out all right. We felt sure that once Owen walked, everything would start getting better, once he was fitted with special orthopedic shoes or a hearing aid, had that eye operation, learned sign language, got vocational training, things would improve. However, final acceptance (if it ever really comes) comes after we have reconciled all the alternatives, in different ways and at different moments for each of us. For some it can come through religion. The church, both intellectually (through the answers it can supply) and socially (through the support system it has to offer), can be a real anchor in the storm. Unfortunately, it wasn't for us. For Mary and me the "wait till" period ended the day we acknowledged our son had reached the age at which, no matter what revolutionary medical breakthrough might develop, it would be impossible for him ever to catch up developmentally or even attain a minimal noncustodial functioning level. That day it was obvious to us that any kind of independent life was no longer in the cards for him or, in a way, for us as well. Acceptance isn't easy; it means the final, irrevocable end of many dreams—sometimes little dreams like having a son you can take fishing.

If you have confidence in your medical advisers and have managed to become a mini-expert in your child's disability, you will be less inclined to nurture false hopes about those miraculous, quick cures you hear about or, for that matter, to ascribe unrealistic possibilities to medical procedures that, although helpful, offer limited potential. Don't set yourself up to be let down. This is not to suggest that you ignore any procedure recommended by competent sources that offers the possibility of improving your child's condition, or that you abandon efforts to build a brighter future for your child. Mary and I have never given up looking to the future. We have just changed our goals and have found it helped to break our hopes (objectives) down into small, realistic steps. This way, progress, however slight, is more easily measured, and we can look forward to more frequent celebrations when Owen succeeds, and we are less disappointed when he fails.

Chronic Sorrow

Unfortunately, a few parents are never able to reach a final acceptance of reality but continue to live in a half-world without either hope or laughter. In its extreme form this inability to cope takes the form of continuing depression, when feelings of guilt or loss of self-esteem are so profound that such symptoms as insomnia, loss of appetite, and psychosomatic illness take over. Some briefly enter the periphery of this stage and feel its influence, but most of us quickly work free from its depths. It's crucial, if this point is reached, that professional help be obtained from one-on-one counselors, through a mental health center or state or local mental health association; peer-support groups can sometimes also provide assistance. More and more, centers that provide diagnostic or treatment services for the child also offer psychological support for family members, since it's increasingly recognized that the parents' ability to provide acceptable care for their children depends upon their own mental health.

Another possible consequence of parents' continuing inability to adjust is that in their frustration they may give up entirely on their child. Although many, many other factors can be at work in such a decision (financial concerns are often overwhelming), some of our friends have, in apparent desperation, let the state take over completely. In this situation a child can receive a bleak message; viewing the result of this "abandonment" and following his parents' lead, he may give up on himself. Fortunately, if parents decide they must institutionalize their youngster, there is a variety of ways they can keep on providing the continuing supervision and emotional support that monitors his physical well-being and constantly reassures him that he's still loved and part of the family (see Chapter 23).

The Role of the Family

Friction within the Family

Trying to deal with the problems of caring for a handicapped child generates tremendous pressure on a couple, particularly if they are young and inexperienced, and especially during the infant's first few years of life. The experience can strengthen their relationship or break down the marital structure entirely.

In the ideal situation, both father and mother cope with stress in a similar fashion and view fundamental issues from commonly held points of view. When this is the case, it's easier for each to support and understand the other and to maintain family equilibrium during potentially divisive moments. When this is not the case, stress can feed on itself and become a negative factor, affecting many aspects of family life. If a father believes in the stoic approach, that it's "unmanly" to show emotion or seek help, it will be difficult for him to understand and support a wife whose approach is to "let it all hang out." Communication and mutual accommodation are important in any marriage, but with the added complication involved in parenting a special child, they become critical.

Although it's unrealistic to suggest that parents can or should try to change their basic personalities, it is realistic to hope that they will communicate and try to be flexible when they need to make decisions dealing with common but potentially controversial questions. Here are some typical "hot" issues: What kind of disciplinary guidelines should be established—if the child is to be disciplined at all? With whom and under what restraints should he be allowed to play? Do you protect the disabled child and, by keeping him away from the rough and tumble of the neighborhood playground, risk limiting his development? Or should you let him take his licks? Most parents walk a tightrope between encouraging activities that develop independence and catering to the limitations imposed by the handicap. However, all parents should check with their physician early to determine what limitations are medically necessary.

> Parents of disabled children need to be counseled about disciplining their disabled child. They are often reluctant to reprimand their disabled infants and toddlers, to train them, as they do their other children, to teach them realistic limits. Their rationale is that the child already has enough to contend with. Perhaps so, but the child must also learn to live with the family and in the world. During his infancy he must learn, as other children, to avoid injuring himself and others as well as to gain a respect for another's space. He must, unless for some special dietary reason, be put on the same feeding–sleeping schedule as are normal children. Later he, too, must be helped through the process of toilet training. It is not uncommon to have children with disabilities, for whom there is no reasonable excuse, come to school without having been toilet trained and with no knowledge of a sense of self or others.[2]

One question Mary and I never had trouble answering is whether it is "right" for parents to go on vacation all by themselves. We found that sometimes we had to get away from Owen and we never apologized for it. We suggest that a vacation should be a high priority for all parents if it's at all possible. Another issue, the extent to which a child's appearance should be a cause for concern, is, in my opinion, more problematical. We decided against long and involved orthodontic work of a strictly cosmetic nature to correct Owen's buck teeth. Some of his ancestors had buck teeth, too. It was a family trademark, and they did just fine in life. They got married and had children. Some were smart, some were wealthy, and some were both. Buck teeth didn't seem to hurt at all; it's one genetic trait I never worried about. We feel differently about seeing that Owen is well groomed. Many parents (as well as institutions) pay far too little attention to this area. In addition to reinforcing an unfortunate stereotype, the child's appearance conditions the family's psychological reaction to the handicapped sibling or child.

In addition, if institutionalization is a viable option, no decision is more potentially destructive to family harmony, because it brings into conflict two basically opposite views of how to deal with a disabled child. It strikes at the heart of a parent's concept of responsibility and the emphasis he places upon his ability "to take care of his own"—to be self-sufficient. It's not always easy to decide on priorities. Should they be the interests of the child or the family or society? Unfortunately,

2. Leo Buscaglia, *The Disabled and Their Parents* (Thorofare, N.J.: Charles Slack, 1975), p. 33.

it's not uncommon for one parent to argue adamantly in favor of sending the child away, while the other insists, just as adamantly, that the
youngster should remain at home. Both parents are convinced that their
position is for the "good of the family." Both believe the other is "unreasonable" and/or "heartless."

The father's role is another source of family stress. The past decade
has seen a dramatic change in attitudes toward parenting and the traditional mother-father roles. Life styles not mentioned in polite society a
generation ago are socially acceptable today; single parenting is common, and in many conventional marriages the father is an equal partner
in the child-rearing process. This change not only has made household
burdens more equitable for the mother, but also has often served the
father's interests and opened new horizons to many men.

Although there is disagreement about the specifics of the father's
emerging role in parenting, there seems to be a general consensus that if
the father is to play a constructive role and feel positive about himself
and his handicapped child, he must be accepted as an equal participant
by both the mother and professionals. (And, of course, he himself must
be a willing participant.) Such accommodation isn't always easy, since
problems can arise in what are often new relationships. Some common
sources of tensions are:

1. Either parent can become distressed because he/she (usually
she) gets stuck with all the unpleasant responsibilities. If you feel misused, talk things over. You may find the offending parent feels insecure
or unwelcome in the relationship. Often your spouse wants to help, but
doesn't know how and is afraid to try, fearing he/she (usually he) may
make a fool of himself. One obvious solution is to help him learn, but
be gentle; if you make him feel like a klutz, you may make your point
and lose a helper. In the past, the father's primary role—and one from
which many men derived satisfaction—was to be provider for both
mother and child; caregiving was not his field of responsibility. A father
of the old school, who is not completely comfortable in his new role as a
partner in caregiving responsibilities, may be more responsive if his
partner is sensitive to his needs. I'm sure that with our last child, Mary
encouraged me to take care of some things, and to feel important in
doing them, that she could have handled herself perfectly well.

2. In dealings with professionals, the father is often treated as an
apparent nonentity, and is left to shift uncomfortably in office corners,
inspecting the doctor's wall-mounted diplomas. One friend spoke of
such a meeting, which began with mother and doctor engaged in a limited two-way exchange. Her spouse, however, proved to be of the new
enlightened generation and refused to be left out. After several moments of frustration he placed a firm hand on the doctor's shoulder,

looked him in the eye and said, "Hey, remember me? I'm part of this deal, too. I'm the father." He refused to accept what I call "the father as fifth wheel" syndrome.

3. Husbands are too often unavailable because of alleged work pressures. I plead guilty to this charge, but argue that I was part of the old school. Although times have changed, old attitudes persist, and women remain the major participants in parents' support groups and on the pediatric floors of hospitals. Often at critical moments I sat with mothers who were waiting for a father "who couldn't get away from the office." In my opinion "pressures of work" can be nothing more than a father's excuse to avoid a situation in which he feels himself unwelcome or with which he feels unable to cope. But to be fair, some fathers encounter additional stress because of increased demands, both financial and emotional, generated by their special circumstances, and feel their career opportunities are thereby limited. Whatever the cause, everyone can be a loser.

I remember one afternoon when I was the culprit. Owen, four at the time, was unmanageable. I was working on some overdue paperwork, and he was getting more and more under my skin. Finally, completely exasperated, I snapped at Mary, "Will you get that impossible kid out of here?" She responded instantaneously and in kind, "That impossible kid is your kid too." This quieted me down and gave me something to think about. It's easy to lose perspective and to pass your frustrations on to those closest at hand, forgetting that the child is "your kid too." But times are changing and fathers are pulling their own weight more and more—not only because they should, but also because they want to. Mothers and professionals can help by making them feel welcome, by being patient with their shortcomings, and by helping them learn the skills required.

One Mother

If there can be such a thing as a heroine in a book like this one, it would be Mary. And, although it's difficult for us other family members to imagine such a thing, there are many other women like Mary in the world, mothers of handicapped youngsters who, without heroics or concern for themselves, everyday do the best they can to improve the lot of their special children. I know. I have seen them in the hospitals and the schools, at the parents' meetings and in the doctors' offices, where they too often keep lonely watch. Each mother, of course, is different, but no consideration of the emotional impact that having a handicapped child has on a family unit could be complete without some recognition of what it is to be in the mother's world. Many find it difficult or impossible to talk about their feelings, and many never are asked. It was difficult for Mary:

> How to capture in a few short paragraphs my life with Owen? Twenty-eight years of joy and tears, hope and despair, enthusiasm and frustration, love and hate. The emotions tend to make wide swings. When dealing with Owen, there has been no middle ground.
>
> The early years were a time of fierce, almost all-consuming love. Owen was a beautiful child—blond and blue-eyed with a constant smile. Once I became aware of his handicaps, all my energy was focused on protecting and nurturing my precious little boy. I loved rocking him every night before tucking him into bed. He enjoyed the motion and would press his ear close to my mouth as I hummed softly to him. When he graduated from his crib to a regular bed, he would climb out as soon as I left the room and curl up on the floor next to the gate across his doorway. I had to buy a woolly carpet and bundle him in heavy sleepers to keep him warm.
>
> I remember the first time Owen got lost. It was at a school fair jammed with people. How my heart thumped with fear and panic until someone found him wandering in the woods nearby. I remember how difficult it was to send him off on the school bus for the first time. But I was surprised at the new sense of freedom I felt—three whole hours without Owen! Even then I had to stick close to home, since the school would often call for me to come collect him when he wet or soiled his pants.
>
> But, oh my, the triumphs we shared and celebrated together during those first school years! Owen learned to sit in a chair and at a desk. He began to learn the alphabet and mouth the sounds and even to vocalize a few words. He could copy his name, write "cat" and "ball." I'll never ever forget the day I saw unmistakable understanding light up his eyes when I showed him the word "house" for what seemed the thousandth time. He grabbed my hand and tugged me out the front door and down the path to the street. Then he turned around and pointed back to our home and said, "HOWSS." I cried. Great strides were made that year, but it proved to be the high point, and in the years that followed the potential I saw in his eyes that wonderful day has never been fulfilled.
>
> I'll also never forget the day we took Owen to Pennsylvania to leave him at the first of many residential schools. It was the worst day! He was only nine years old, and leaving this beloved son of mine in the care of strangers was a tremendous wrench. But the time would eventually come when an entire day would pass without my thinking of or worrying about him. And gradually my life without Owen began to brighten. The heavy pall of gray guilt slowly lifted, and I felt a sense of freedom

and independence which was overwhelming (but a little disquieting). No longer did I spend every waking hour with Owen tucked at the edge of my consciousness—where was he, when must I collect him, how could I manage, who would be watching him? It was a new life and different relationship for both of us.

Since then my time with Owen has been a series of visits—periods of two weeks here, a month there, and one frustrating six-week episode with him living at home again as we desperately tried to arrange new schooling and residential facilities in Maine. Visits are bittersweet experiences—joy at seeing him again and watching his eyes light up as he comes for a welcome-home hug, fixing his favorite foods, arranging excursions he will enjoy, stocking up on new puzzles for him to put together, buying him new clothes and mending his old ones. Once again I have the chance to mother him, but I fuss and worry and agonize over him, too.

Though we often have good times together, it is also a relief when we put Owen on the plane for his return to school. I always go through a down period for a few days after he's left, when the feelings of guilt return, but they don't last long and once again I settle back into my comfortable life without Owen. He is 29 years old now and has his own life to lead; that is as it should be. And yet, inside that lanky and somewhat awkward man's body, there still is the small chubby boy I held close in my arms many years ago, the son I had to protect and nurture and love with a special strong love because he was so different. Despite our separate lives, the bonds of this love still hold me fast and console me. But I still sometimes wonder what might have been.

Siblings Are People, Too

Being the brother or sister of a handicapped person adds one more challenge to the difficult business of growing up. For many, this is a stage—unlike acne—they'll never outgrow. Whether it turns out to be a challenge from which much can be learned or a debilitating problem depends upon too many variables to make any generalization reliable, but it is obvious that parental attitudes are pivotal. Unfortunately, many fathers and mothers forget that the very pressures that frustrate and anger them can affect their children even more, since they are a captive and impressionable audience. On the other hand, in many instances, problems can be converted to opportunities and final results made positive ones.

It has always been interesting to me to see how Owen's brothers and sisters evaluated his impact on their formative years. Reid, Owen's oldest brother and in many ways the leader of the younger generation, looks back on life in a special family in a very positive way:

> One's memory has a way of softening the rough edges of the past, and so it is that in my memories of growing up with Owen I have blocked out many of the frustrations, the heartaches, and crossfires of our years together. From my perspective now at 36, I view my relationship, past and present, with Owen only as a positive one. What I do remember, as a member of our family, is that Owen created special problems for all of us to deal with and to overcome. For me these special problems were never overwhelming nor a serious burden. Perhaps being the eldest of six prepared me for Owen's arrival as the fifth. By then I had become well versed in the art of sibling tolerance. Parental attention, as you would expect, was sent Owen's way. But once again, being one of six helped to soften the lack of the attention we all might have received were it not for Owen's special nature.
>
> The most difficult times came from the frustration of not being able to communicate with him. When Owen was doing something he wasn't supposed to or you didn't want him to, and communication or logic would normally be called for, he couldn't hear or make sense out of our explanations. But you learned from these limitations to use other forms of problem-solving. For example, you might distract him from pushing the cat out the window by interesting him in a toy he hadn't seen in a while. Owen's presence in our family offered me a wealth of opportunity to develop patience and tolerance towards someone so different and so disadvantaged. For, once you leave the relative security of the family structure, you are confronted with a world of people different from anything you have known before, and you must be able to tolerate and make some sense out of their differentness. In this respect Owen was a great teacher.

Reid's sister Martha recalls those years from a different perspective, a point of view that reflects her interest in what lies beyond the senses:

> When I review the years I spent living with Owen, I remember myself having little patience or tolerance for him and his behavior. I was often embarrassed by the way he acted when we were out in public together, wary of the inquisitive stares of strangers, afraid that I might be judged as handicapped myself, or seen as less than perfect because Owen was my brother. I was frustrated by my inability to communicate with him, and more often than not, my frustration would turn to anger and I would cease further efforts to connect with him, having decided that the situation was hopeless.

To this day I feel a wall between us, and I sense that I have failed him somehow. At the same time, however, I envy the sense of peace and calm acceptance that Owen has, joining with others in my family in the belief that behind that wall lies a soul that is light-years beyond me in evolvement—as though he has seen the truth that we normal people struggle so hard to reach. I envy his ability to laugh and totally accept himself and all of us with love and without judgments.

Tom, who once hid in a hillside cave above our home to escape our family's move to Baltimore in the first leg of our journey to get help for Owen, seems to bear no scars of resentment, as he speaks of acceptance:

I was five when Owen was born, and, because he didn't at first look or act any different from other babies, I treated him just as I did my other brothers and sisters. When Owen got to be five years old and still wasn't talking or understanding much, it was frustrating. I was always wanting to play something new, but Owen moved in a narrow groove and could understand only a few simple games. He was good at puzzles and knew the rules of tag and hide and seek. That was it! Now that Owen's twenty-nine those are still the only games he knows, and today, I'll play them with him. But at ten, it was as if I was incapable of repeating those games more than once. Unfortunately, Owen was left behind.

Mom and Dad put no pressure on me to continue to play with him. They realized that to do so would have caused me to resent him, and perhaps because of this, the love between him and me has remained unobstructed. There were, of course, times when I would lose patience, but never would I lose my love. That has, perhaps, been Owen's greatest gift to all of us. He has always been a happy kid, always smiling, always joyous. And if I'd get mad and scream and yell, he'd just look at me and grin. He didn't seem to absorb any of my anger; it was as though it would reflect right back onto me, and I'd see the anger and frustration for what they really were—my attachment to the way I wanted things to be.

During my teenage years I was trying so hard to be cool and be accepted by my peers. There were times when I'd be in public with Owen and he'd begin to wave his arms and act weird. People would stare, and, instead of feeling cool, like I so desperately wanted, it made me feel like a leper. Sometimes I'd try to quiet him, scold him, grab him and try to make him stop. But he wouldn't understand. He'd just smile and continue waving his arms around. There was nothing I could do. Eventually it became evident to me—and to everyone around me—that my embarrassment and the frustration I directed at Owen were really the result of my own insecurity. Eventually, I came to accept Owen, not only as my brother but also as a part of who I was. It's a bit like growing up with a crippled hand. It's something you can't manipulate, change, or deny, no matter how you try. Eventually you come to accept it, and move on from there to an acceptance of who you are—including your limitations. It was impossible to play the "appearances game" as long as Owen was around. I guess it was through him that I was able to see appearances for what they were.

All of us Callanans have grown up with a certain confidence—an ability to go our own way even if that isn't the convention. I can't help but think that Owen has something to do with this.

It's naive to assume a parent's peculiar responsibility to intercede between the siblings and the special child will expire automatically with the end of their childhood years. Actually, the relationship is more a continuum that begins with the birth of the disabled youngster and, often, ends only when the parents have made final arrangements for the handicapped youngster and passed on the responsibility for his care to someone else (in our family it will be to Owen's brothers and sisters). With time, the stresses that siblings are exposed to change, but they never completely disappear unless the family relinquishes its responsibility to someone else, usually some governmental agency. (See Chapter 27 for "after we're gone" planning.)

Many factors affect how a sibling will be influenced by this unusual childhood experience: the number, sex, physical condition, and age of his other brothers and sisters; the economic status and ethnic background of the family; the geographic location of the home; and the disability involved and its prognosis. Little can be done to alter most of these characteristics. However, other factors—parental attitudes and behavior, for instance—are sometimes controllable and have the potential to improve or exacerbate conditions, sometimes even determining whether the overall impact is positive or negative.

Owen's sister Sarah, our fourth child, had this reaction to being a part of a large family with a handicapped brother:

> Growing up in a family of six children is quite an experience. We are all so different from one another. When friends find out I've got a retarded brother, they get that awful look on their faces that's both sorrowful and apologetic—as if they know they should say something but don't know what to say. Sometimes I'd like to help them out. Actually, I feel lucky to have a brother like Owen. This was particularly true when I was young and growing up.
>
> Owen is number five in our family line-up, and I wasn't far ahead at number four. That meant that ahead of me were three older siblings, and if any of you have older brothers and sisters, you know that means

trouble! I was a prime target for both physical and mental abuse, as younger sisters usually are, and having long, pullable braids didn't help the teasing much.

On the other hand, Owen never gave me one bit of grief. He couldn't talk, so he never snapped back at me, and, since he isn't very coordinated, he never was able to tackle me going down the dark, upstairs hall. On top of that, he always had a big smile on his face which made it impossible to get mad at him—at least for very long.

The most difficult part of living with Owie—and the part that kind of hurt—was the total lack of communication. Even now he can't tell us what he's thinking about, and we all get frustrated trying to make him understand our language, our world. Who knows what goes on in his head hour after hour? I feel bad for him and for us. I feel he's missing so much from a life that's been great for the rest of us. Do you suppose he has any clue to what's going on around him, or do you suppose he just goes around all day like a robot, without any thoughts going through his mind at all? I just can't believe that. Do you suppose he's ever happy?

Miss Mary, our youngest child, remembers Owie only from vacation time. None of the kids has seen what the others wrote, and it's been interesting for my wife and me to compare their perspectives.

Owen

When I was young and growing up, Owen was not living at home. I would see him only a few times a year. Because of that, I guess I really was never close to Owen like I was to my other brothers and sisters.

One of my earliest memories of Owen was watching him do puzzles. I used to take a few of the puzzle pieces and hide them. He would finish the puzzle and point to the spaces that were empty and kind of grunt. I wanted to try to get him mad. I was trying to get some sort of reaction from him. When nothing happened I gave him back the puzzle pieces. Owen never really reacted strongly one way or the other.

I remember going with Owen to the Fourth of July parade in town each year when he was home on vacation. He used to get all excited when the fire engines and police cars came by flashing their lights and screaming their sirens. He used to wave his arms and open his mouth wide and yodel. I did not think his behavior was particularly unusual. That was just the way Owen acted. I had accepted that. People used to stare at him, however, and people still do sometimes. Having a brother like Owen had taught me to accept people for who they really are.

Here are some lessons we learned, occasionally the hard way: Siblings can feel deprived of love and attention because of a handicapped family member, and miss out on treats such as movies, having friends over, or other special events. Even Christmas and birthday presents may seem unfairly distributed. The special child often becomes the focus of attention, regardless of the needs of the nonspecial children. This excessive emphasis is apt to work to the disadvantage of all concerned: siblings, especially, feel their interests are unfairly sacrificed, while at the same time the handicapped child's goal of eventual independence is undermined by their very sacrifice. Brothers and sisters may act out their displeasure with disruptive or attention-getting behavior, become depressed, and develop severe headaches or other physical symptoms. On the other hand, older brothers and sisters may seek their share of the family spotlight by making excessive efforts to excel. Whatever the response, if the children are school age, keep their teachers advised of the home situation and educate all the kids so they'll be able to answer the kinds of questions their classmates are bound to ask.

A parent who is aware of the potential for stress can minimize it by making a conscious effort to avoid playing favorites and by being sensitive to such things as birthday presents and special dinner-table treats. Equal time for everyone, often logistically difficult, may be made possible by respite care and babysitting services and as more facilities like special preschools and summer camps for the handicapped youngster become available. Parents should use these resources for their children's sake if not for their own. We reserved Friday nights for family activities. The other kids counted on this outing, a treat everyone could look forward to and enjoy. We learned that family routines have a remarkable capacity to reduce stress and increase stability, particularly during trying periods, while an interruption of a familiar pattern can be threatening.

Another option often overlooked is that older siblings will usually feel better about themselves if they are taken into the parents' confidence and encouraged to participate in their brother's or sister's treatment. Sometimes they can act as "home teachers," reinforcing subjects taught in school. In addition, going along on visits to the clinic can be instructive and help imaginative siblings separate reality from fantasy.

Siblings, particularly adolescents, can become exquisitely embarrassed by the appearance or behavior of a family member. If a teenager is devastated by his own facial blemishes, it's easy to imagine his reaction when his buddies meet him on the street in the company of his acting-out handicapped brother. Owen's contortions are so strange that even Mary and I, after years of experience, can be thrown off stride by them. No wonder that our kids, when they were younger, sometimes felt like sinking into the ground. On the other hand, siblings may become overly protective. All our youngsters stuck up for Owen when they thought he was being made fun of, no matter how angry they might get at him at home, but then protectiveness is apt to be typical of a large family's behavior. In general, our children seemed to follow our example; if we were calm, patient, and sympathetic, so eventually were they.

It's surprising how quickly and easily the very young will naturally accept a person's abnormality. Sometimes I feel they can be more understanding and, in a way, more realistic than their parents. I remember how one of our youngsters introduced Owen to his friends by saying offhand: "This is my brother Owie. He doesn't talk and can't read but he's O.K." And that was all there was to it—all that needed to be said. The kids went about their business and accepted Owie for what he was. My advice is not to worry too much about your children's intrafamily relationships except to try to be fair and straightforward and to set a compassionate example in your own dealings with the handicapped child. As your children grow older, see that they become knowledgeable about their sibling's disability. Talk about it in a free and matter-of-fact way; if you don't, the family will have every reason to feel it is something to be ashamed of. Information, even concerning a painful subject, is preferable to ignorance distorted by imagination.

It's only natural for brothers and sisters to grow resentful if they are required to shoulder what seems an unfair proportion of home-care responsibilities. As we have seen, family teamwork is essential; however, cooperation will be difficult, at best, if chores are not assigned equitably and if parents, as captains of the team, fail to exercise leadership. For example, there is no justification for sisters being expected to carry more of the babysitting load than brothers.

Sometimes in their late teens or early twenties siblings may develop other worries: Are they themselves all right? Must they assume responsibility for their handicapped brother or sister after their parents are gone? Might they, too, have a handicapped child when they get married and begin a family? These questions, the silent ones that can prey on the mind of a young person, are among the most difficult for parents to handle. If information is available and facts are known and non-threatening, why not choose an appropriate time and explore the situation honestly and in as much depth as your children can understand? Before you launch into a medical dissertation, however, I strongly suggest you get advice from your family doctor so that you're sure of the facts. It would be unfortunate to create fears before any exist. Sometimes, if he is good with children, your doctor can be the ideal person to lead the discussion, since he can provide specific, authoritative answers.

Questions lacking definitive answers are more difficult to address. In many instances it's better not to initiate a discussion until more facts are known. Unfortunately, some information may never be available, as is the case with Owen; lack of a definite diagnosis has left many questions unanswered. Typical of the stress created when this happens is the crisis we experienced when, as expectant grandparents, we learned Owen's problems might be caused by what is known as the "fragile X syndrome," a genetic condition affecting some children of female siblings. At that time one of our daughters had just given birth to a son, apparently normal, and another was contemplating marriage and raising a family. Fortunately, Owen's tests were negative, but we lived through many anxious months waiting for the results, imagining all sorts of things and not wanting to worry our daughters needlessly before we had more information.

If parents desire more information on sibling relationships with the handicapped, I recommend *Brothers and Sisters: A Special Part of Exceptional Families* (see Resources: Support Groups). In addition to normal intrafamily help, sibling support groups are becoming more common, but they ordinarily are found only in large urban areas. If he's interested, help your teenager organize a local group (see Chapter 12). It may be easier for him to discuss some problems with peers whom he feels understand him.

Frustrations from Outside

Well-meaning friends can be supportive and helpful, but some can add to your anxiety level. They are the ones who feel compelled to confide, "for the good of the child," that the professionals you have engaged are known to be incompetent, are using inappropriate medications, and/or are apparently unaware of a new and miraculous cure developed by a faith healer in Central America. (Your friend is sure of the facts because she read the headlines at the supermarket check-out counter.) This kind of "free assessment," when taken seriously, is not likely to reduce your anxiety level or to improve the medical situation, no matter how outraged you may be with your doctor.

In Chapter 9 I discussed patient–doctor relationships and possible areas of conflict. When things go wrong it's natural to blame the person in charge. It's always been that way. In Italy, when they get disgusted, they change governments. In ancient Greece they killed the messenger who brought the bad news. This alternative is normally not available to the parent, and of course, it's just as well, since it's often the professional who is the nearest nonfamily member in sight when things go haywire.

Although parental complaints about caregivers cover a wide range, I have been struck by a remarkable consistency in parents' pet frustrations and in what bothers them most. Complaints tend to be concerned with two general areas.

First, especially among young parents, is the charge that professionals either have unrealistically high expectations of the workload parents can handle at home or are not inclined to take any such limitation into consideration when they make home assignments (physical therapy exercises with their child, for example). Parents complain that if a doctor's instructions involve more than they can cope with, their options are limited and almost sure to induce anxiety. They can appear to challenge the doctor's judgment by questioning the prescription; they can question their own competence, on the assumption that the prescription is reasonable for most people and they are incompetent and/or selfish, or they can do the best they can and neglect whatever part of the therapy they can't get to on a hit-or-miss basis. The last approach is chancy, since parents may not know what can safely be reduced or eliminated.

However, even if the doctor fails to communicate, that doesn't excuse the parent. Speak up! Describe your home circumstances, particularly any unusual limitations or problems. Where overly taxing medical responsibilities are required, ask the doctor to visit your home to see for himself what you're up against. That may increase his anxiety level. Be sure that when the doctor originally prescribes home-management duties, you understand them. Your feelings of anger and frustration will only increase if you discover, after the fact, that you misunderstood and are performing unnecessary or needlessly complicated jobs. Ask how you can operate more efficiently or if any of the requirements can be altered or reduced. If you are discontented, bring your discontent out in the open. It may be emotionally taxing but better in the long run. It gives the doctor an opportunity to make corrections before pent-up emotion blows a minor concern out of proportion.

Avoid an adversarial relationship with professionals, but not at all costs—not at the expense of your peace of mind. Many parents, one way or another, look to the doctor for emotional support. If you have a personality conflict with the doctor, it's often possible to maintain the same professional relationship while shifting your personal relationship to some other member of the team with whom you feel more comfortable, such as the physical therapist or the nurse. If this is unrealistic, consider approaching a lay support group, your minister or rabbi, or a professional counselor. No doctor is omniscient, and his basic responsibility is, after all, not to you and other family members but to your child. If he is realistic, however, he understands, better probably than you, that he can't treat one without influencing the other. And be realistic yourself: many potential sources of conflict will never materialize if you choose a doctor whose style is compatible with your needs and if you are sensitive to his.

Another common parental complaint is that many doctors tend to be patronizing, appear to "talk down" to parents, and are sensitive neither to their needs nor to their concerns. The situation is not improved if the physician is frequently unavailable for face-to-face conferences, one of the few opportunities when mutual understanding can be developed, or if his secretary is more concerned with "protecting" her boss than with being sensitive to patient needs. Unfortunately, many doctors appear to be unaware of such dissatisfaction. Let yours know! Whether these concerns are justified shouldn't be as important to either you or the doctor as finding ways to eliminate them.

Before you are too hard on the doctor, be sure you are realistic about your own priorities, that you are using your time wisely and aren't taking on too much. One obvious solution is to adjust your life style. That's not the end of the world. There's an old saying, "Cut the suit to fit the cloth"; the cloth in your busy life is the time you have available. No matter how organized you are or aren't, you can do only so much. Even parents of nonhandicapped children must set priorities to bridge the gap between aspirations and reality. For special parents this problem is compounded by the fact that they carry a heavier load than their neighbors, but are limited by the same finite resources of time, energy and finances. Eliminate the nonessentials from your daily schedule, at least until your feet are on the ground. But don't make the mistake of thinking that recreation and relaxation are nonessentials; they are one of the best investments of time you can make.

Curtailment of a family's normal life style need not have a negative impact, and often good things can result. The realignment may be temporary and necessary only until you learn to what extent normal family activities will have to be permanently altered to make room for the added responsibilities. Common sense and experience will be your best instructors. Since you will have less time available, see if your extended family and friends can help temporarily with the shopping, cleaning, and normal household chores. People who care about you will welcome the opportunity to help in other ways than just offering a shoulder to cry on. It will make them feel good to pitch in, and since it's only for the short term, you shouldn't feel guilty.

In conclusion, some general principles should apply to almost everyone: when tensions build, talk things over—get complaints off your chest. Don't be so foolishly proud you can't accept assistance. When the going gets tough, seek professional help and take a break, even if it's a short one. Try to keep your sense of humor, and laugh at yourself; it's cheaper than going to a psychiatrist. Get regular exercise, maintain family routine, and plan your work so you're not frustrated by time wasted. All these suggestions can help; however, I feel the most effective way to reduce stress and keep it at manageable levels is to learn what specifically you can do to improve your everyday effectiveness and hence your child's chances for success. It's possible for you to be despondent, anxious, and depressed even after you have eliminated most stress-generating problems, but it isn't likely.

12

Support Resources

The Support Group

Under most circumstances the family is the best support system known to man. When it's working, it's hard to beat. But no matter how independent you are—or think you are—there will be times you'll benefit from moving outside yourself, beyond the predictable responses of your own family. If you're lucky and receptive, you can learn from the diverse perspectives of your peers, others in the same boat as you, people knowledgeable about resources locally available. They can be objective in their reaction to you and offer insights gained, not second- or third-hand, but by having already grappled with the problems you face now.

Peer support (sometimes called "self-help" or "mutual aid") offers this potential. Support groups are collections of individuals with a common bond who get together to help one another. Although groups are often composed of parents, grandparents, siblings, professionals, and the handicapped individuals themselves (or a combination of these groups), this book is concerned primarily with parent-centered organizations. Many mothers and fathers will feel right at home, since a support group functions very much like an extended family. However, it's not for everyone. How can you tell if it's right for you? What are its characteristics, its pluses and minuses? The first part of this chapter considers these questions.

Any day of the week, outside operating rooms and in the corridors of hospitals and institutions across the country, you will see informal and spontaneous support groups in action as parents wait for their kids —or for news of them—and "pass the time of day." You yourself may have participated, helping or being helped by someone—someone you hardly knew. Even with the occasional sad moment, it's a satisfying experience and makes you feel good to see people supporting one another without thought of personal gain.

The more formal, "institutionalized" support groups in which you may be interested take many forms. Organized originally by a parent, social worker, or some other professional, and sometimes centered on one particular institution, they reflect a wide range of approaches.

Groups reflect the needs and goals of their membership, but no matter what form they take, they will reassure you that many share your problems and that your frustrations and concerns need not be unsolvable or signs of unredeemable failure. The organizations can be many things: informal, self-help (with little or no professional direction), independent, and locally oriented or more structured and affiliated with a national association. In our family's experience with various groups, we found that, although some structure is necessary if an organization is to continue and thrive, the benefits to be gained by the individual parent spring not from bylaws and parliamentary procedure but from parents' willingness to share experiences and to give and accept help. Remember this if you are tempted to get involved in arguments over protocol; such confusion of priorities can ruin a meeting for others.

As our family learned the hard way, accepting help can be more difficult than giving it and is a valuable skill to acquire. Judging from the body language obvious at meetings, I'd say those helping often benefit as much as those they help. Parents I know have joined support groups primarily to help them combat emotional pressures that sometimes seemed to be almost beyond their control. One usually quiet father surprised me by saying, "Listen, other parents are the best way I know of to get help when things go sour. Hey, they know what it's all about. They've been there and understand and don't look down their nose at you. You'd be surprised at how much you can learn. And it doesn't cost anything, either." A young mother of a son with Down syndrome made a point I have heard time and again: "Parents of special needs kids have special needs themselves, and there are lots of professionals who forget the parents or talk down to them. Parents understand other parents—usually."

Unfortunately, support groups are not universally available, particularly in rural areas, and the need often exceeds the supply. One solution is to form your own group. Mary and I once began a short-lived parents' organization, and it's possible sometime you will, too. (Later in this chapter I discuss the mechanics involved in such an undertaking.) Fortunately, most parents will be able to locate one or more groups already meeting locally and will need only to determine which, if any, meets their needs.

Support groups usually either limit their membership to parents and professionals concerned with only one type of disability (cerebral palsy, for example), or are all-encompassing, such as groups for parents of chronically ill children or any special needs children. Membership consists primarily of parents, although often the handicapped persons themselves or various professionals join the group, as leaders, guests, or regular participants. The greatest potential advantage of group participation is its warm, experienced, and nonjudgmental forum of peers in which a parent's concerns will be respected and understood (you can get things off your chest). This potential, of course, is not always realized, since a parents' group, like any organization, is made up of people, with all their strengths and weaknesses, and it would be a mistake to assume individuals cast aside their human frailties automatically upon gaining membership in the group. Don't be surprised to find a chronic talker or complainer or objector in your organization. Don't expect saints. (They're there, but you have to look for them.)

As important as emotional support is, a group of experienced peers can also offer much more specific help by providing feedback, both objective and subjective, on the availability and characteristics of local health-related services. This often-informal process may be the most effective way—sometimes the only way—of obtaining answers that are difficult to obtain through conventional channels (for instance, information about doctors' personalities, or about their comparative billing practices). A peer group can provide practical parent-to-parent tips on efficient and economic handling of both medical and nonmedical home-management problems. In most groups you will pick up information on state and local political issues affecting you, particularly those dealing with the rights of handicapped persons; in some meetings a specific time is set aside for announcements and a regular newsletter is published. Some organizations are more action oriented than others and provide a ready-made structure by which members can work as advocates in areas of particular concern—for example, converting all municipal transportation to handicapped-accessible vehicles. Other organizations make parent education a top priority and provide extensive programs, many of which concentrate on training parents to teach other parents, so that those taught become more self-sufficient and eventually become teachers themselves, to form a continuing, ever-lengthening, and renewable chain of support.

If your group consists exclusively of parents from one institution, you may want to request a regular opportunity to present constructive feedback to management, and to join together in activities to benefit the institution. Although it shouldn't be the sole basis for your motivation, often your own child will benefit from your efforts. You can raise money to support a favorite project or organize fellow parents, as we did, for regular "field days," during which grounds are spruced up and windows reglazed. You can repaint shabby classroom walls with bright, cheery colors or act as chaperones for trips that, without such help, might not have been undertaken. In most support groups, your self-education program can benefit from activities organized to address issues affecting handicapped persons, utilizing outside speakers, role-playing techniques, slides, and movies. Or the membership itself can provide a resource pool from which to launch programs into the community, as this book often suggests (for instance, a puppet show dealing with sibling rivalry, produced by a group of talented mothers). In a number of public elementary schools, I witnessed excellent educational units sponsored and entirely organized by parents dealing with "Understanding the Handicapped Person." And last, but, for some mothers and fathers, most important of all, belonging to such a group offers the possibility of establishing contact with a "veteran" parent who can act as your mentor to help you through the rough times until you, too, become seasoned.

National Organizations

If you are interested in the larger picture and in the advantages that a broad membership base and a more formal staff support system have to offer, consider joining an affiliate of a national group, such as the Muscular Dystrophy Association, the Epilepsy Foundation of America, the United Cerebral Palsy Associations, and the Association for Retarded Citizens. (However, joining *only* the national organization, if it has no local affiliate, does not offer the personal support and peer interaction that, in my experience, are the most important benefits of any membership organization.) In addition to the locally oriented activities just described, these national organizations can offer some advantages unavailable to unaffiliated groups, such as a nationwide political base for advocacy activities. If you are interested in national change or improvement, 100,000 votes are better than 1, and such organizations have in fact exerted significant influence at both the state and national levels, by helping to obtain needed services and by ensuring appropriate education and equal access to buildings and transportation facilities for handicapped persons.

Largeness can have other benefits—for instance, some associations offer group discounts on both prescription and nonprescription medicine and provide medical and self-help equipment. The Easter Seal Society, with "more than one million clients" and 800 state and local affiliates, is an example of the potential benefits of size. One year the society indicated that it committed more than 70 cents of each dollar raised to providing "direct services to people with disabilities," and that among the services offered were "physical, occupational, and speech-language therapies; vocational evaluation and training; camping and recreation; and psychological counseling and speech therapy."

Many national organizations fund significant research and professional education programs that, through conferences, postresidency training, and scholarly publications, seek to improve professional standards in the field and help health practitioners keep up to date on current developments in their fields. And some associations, either nationally or through their local affiliates, support clinics that provide many different services, including diagnostic, therapeutic, and rehabilitative follow-up care as well as social service counseling. Other national organizations, such as the Association for the Care of Children's Health (ACCH; see Resources: Associations), which I have previously recommended, are primarily concerned with research and the distribution of information, but ordinarily do not offer a wide network of local support-group affiliates. Of course, they are indirectly very supportive through the materials and knowledge they furnish.

Although smaller, unaffiliated local support groups may circulate an informal newsletter, national organizations usually publish a professionally organized newsletter or magazine presenting current national and international developments and information of a general nature about the disease or handicap with which the association is concerned. They often sponsor other, more specialized publications dealing with specific technical concerns, and sometimes they maintain a handicapped-centered clearinghouse—sometimes with a WATS hotline to answer members' questions and identify resources. In the final analysis, the type of support group that most appeals to you may boil down to a matter of size and everything it represents (i.e., whether you want to be a little fish in a big sea or a large fish in a local swimming hole).

The Obligations of Membership

With the exception of dues, which may or may not be required (find out early), ordinarily only as much participation and regular attendance is expected of parents as they are willing to give. But since the effectiveness of local parents' groups depends upon the willingness of the membership to exchange ideas, share experiences, and support one another, the program will be strong only if parents participate on a regular basis. Mary and I found that erratic attendance was a major weakness of many groups, and I would steer clear of any with a poor track record in this regard. If you are interested, attend a few meetings as a visitor to see if you feel comfortable with the group's climate. The whole idea may not be your cup of tea. Some people are just not comfortable with the public sharing of personal experiences and the give and take of group interaction, no matter how warm the environment or well-intentioned the members. Take your time in deciding whether to join any support group. If you decide you want to give it a go, make it an informed decision, and once you're in, participate as fully as you can.

Selecting the Right Group

Your child's pediatrician, assessment team leader, and visiting nurse are usually reliable sources of information about local support groups. The hospital social worker, the play therapist, or a representative of the local department of human services, as well as parents you meet and become buddies with in the waiting room, may also offer good feedback. If your child has a specific illness, a natural starting point is the nearest office of the applicable national association or its state affiliate. The State Resource Sheet, available from the National Information Center for Children and Youth with Handicaps (NICHCY), lists the names and addresses of some supportive organizations, along with other state agencies concerned with the handicapped. The following randomly selected examples are typical of the kind of resource you may find listed for your state: the Washington Association for Retarded Citizens, the Vermont Chapter of the National Association for Children and Adults with Autism, the Utah Parent Information and Training Center, the New York State Head Injury Association, the Easter Seal Society for Crippled Children and Adults of Nevada, and the Missouri Association for Children with Learning Disabilities. Send for your own state's Resource Sheet from NICHCY (see Resources: Clearinghouses/Databanks/Information). Another particularly well done publication is *The Self-Help Sourcebook: Finding and Forming Mutual-Aid Self-Help Groups*, compiled by Edward J. Madara and Abigail Meese (see Resources: Support Groups). This book will also be helpful, later, if you decide to form your own group. In addition, your state's Developmental Disabilities Council should be a particularly helpful source of information on local parent activities. All these organizations may also have information on the more specialized sibling and grandparent groups, which often are centered only in large urban areas. For example, the King County (Seattle, Washington) Advocates for Retarded Citizens (ARC) operates programs it describes as intended "to help grandparents meet each other and professionals, and obtain support and information. . . . New grandparents can contact the ARC for a match with a trained helping grandparent."

Don't be discouraged if there is no group nearby concerned exclusively with your child's particular handicap. Other, more diverse organizations can be equally valuable but in different ways. You may find some groups, often sponsored by local hospitals, that are concerned with the general problems faced by bereaved mothers and fathers or the parents of chronically ill children. Chances are there will also be "umbrella" statewide organizations—sometimes called "federations" or "alliances"—that welcome parents of all handicapped children in your state, irrespective of the handicapping condition. (One example is the Parent Advocacy Coalition for Educational Rights [PACER] in Minnesota, an active organization whose excellent publications, *PACER* and *PACER Advocate,* are of interest to all mothers and fathers, no matter where their home.) Recently the federal government has become active in sponsoring parent projects. The U.S. Department of Health and Human Services, Bureau of Maternal and Child Health, sponsors a project called Collaboration among Parents and (Health) Professionals (CAPP). Through this organization the department encourages communication and understanding between parents and health-care providers by means of a nationwide information system that assists parents in assuming a prominent role in their children's home health care. One of the priorities of the program is to encourage coalitions and federations of parental groups to maximize their efforts and to provide more stability for the various small local groups. Particular emphasis is given to parent participation and training.

Another area of parent concern is addressed by the Education for All Handicapped Children's Act (P.L. 94-142), Amendments of 1983, P.L. 98-199 Sec. 631 (c), which provides for an umbrella organization called the National Network of Parent Centers, as well as authorizing grants to support parent-to-parent efforts to help mothers and fathers "participate more effectively with professionals in meeting the educational needs of handicapped children." The Federation for Children with Special Needs located in Boston, Massachusetts, which is the overall coordinator of the National Network of Parent Centers, publishes a first-rate newsletter called the *Newsline* as well as monographs—for example, *Some Suggestions for Communication with Medical Personnel*—and annotated bibliographies, such as *Personal Accounts of Disability and Illness* and *Attitudes Toward Handicaps and Chronic Illness and Strategies for Coping.*

Interwoven in the educational orientation of this legislation is another, even more basic emphasis: "All activities of the National Network of Parent Centers are committed to transforming expectations about people with handicapping conditions, shifting the emphasis away from deficits and limitations toward an emphasis on their strengths and abilities, their potential contributions as citizens and taxpayers." An organization called Technical Assistance for Parent Programs (TAPP), operating through four regional centers, was created to transform these worthy sentiments into services, such as assisting groups planning to organize parent programs. Since the benefits offered by both CAPP and TAPP are diverse and may change, I suggest you write or call both CAPP's national office, asking what resources they currently offer parents in the area of home health care, and your TAPP

Regional Center for information about special education. You might adapt the form letter included in Chapter 8. (For the addresses of all these organizations, see Resources: Support Groups.)

Another resource with which you should be familiar both as an individual and as a member and perhaps founder of a support group is the research community. Although much of the work it does is presented in technical terms, some academic professionals bring a warm understanding to their efforts and dedicate much of their activities— writing, research, teaching, workshops—to parents. Ann and H. Rutherford Turnbull, university professors and themselves parents of a developmentally disabled child, are outstanding representatives of this group. (I attended an excellent workshop they gave dealing with all aspects of parent support.) Your state university's department of education should be able to give you information on how you can keep current on what is happening in research/academia, and many national associations publish calendars of workshops and lectures that might be of interest to you or your support group. Perhaps a number of smaller groups could combine to sponsor a program featuring a nationally recognized expert—but be sure he speaks well to laypeople (the Turnbulls do).

Joining or Starting a Support Group

If several organizations are already established in your area from which you can choose, you're fortunate, but you need information to decide which, if any, you will eventually want to join. If no support group is available or those that are don't suit you, you may want to start one from scratch. In either case, before you get to the decision-making stage, think through some critical questions: How should time, frequency, and location of meetings be arranged for maximal member convenience and program effectiveness? Do you feel comfortable with a professional staff member acting as a kind of executive director or do you favor a more laissez-faire completely parent-controlled approach, with parent volunteers running the show? I have found that a good professional staff member is almost a prerequisite unless a volunteer parent has the skills necessary to organize such a group and the time required to keep it going. A variation of Murphy's Law states that any job that appears easy will be twice as difficult as you predicted. One caution: if you involve nonvolunteer staff, make sure that you, the parents, determine group policy and not the staff member.

Another matter to consider is whether you prefer an established organization with a proven track record (that might give you security) or the excitement of a fledgling group just trying its wings (that might make you break out in a rash). Would you welcome local institutional sponsorship—a hospital or state agency, for instance—or do you fear the sponsor might set the agenda and exercise control? Would you prefer a group made up exclusively of parents whose children have handicaps similar to your child's? (One obvious benefit of this arrangement is that group homogeneity offers a maximal opportunity to concentrate all the group's energies and experience as well as the resources of a sponsoring national organization, if one is involved, on common concerns.) Finding a large enough group of interested parents to support such a restricted focus, however, may be difficult, particularly if a rare syndrome is involved. But when it is feasible, organizational support— including a local staff member to help at least in the initial stages—may be made available by the national sponsor.

A mixed group, made up of parents whose children suffer from many different disabilities, offers its own unique pluses and minuses. Although the diversity means you will have many different problems with which to contend, this very diversity offers its own advantages:

- No parent need be excluded.
- A wide range of perspectives inevitably results, offering each member an opportunity (sometimes almost forcing him) to expand his horizons and better understand the problems and potentials characteristic of other handicapped groups.
- Despite the diversity, many problems common to one disability are, in varying degrees, chronic and common to all, e.g., the inaccessibility of vital facilities, the lack of public understanding, and the difficulties inherent in securing an appropriate education or gaining satisfactory employment.
- Not being affiliated with a single national sponsoring organization may make it possible to secure assistance from not one but several national organizations.
- Diversified groups, because of their broader focus, are often more effective in their efforts to influence and cooperate with other community organizations, such as schools, the bureaucracy, and social service agencies.

If you find the idea of a support group appealing, attend a few meetings of representative organizations. Even if you must travel some distance, the effort will help clarify your thinking. Take time to prepare, so that you'll know what you're looking for and get the most out of your visit. Here are some suggestions: Try to make arrangements ahead of time to go with a member or the staff leader. He can see that you don't get lost, fill you in on the way to the meeting as to "who is who," and, once there, introduce you to members as they arrive. Through this kind of introduction, you will be off to a good start and less apt to be left abandoned in the corner, wondering where the bathroom is and why you came. (Once I drank coffee and chatted with some delightful people for fifteen minutes before the conversation turned to hydraulic presses and I discovered that I was at the wrong meeting!) If minutes are regularly kept, ask if you can look over some back "issues." This can be a good way to get a feel for what goes on.

Listen carefully, make notes if that helps, and remember to take a pad and pencil along. Above all, at least at the first meeting, resist the temptation to talk too much yourself, although be prepared to explain who you are and the nature of your child's disability. Self-introductions may be a normal part of the meeting's opening—and people will be genuinely interested. Most important of all, get a sense of the spirit of the meeting and the attitudes of those present. Find out if you relate to at least some of the members and, in general, if the concerns dealt with are the kind of issues you find important. See if someone is there who you feel has been through experiences similar to yours and who might help in the future. (Don't, however, enter into close confidential relationships on the basis of first impressions—they may be much easier to get into than out of.)

If you decide to start your own group, locate a good "how-to-do-it" manual to help you. *Learning Together,* by Debra Haffner, is an excellent resource (see Resources: Support Groups). If you do your homework, the questions you should be able to answer are:

- What kind of initial planning group is most effective, and how can you gather it together? Although you may have a clear idea of the nature of the "sounding board" you want—perhaps two or three parents whom you know and respect—be flexible and be prepared for the possibility that others might not agree with all your preconceptions.

- How can you identify potential parent-members? The same resources useful in the past—the hospital, your doctor, the visiting nurse, the school system, and social service agencies—should be helpful, but don't overlook local churches and synagogues, the PTA, national organizations that have no local affiliate, or state advocacy groups. Ask if you can use the organization's mailing lists, but don't be hurt if they say no. Would advertising through public-service announcements on local radio and TV stations or in the newspaper be appropriate?

- What's the best way to set up an initial organizational meeting of all interested potential members? Where and when will the meeting be held? Who will write the invitation letter? What information must be included? Who will chair the meeting? Who will take notes (don't assume it will be a woman)? Will an attendance sheet be passed around, with space for names, addresses, phone numbers, and possibly the nature of the child's disability? What should be discussed at the meeting? What decisions should be reached?

- What is your role as organizer? Even though this first meeting may be critical, don't be directive or pushy. It's vital that everyone has a say. If the meeting appears to be steamrolled, you will lose your members before you have started.

- What details must you attend to which, if mishandled, will result in chaos and affect the tone of future meetings? Take nothing for granted. Be sure that the doors to the meeting room are—and remain—unlocked till the meeting is over. See that directions to the site have been clearly given and arrangements made for those who need transportation. Check calendars to avoid a conflicting meeting, if possible.

The leader walks a narrow line between being too relaxed and "laid back" on the one hand and being organized to the point of officiousness on the other. Since you are convinced—I hope with an evangelical zeal—that the support resource you are trying to establish will make a valuable contribution to your community, be certain in your attempt to provide it that you have given the effort your best shot.

Professional Counseling

Although many parents who might benefit from counseling don't take advantage of it, it's a valuable and often misunderstood support resource.[1] Some have reservations about anything connected with the mental health profession, and others worry that the costs will be prohibitive. Reactions of our parent friends have ranged from "Do you think I'm crazy?" and "I'd worry what my friends would think," to an unusually positive, "When our child was born [severely retarded], the impact on all of us was devastating. I'm convinced that therapy saved our family." Unfortunately, the multitude of mistaken stereotypes combined with a lack of readily accessible facilities have tended to blunt the effectiveness of an extremely valuable resource for a host of people, many of whom live under constant and often extreme emotional pressure.

1. Some of the concepts that follow are drawn from "Who Needs Psychiatric Help?" a leaflet distributed by the American Psychiatric Press Inc. (Department 505, 1400 K Street NW, Washington, DC 20005), the publishing affiliate of The American Psychiatric Association. Contact them for information on available material.

Some circumstances for which you might consider professional counseling are:

- You are seriously concerned about your ability to cope with the situation and feel you need help. You may be experiencing one or more of these symptoms: frequent depressions and deep unhappiness, severe anxiety, panic or fear, extreme emotional swings, excessive worrying, an abrupt change in weight or in sleeping or eating habits, frequent loss of emotional control, difficulties with concentration, overuse of alcohol or drugs, sexual problems, or feelings of emptiness, worthlessness, and loss of self-esteem.
- No parent-initiated support group is available in your area, or, if there is one, it hasn't provided adequate assistance (for example, it may not meet often enough, a common parent complaint).
- You feel extremely uncomfortable in a group situation and find public discussion of your concerns unprofitable. Fathers, for example, sometimes are ill at ease in a predominantly female environment but could benefit from emotional support.

Bear in mind that, almost by definition, being a special parent involves exposure to extraordinary pressures. The natural grieving process is emotionally draining, and most of us have suffered the physical exhaustion that often results from frequent loss of sleep, the disruption of regular routines, and the strenuous physical therapy regimen involved with our children's care to which our bodies aren't yet accustomed. (In pre-aerobics days and while Owen was nonambulatory and still careening around on his knees, Mary maintained her muscle tone by lugging her son around the house and hoisting him in and out of our 1955 Dodge coupe.) You and your family will be worn to a frazzle; you wouldn't be normal if you weren't. A young and attractive friend of ours looked at it differently. She said, "I get more good exercise from giving Timmy his physical therapy than I ever got at the YWCA."

You may be eliminating one important helping hand if you arbitrarily reject the possibility of counseling, whether it be for yourself alone, for you and your spouse together, or for the entire family. One mother who got professional help said, "The pressure on my family was beyond anything you would believe. The roof could have fallen in and we wouldn't even have looked up. Our once-a-month support group was better than nothing but not a whole lot. Our pediatrician played God. What he didn't seem to understand was that we were left to handle the results of his divine edicts. Counseling helped us sort things out. It helped us see what was going on and made all the difference in the world."

Almost every community offers counseling services, although you may be unaware of their existence. Many provide crisis counseling for families disrupted because of bereavement or the impact of a handicapped child. Some sponsor their own support groups and offer workshops dealing with such topics as single parenting, stepparenting, and coping with terminal illness. Look in the phone book in the "Community Services" section under "Family Services and Counseling" or "Mental Health." Many of the organizations are members of United Way or receive public support and offer free or reduced-charge service for qualifying individuals. Check also with local affiliates of national associations, which sometimes offer counseling services. For example, the Baltimore Association for Retarded Citizens says it "is charged with helping people solve their problems through the process of a structured, therapeutic experience. Counseling is available to and for the retarded person experiencing either personal problems or poor adjustment—whether at home, in the community or on the job. Counselors provide individual, family and group services to both the retarded citizen and the family." Your doctor, visiting nurse, or social worker should be helpful in locating local resources.

If your discomfort is severe, a consultation with a psychologist or psychiatrist may be helpful. Be sure to clarify any financial commitment involved, since these services can be expensive and are ordinarily covered by third-party payers only under very specific circumstances. Check with your insurance carrier!

Respite Care

As effective as any kind of external emotional support may be, it should never be considered a substitute for practical action that reduces stress by removing the problems that caused the stress in the first place. Improving the lot of your child through more satisfactory educational or medical intervention is the most obvious move in that direction. Another approach is to give yourself a breather while you regroup. Arrange for someone else to assume responsibility for your child so that everyone in the family can enjoy a break—both from one another and from the frustrating limitations of their demanding routine. Such practical therapy is called "respite care." (The dictionary defines *respite* as "an interval of rest or relief.") When everything seems to be going wrong and you need to catch your breath and put your problems temporarily on hold, respite care can bring color back to your cheeks and a spring to your step. It certainly helped us.

Acceptance of respite care, which is usually given by someone outside the family, has been slow. Such services are still often difficult to obtain, and, even when they are available, families who most need them often consider their need to be a failure—an admission that they are unable to "take care of their own." This position is usually unfounded and counterproductive. Fortunately, the situation is rapidly improving.

Rest periods generally do not need to be long to be effective. Frequent and brief breaks can offer wonderful relief from the constant responsibility of being a 24-hour caregiver and allow family members to attend to activities that otherwise might be neglected—shopping, running errands, or even going out for a night on the town. Sometimes periods as long as a month can be arranged to allow mother and father to attend to an emergency or go on a much-needed vacation. One advantage of organizing respite care on an ongoing basis is that, once a relationship has been established, arrangements can more easily be made if the unexpected happens. Regularly scheduled "intervals of rest" were particularly important to our family, since they not only gave us something to look forward to but also broke time down into pieces we felt we could handle.

Everyone suffers when a family's life is so restricted that contact with the normal outside world is either limited or, in some instances, eliminated entirely. Even when Mary and I finally swallowed our false pride, it took months to locate help. But once we found an appropriate home and saw how valuable a change of scene could be for everyone, including Owen, it became an almost guilt-free part of our regular family routine. Respite care has the potential to be far more than a crutch to be used only to support a family in emergency situations, as important as that may be. At best, and on a regular basis, it can allow a disrupted group to function normally once again; it can provide parents the luxury of being able to plan; and it can help restore the feeling that, at least to a degree, family members have some control over their own destinies. For the handicapped individual, respite care can introduce a new face, a fresh personality (the professional caregiver) into his life and open up the possibility of social experiences and friendships beyond the family circle. It can begin to loosen his dependency on the family and initiate the process that must take place if some independence is ever to be achieved.

Respite care came into its own in the mid-1970s, along with the policy of mainstreaming and deinstitutionalization, under which handicapped citizens were to be integrated as much as possible into society and no longer isolated. But this movement, however well intentioned, had problems, and many local communities and school systems were not prepared to handle the challenges the new policy created. Many children who otherwise would have been cared for in an institution had to remain in homes ill equipped to care for them either emotionally or physically. There wasn't suitable public respite service available, and many parents who couldn't afford expensive private care had to fend for themselves.

Respite care is now provided in many locations. It may be offered at a distant institution, right in your own community, or even in your own home, with friends, volunteers, or professionals coming in to take over. In another approach, a group of parents forms a cooperative or swaps babysitting responsibilities on an informal, nonpaying basis. Such arrangements are economical and flexible, but be careful! This kind of intimate sharing requires a very special relationship between families. It can turn out to be like lending money to a friend, with each party losing both a convenient arrangement and a friendship. Another possibility is to ask a relative or a specially trained babysitter to take over for a short interlude. (Be sure the relative is calm by nature, well instructed, and not expected to leave you a large inheritance.) Older siblings may also fill in occasionally, but don't overdo this responsibility, since they, in their own way, need respite as much as their parents. When your children grow up and start their own families, they may be glad to invite their handicapped sibling to their homes for brief visits to give you flexibility, particularly around vacation time. Our kids have.

Some commercial organizations offering other kinds of home-care services will also take charge of the procurement and supervision of respite care workers for in-home duty, but be sure that their employee is a person in whom you have confidence. Ask for a pre-employment interview; otherwise you'll spend all your time away from your child worrying. Out-of-home service can be provided in several ways. Some institutions that serve full-time residential clients also reserve a few rooms or beds for the occasional respite use of individuals ordinarily cared for at home, and a few organizations specialize in respite placement. Several associations, both local and national, provide comprehensive respite-care programs that go considerably beyond the mere furnishing of temporary supervision. For example, the Shoreline Association for Retarded and Handicapped Citizens of Guilford, Connecticut, offers a 24-hour emergency system, licensed respite homes, in-home health-care aides, a registered list of sitters and companions, sliding-scale fees, and a respite-provider training program. This wide coverage should be a model for other communities. Does your community offer anything like it? If not, why not?

Sometimes a provider will take children into his own home, serving as a short-term foster parent. We eventually discovered such a person, a woman who worked at the local state institution for the mentally retarded and accepted special youngsters into her family as a source of additional income. She was knowledgeable and competent, and after visiting her home, checking references, and meeting the other temporary resident, we began what turned out to be a very satisfactory relationship.

Today, many local nonresidential programs, such as special-needs day care and preschool centers, routinely cater to handicapped children. More and more, they and other facilities are being established by church groups as well as other private and public service organizations. Some individual parents and support groups have been instrumental in forming their own programs, which can provide a superb service to any community, but it's a demanding job, since you must learn to cope not only with a wide range of disabilities but also with the bureaucracy. At one time I investigated the possibility of starting a community group home but finally gave up in frustration, convinced that the handicapped youngsters presented fewer problems than the politicians and bureaucrats who created and interpreted the regulations.

Actually, regularly scheduled programs designed for the entire community that accept and are qualified to care for disabled kids can offer parents a kind of respite care in many ways more effective than services designed exclusively for handicapped children. Summer recreation activities, which are often sponsored by community adult education agencies, are a good example of programs ideally suited for this kind of mainstreaming. The advantages of such programs are twofold: they give the handicapped child the wonderful opportunity of living for a time in the "outside world" under somewhat sheltered conditions, and they offer the nonhandicapped students and their parents an equally wonderful opportunity to expand their own horizons and understanding. Mingling the two groups in a common activity is the most desirable respite program. As more and more community programs make provision to accept special kids, the need for separate respite facilities will decrease. This is a good reason for you to be active in community affairs at the town council and school board level, where such issues will be considered.

Respite care can be a godsend, but it carries with it certain responsibilities, for whenever you entrust your child to someone else, even for short periods, you will want to ensure that the arrangement is safe and the placement is the one most likely to meet your child's needs. Your methods of checking out the care provider will vary, depending upon the nature of the resource, be it babysitter, day-care facility, summer camp, or residential facility. What do you look for when you consider such placement? Although each situation is different, some concerns are common to all arrangements. First and foremost, you must be convinced it's safe. Is the responsible person humane and competent? Are the other clients appropriate companions for your child? Does the institution or care provider come recommended by a number of references? Is communication satisfactory?

Locating and Paying for Respite Facilities

A logical first step in locating nearby respite services is to consult your regular sources of health-related information (visiting nurses, social workers, and community counseling services). The department of human services and/or other state or city agencies should operate a registry of qualified local providers. Depending on state regulations, they may or may not be certified. The Maryland Developmental Disabilities Council, for example, publishes a state guide. But although our own applicable state agency maintained such a list, Mary and I, in our hour of need, apparently felt more urgency in acquiring the information than the agency did in providing it. The staff person responsible for this service was replaced while we were seeking help, and the replacement was frequently away at conferences, "away from her desk" (this expression will be familiar to many), or just plain away.

We were eventually successful in obtaining information, but only after we retained a consultant to represent us—a psychologist who knew Owen and who also knew "the system." Even though the situation is improving, a personal consultant or ombudsman can sometimes be helpful, if you can afford one. The discouraging aspect of this situation is that there is no reason why such representation should be needed in the first place. Some state laws now provide that under certain circumstances personal representatives must be made available to help and represent parents. Check with your human services department. (Part Four describes federal legislation that requires the formation of state advocacy groups, which in some ways can perform the same function.)

In some respite facilities services are free, or charges are based on the parents' ability to pay. There are, of course, limitations. For example, the Owarii Respite Care Program, in Baltimore, Maryland, supported by United Cerebral Palsy of Central Maryland and various public and private agencies, provides subsidized service with charges adjusted depending upon income level and family size. However, the cost subsidy is limited to fourteen days of care in any fiscal year. Paying private facilities for services may present a problem. Perhaps your insurance carrier will cover part of the expense or, if no public facilities are available, a state agency may be responsible for part or all of the expense involved. Logically, respite help is a justifiable medical cost. Not long ago most multiply handicapped youngsters were institutionalized at heavy, usually public, expense. But now many of the old facilities are either closed or drastically reduced in size, with resulting savings to the state. Some recognition of this shifting of responsibility from the taxpayer to the individual parent must be made; indeed, several federal incentive grants are now available to help initiate respite programs. If your state doesn't provide financial respite support, perhaps you will wish to urge your support group to become involved from an advocacy point of view.

Summer Respite

More and more vacation activities, such as community summer programs and camps, both day and residential, are becoming available to the disabled population. They serve both as respite service for the family and as a recreational activity for the child (see Chapter 26). Sometimes parents are included, too. The Southern California Children's Cancer Service, for example, operates a residential summer program for children with cancer and their families. Camps specializing in programs for handicapped children may be run by the state, some churches, private for-profit organizations, and civic groups. On the other hand, occasionally regular Boy or Girl Scout or YMCA/YWCA camps catering to the nonhandicapped population accept special kids as well. A few private resorts and camps now open their doors to special children and their families either early or late in the season.

The kinds of camping experiences available vary widely from one location to the next, and it's difficult to generalize except to say there is reason to expect an appropriate program will be available somewhere in your state, although you may have to bear the expense yourself. Camps accepting severely handicapped kids exclusively are generally custodial in nature, while other camps, catering to less seriously affected children, generally place heavy emphasis upon skill development, social interaction, formal activities, and an activity-filled, structured day.

Our primary goals with Owen were to provide him the opportunity to be among new friends and to be exposed to a variety of exciting experiences in a warm, understanding environment. We were hopeful he could be drawn out of his shell and were heartsick at the long periods of time he spent sitting at home looking into space. Unfortunately, neither camp nor any of our other efforts succeeded in breaking into his isolation. However, his summer-camp experience was a success in one critical regard—it offered him a change from his normal routines. Unfortunately, as we have seen, Owen never communicates any but the most extreme reactions. His body language tells us when he hates something (an enema, anything he has to chew, heights, or slippery or uncertain footing) or when he particularly likes something (applesauce, a screeching buzzsaw, hammering nails, his father bumping his head and getting mad). All his emotional responses in between must be guessed at. We are confident, however, that he enjoyed his camping experience and enthusiastically recommend a summer's activity away from home for most disabled youngsters.

For children not as limited as Owen is, camps offer benefits not always associated with respite care: They can instill in a child hope for a better world for himself, and prove to him that he can function away from the people he depends upon most. They can be a bridge to the beginnings of independent living, as both parents and child see that it can be done and learn that separation for extended periods is possible without disaster. The child may develop increased self-confidence, learn new skills away from the academic classroom, where he has often met defeat, and develop a spirit of group identification. Children who never could have endured being different (such as being the only child with a prosthesis or catheter) have an opportunity to enjoy the benefits of outdoor life and to prepare themselves for a more mainstreamed environment at camps where many are in the same boat. If your child has the potential, it is important that you select a camp that offers some decision-making opportunities. For some children whose handicaps are basically physical, the computer camps run by the Easter Seal Society are worth considering.

The same community sources you would approach for medical information should be helpful in locating an appropriate camp, particularly social workers and local health and human services agencies. Your church and the organizations that regularly operate community summer activities, including the Salvation Army, may also be helpful. Camps occasionally advertise in *Exceptional Parent*, and *The Parent's Guide to Accredited Camps*, a publication of the American Camping Association (ACA), lists several camps accommodating children with disabilities (see Resources: Recreation). A source of brief but valuable information is the National Easter Seal Society's pamphlet *Camps for Children with Disabilities*.

When you locate a program that sounds appropriate, write and ask for a brochure describing the camp, particularly the exact nature of the program offered. Easter Seals and ACA have collaborated in developing "standards for persons with special needs" as part of ACA's accrediting process. Find out if your prospective camp is accredited. The information that could be important to you includes: What is the minimal functioning level required of campers? Are any nonhandicapped children included? What is the nature of supervision? The National Easter Seal Society recommends counselors be at least eighteen years old, preferably with an educational background in and prior ex-

perience with special children. Easter Seals also suggests a minimal
ratio of one counselor for every two or three severely handicapped
campers. In my dealings with all kinds of institutions and activities, I
have always been interested in the personnel turnover rate and would be
concerned if there did not appear to be a substantial core of professionals associated with the operation for a significant period. The director's background is particularly important. Has he had experience
working with special needs children? If your child can communicate,
include him in your planning and find out if he is enthusiastic about
going. Also, consult with people who have worked with him to get feedback on the kind of camping experience they believe would be most
appropriate.

All parents will want to know what provision is made for medical
care—is there a nurse, an infirmary, a consulting doctor, an arrangement with a nearby hospital emergency room? Each parent will also
have his own particular concerns. Mary and I were especially interested
in meeting the nurse to talk about Owen's medication and seeing to it
that the counselor assigned to Owen could "sign." And, of course, we
spoke with several parents of former campers.

Costs should be a matter of concern. Does the tuition cover all expenses? Are there any extras? Some expenses may be covered by your
local school system if the system feels a structured summer experience is
necessary to maintain your child's academic progress. Our system did this.

Religion: For Some People, the Ultimate Respite

In Phippsburg, Maine, where we have a summer camp, there's a
small, nondenominational chapel. It's painted white and has a steeple
and looks just like a self-respecting chapel in Maine ought to look.
Owen rings the bell before service, and he thinks that's great. There
aren't many things he can do for others all by himself, and the bell
makes a wonderful sound. The congregation seems to get a kick out of
seeing him heaving up and down, and many smile and say hello as they
squeeze by on their way into the sanctuary. It's a good beginning for the
service.

For a person whose handicap is limited to physical functioning,
integration into the religious community doesn't present the same conceptual problem faced by those with mental limitations and is usually
concerned primarily with seeing that the church provides access in the
broadest sense of the word. But how do you evaluate the impact of spiritual life upon a disabled person who is profoundly retarded or who
can't communicate? What responsibility do parents have to provide religious instruction, or if that is not possible, at least religious exposure?

Years ago, when Owen was a baby, I approached a close friend—also our family doctor—with questions like these. I can still recall his reply: "Those are deeper waters than I dare to swim in." Today, still struggling with the same questions, I come to a similar conclusion. Theological waters are much too deep for this book to plunge into. Families must work out their own solutions based upon their view of God and His universe.

Many families, however, gain tremendous reward from their religious belief, which during crises represents the stability that holds life together, and the strength that comes from a deep faith enriches and makes meaningful the lives of many of the severely handicapped population. We always took Owen with us to church, even though he was apparently oblivious to the significance of the service. He obviously enjoyed the sounds, the colors reflecting from the stained glass windows, and the excitement of the service. For us that had to be enough, or at least we thought so. On the other hand, some mildly to moderately retarded youngsters obviously take comfort in the routine of the service, of knowing what comes next, and of being able to join with others for once on an equal footing, even if it's only rising and sitting and kneeling all together.

Religious instruction for Owen never seriously entered our minds. During the early years, when we couldn't teach him to talk or walk or even chew his food, our attention never moved from specific, concrete objectives. Perhaps we should have tried, but that is only one of the many "what ifs" that crowd our minds. There are, however, many specific concerns linking the handicapped population with the church or synagogue that don't involve matters nearly so subjective. The organized church offers other resources in addition to the spiritual, but sometimes parental initiative is required. (In this chapter the word *church* refers to any place of religious worship, and *minister* designates the church's religious leader.)

The Church as Educator

Most organized religions have become actively concerned with their disabled constituency. The Special Education Department of the Catholic Educational Association is a force in its parochial schools and publishes a special education newsletter, which includes information on resources, recent publications, and meetings. The National Catholic Office for Persons with Disabilities publishes a quarterly newsletter (including a resource section), and the National Council of the Churches of Christ, seeking better ways to serve its congregations, organized a Task Force on Developmental Disabilities. In 1982 the National Council of Churches published *Resources: Persons with Special Learning Needs*, a collection of input from congregations of many denominations from all over the country. Their purpose was to help one another better understand and welcome men and women who happen to be handicapped into their various church communities. This brochure lists books, pamphlets, audiovisual materials, newsletters, and agencies concerned with the disabled population, categorized by disability. It is annotated in understandable language and combines a comprehensive overview of what is available in current "disability literature," expanded to include material dealing specifically with religious concerns. I found it extremely helpful (see Resources: Religion).

Although the details of individual church participation are too numerous to mention, nationally, many denominations include disabled persons as participating members of the church and offer curricula and teaching methods appropriate for use in religious schools. If your congregation offers little in this area you may wish to pitch in and help promote such services. If they are not available from your own church organization, perhaps teaching materials can be adapted from those produced by other churches. Contact your minister to find out what resources are available. He could probably use your help in generating interest. Bette M. Ross devotes a section to religion in her excellent book, *Our Special Child* (see Resources: Disability: Down syndrome). She found a personal solution to the problem faced by many parents when her son was too old for Sunday School but not yet ready to join the adult congregation. A sensitive teacher suggested that he help out with the prekindergarten class, where he worked as a teacher's aide, serving juice, moving furniture, putting away blocks, etc. In time there proved to be other ways in which he could be helpful. Like Owen's ringing the bell, there are ways your child, too, can participate somewhere in your church community. Your youngster can help decorate for the youth organization's dance, pass the collection plate, or participate in some part of the service. The details of the task will vary depending upon circumstances, but the opportunities should be there.

The Church as Service Provider

For generations, religious organizations have provided services for handicapped persons. At one time they offered practically the only compassionate care available (the Catholic Church is a leading example of this commitment), and church-sponsored institutions still constitute a significant proportion of the country's independent residential facilities. Although recent deinstitutionalization policy has shifted emphasis elsewhere, these total-care residential facilities still fill a vital function in the spectrum of services. Today, many daytime centers for various handicapping conditions are also church sponsored and offer an alternative to public facilities.

The Church as Halfway House

Although one of the results of P.L. 94-142 has been mainstreaming, this integration has not been easy. The church setting can help soften this transition, for the church is naturally suited to provide a noncompetitive, nonmaterialistic, sympathetic environment in which disabled persons can be accepted as the human beings they are. The emphasis is on their humanness, not their handicap. Sunday School, youth groups, church committees, and participation in the adult congregation all offer appropriate opportunities for disabled people to learn to function in a community setting.

In small congregations with few handicapped members, the initiative to create such opportunities may have to come from you. Don't be bashful; the congregation will expect it of you as a parent. Make an appointment with your minister to discuss ways your child can become a member of the congregation in fact as well as in theory. It's important for everyone to remember that such interaction has precedence in the teachings of every religion as well as reciprocal advantages. Benefits are not limited to handicapped parishioners; the entire congregation can be expanded and enriched.

The Church as a Clearinghouse and Support System

More than most of society's organizations, the religious community is in a position to provide needed resources to its membership and to the community at large. Organizing respite care, locating appropriate employment possibilities, and providing transportation all fall within the natural consideration of a religious community, and many churches actively involve themselves in these concerns. Often all it takes to galvanize a congregation is the spark that one parent can light. The minister, because of his training and experience, should be able to act as a link with the outside community and become familiar with available sources of help.

In those inevitable moments when parents could benefit from professional counseling or a sympathetic listener, the minister can, and should, be a valuable resource. Many denominations provide formal counseling instruction for their clergy, and your minister may have had training as well as practical experience. If not, your church community could see that funds are designated to finance his instruction. Possibly no professional skill can be of more value to a congregation.

The Church as an Accessible Instrument of God

Making sure that both the physical facilities and the printed and spoken word are available to everyone in the congregation is essential. Many national organizations have responded to the problems of church barriers. The American Baptist Church offers a barrier-free facilities loan program. The Protestant Episcopal Church has created a special task force on accessibility, and the United Methodist Church publishes an *Accessibility Audit for Churches* (see Resources: Religion), which assists in identifying physical barriers and suggests specific ways they can be eliminated. (It is a comprehensive document and should be applicable to most churches.)

The fight for true accessibility can also involve Braille texts, talking books, and "readers" for the blind, and specially amplified pews and signers for the deaf. Although the nature of the adaptive equipment will depend upon the local church's circumstances, all these resources have today become part of routine efforts to make the church available to all the congregation. The important point to remember is that your church can and should make provision so that the total religious experience is denied no one.

Finally, I quote here the comments of Mrs. Charles Moser, a friend of mine, about her life with her son John, who has Down syndrome and lives at the same school as Owen in Kentucky. A deep faith in God and the supportive human resources of her church congregation have provided Mrs. Moser with the strength to persevere and to build a remarkably happy and fulfilled life for herself and her son, despite setbacks and losses that would have crippled most others. Her comments naturally reflect the sources of this strength and they are to me moving and significant.

> Soon after our move to Greensboro I joined the Starmount Presbyterian Church. The way into this particular church, unknown to me at the time, was opened by the minister in our Tennessee church, who had been a tower of strength to Charles [Mrs. Moser's husband] and me during his illness and death. In the Starmount Church I soon found a warm and caring church home—a blessing to count!
>
> On the same day that the pediatrician had given me the diagnosis for John, late in the afternoon, my minister appeared for a visit. A coincidence? No one could have told him about the shattering diagnosis, for at that time I had shared it only with my mother. Of course I poured it all out, and as he left us this gentle, caring minister prayed with my mother and me. His petition to God was that somehow good could come from what then seemed only tragedy. . . . Before I came to Greens-

boro, the Starmount Church had done some groundwork for development of a Sunday School class appropriate for young retarded children. In time I accepted the responsibility of chairing a committee to explore this project. Almost unbelievably, a new family came to the church at that time—the wife and mother was a certified special education teacher with teaching experience in another state. When approached she readily agreed to be responsible for such a class.

For several years she guided a class which reached some five to seven children from the area. The two-hour Sunday morning group was geared to their needs. Various members of the church also helped with the group. John profited greatly from this Sunday morning group activity. As a result of positive experiences in this church building, both in the weekday program as well as the Sunday morning group, the body of the Starmount Church became a very happy part of John's life—another blessing to count. . . . As an infant John was baptized in the Presbyterian Church. After our move to Greensboro many of his activities took place in the Starmount church building. This has been a happy place for him to be. He knows many people here and when he is at home, "going to our church" is anticipated with pleasure. Last summer our young associate minister said to me that he would like to talk to John, spend a little time with him when he came home for vacation and prepare him to be confirmed. This was truly a blessing to count, one I would have been reluctant to request, trying to content myself with the fact that my son had been baptized and could receive communion. In August 1982 John was received by the Session of the Starmount Church. Then he stood before the congregation and accepted the charge which the ministers had skillfully adapted for him.

As I sat in the church that Sunday morning surrounded by caring friends, I remembered vividly my prayer of years ago for guidance and for the way to be opened. My prayer now was one of thanksgiving for all the ways opened and for all the people who helped—family, friends, caring and dedicated professionals. I was reminded, too, of the earlier minister's prayer "for good to come of this"—and, indeed, much has for John and for me.

13
Nutrition and Dental Health

Nutrition

"You are what you eat" is a sobering thought for all parents. Battling your family to keep them off the junk food habit requires constant surveillance and the strength of character that permits you to turn a deaf ear to such entreaties as, "But Mom, all the parents in the absolute entire school let their kids eat Sugar-Coated Zaps for breakfast. I feel degraded." That's tough for anyone to handle, but keeping your family healthy while meeting the unusual needs of a handicapped child is tougher. It's possible, but sometimes just barely, and you have to know what you're doing. (For additional information on the subjects covered in this chapter, see Resources: Nutrition, Dental Health, and Feeding.)

Although the handicapped child has the same general need for nutrients as any other youngster, his requirements may vary depending on his individual situation, and certain physical or mental disabilities can complicate ordinarily normal processes with serious results. For example, cerebral palsy, spina bifida, failure to thrive, pica, rumination, epilepsy, Down syndrome, and Prader-Willi syndrome can each present particular nutritional complications. Any behavioral or orthopedic problem that interferes with ingestion may also require special attention (*ingest* is a word doctors use meaning "to take something into the digestive system," usually by eating or drinking). Before mealtime becomes a shambles, learn the details of your child's needs and work with the professionals so that you meet nutritional and medical requirements in ways that benefit your special child while causing as little disruption as possible for other family members.

It's easier said than done! Getting a handicapped child to eat properly can be frustrating and messy (in my personal vocabulary, eating properly means: not too little and not too much of the right foods, at the right time). Don't try to "wing it." Your health professional is your best source of information on special diets, positioning, and administering medication, and should be consulted if you get concerned.

Not surprisingly, nutrition is another area with its own language. Learn the jargon. If your child is developmentally delayed, become familiar with the sequence in which the feeding skills are normally acquired. Your youngster should follow this same progression but at a different pace. Armed with this information, you will know when your child is ready for the next stage and be able to help him move ahead by providing appropriate transition foods. Even if your child is not on a special diet, ask the doctor if he should have any food supplements; if not, remember that a healthy diet, appropriate for his age, is certainly as vital for him as for any child.

In certain instances he may recommend what's called a "feeding assessment," or that a specialist be consulted. A feeding assessment is a process, generally available only at larger medical centers, in which a team of professionals studies an individual's nutritional/eating characteristics and makes recommendations. In addition to a medical doctor, the team may include a speech therapist, an occupational therapist (often a key member), a nutritionist, and even a psychologist, since many feeding troubles have emotional implications. When might a feeding evaluation be helpful? First, don't be overly concerned if your baby specializes in getting more food outside than inside. That goes with the territory. However, if he doesn't seem to be thriving and gaining as much weight as you think he should, or has continuing problems in the mechanical process of getting food into his mouth (and keeping it there), it's a good idea to discuss your concerns with your doctor. A good book dealing with this area is *Nutrition and Feeding of Infants and Toddlers* (see Resources: Nutrition).

For a book that presents wide-ranging insights into common mealtime problems from the perspectives of parents, caregivers, and handicapped persons, I recommend *Mealtimes for Persons with Severe Handicaps* (see Resources: Nutrition).

The assessment team's plan may have included, or your doctor may have supplied, a nutritional prescription, sometimes called a "profile," setting forth all the details of your youngster's recommended diet and medication. Naturally, it will require updating from time to time as circumstances change, but it's desirable that there always be one professional familiar with the situation to whom you can turn for assistance concerning both nutritional content and feeding techniques. Using a feeding tube, central line, or Broviac for the first time can be scary, but parents do handle them successfully every day. What do you do about a child who has a cleft palate? Even the positioning techniques involved in facilitating your baby's eating or drinking may present problems. Go over the procedures often enough with your professional when he gives you the instructions that you become comfortable with each step. To reinforce you even further, certain manuals cover management techniques, including behavior modification for the youngster who refuses to eat because of an emotional problem. *Handling the Young Cerebral Palsied Child at Home*, by Nancie R. Finnie, is an excellent source and has some good practical ideas that are applicable for children with many disabilities (see Resources: Disability: Cerebral Palsy).

Unfortunately, there isn't much written in lay language that deals specifically with nutritional problems and the handicapped population. The Nutrition Division of the John F. Kennedy Institute for Handicapped Children has developed an outstanding book, *A Nutrition Handbook: Eating for Good Health for Caretakers of the Handicapped Child*. I have drawn upon it for much of the nutritional and dental information in this chapter. It is available for a modest charge from the Nutrition Division of the Kennedy Institute (see Resources: Nutrition). I recommend it to any parent whose child has an eating, nutrition, or medication problem. In down-to-earth language and with a great deal of imagination, it offers realistic and humane suggestions that will make living on a strict diet more palatable to youngsters who may not have much besides food to look forward to. There are recipes for a concoction called a "Dandy Bran Bar" (with honey and cinnamon and raisins and walnuts) if constipation is a problem and for "Super Shake," "Super Pudding," and "Peanut Butter Logs" for a kid who needs to gain weight. To the parent whose youngster is fighting obesity, the handbook cautions, "Don't let your child skip meals. This leads to high-calorie snacking. Every little nibble adds extra calories to your child's diet," and "Keep the right foods on hand & the fattening ones won't be as tempting to your child." It tells why feeding problems occur and why some foods or liquids can improve or worsen the situation. The "Drugs and Diet" section contains specific suggestions about how food selection and meal timing, when coordinated with medication, can make drug use more effective and less disagreeable—and it tells you why.

The Food Problem

Over the years, Mary and I have suffered more stress because of Owen's bizarre eating and digestive problems than for any other cause. On one of his recent visits home he and I spent four hours in the local emergency room because of his possibly impacted bowel. The prescription: three enemas and a pint of liquid laxative. Between enemas Owen managed to charm the triage nurse with his smile. (I was pleased. It's nice to give a triage nurse something to smile about.) As a child, Owen would eat only strained baby food and even today he still refuses to chew, a fact that confounds doctors, who are unable to detect any physical defect to explain it. This masticatory irregularity also pushes his digestive system, which must pick up the slack, to Herculean efforts.

Despite exhaustive investigation, we have never solved the problem, just established an uneasy truce with Owen's insides. For a while doctors thought he might suffer from "oral dyskinesia," a term that's enough to set anybody's teeth on edge, but if you know it's a defect in the mouth's ability to function properly, it's something you can deal with.

The Weight Problem

Because of the restricted nature of their activities, handicapped children can be susceptible to obesity. Unfortunately, it is sometimes the direct consequence not of their disability, but of parental overindulgence. Extreme overweight is always debilitating; it can damage self-image, increase the incidence of physical problems, and complicate the management of an ambulatory child. Fortunately, sometimes it can be controlled. Here are some potential problems to look out for:

- A parent can overfeed a child. Often sweets are involved, either as a reward to the child or as solace to the parent. Either way it's the wrong thing to do. When Owen is home and I can't think of anything else to occupy him, I buy him an ice cream cone (it makes me feel good and it's good for Owen). Owen is skinny. Obese children should skip ice cream cones.
- A disabled person often eats to combat stress. The more he eats, the heavier he gets; the heavier he gets, the more stress is created; and so on.
- Some illnesses are characterized by low basal metabolic rates (the speed at which we burn up energy); as a result, the body needs less food than normal.
- Normal appetite regulation can go haywire. In Prader-Willi syndrome, overeating is due to hyperphagia (abnormally increased appetite) and absence of the reflex that tells us when we are full.
- Some disabilities, like spina bifida and spastic cerebral palsy, limit mobility. As a result, calories aren't burned off. Some conditions, such as Down syndrome, result in a below-normal body size, reducing the child's food-intake requirement. Unfortunately, appetite often exceeds need, and again calories are stored as fat, often in unsightly places. Not only is mobility reduced but skin rashes develop and braces become more difficult to fit for the orthopedically impaired youngster.

Correcting the problem is difficult for both parent and child. Appropriate daily caloric intake (energy needs, not wants) should be determined not by RDAs (recommended dietary allowances), which are based solely on chronological age, but on an individualized basis and by a physician. Ask your doctor for guidance, and then help your child work gradually toward his recommended weight. Perhaps you should come up with a target weight for yourself at the same time and compete pound for pound right alongside your youngster. He might get a kick out of it. The general guidelines for dieting used by the nonhandicapped population can ordinarily be followed, but check with your doctor before beginning any weight-shedding program. Since snack times are apt to be bright spots in the day of a disabled child and can be medically necessary, continue them; your child can still lose weight by reducing the size of his three regular meals and by replacing typically high-calorie, low-nutrient snacks with healthier ingredients.

In conjunction with reduced calorie intake, a regular exercise program will lop off excess weight, improve the digestive process, and, when properly supervised by your child's doctor or physical therapist, offer many other health and recreational benefits. The scope of the program is, of course, determined by the nature of the disability. Preoccupied with other worries, a parent easily forgets that most handicapped people can enjoy and benefit from exercise just as much as you or I. *Routine* is the key word. While your child lives at home or if he moves into some kind of independent housing situation, regular physical activity can be neglected if you don't provide supervision and reinforcement. Later, when your youngster is in school, insist he takes part in a physical education program adapted to meet his special needs (called APE). An APE is his right under the law.

Although I was late in realizing how much exercise can mean to a handicapped person, I eventually began to schedule long walks with Owen whenever he was home on vacation. Even today we two make quite a show when we take our morning constitutional. On the way out—striding toward the ocean—he refuses to walk by my side but hangs back, shadowing me by a fixed interval that never varies. If I speed up or change course, so does he. We travel on with the regularity of a precision drill team, despite the distraction of rain, cold, or sociable neighborhood dogs. At least we do until we reach the beach and turn to head for home. Suddenly Owen comes to life and, shifting his loping gait into overdrive and looking back over his shoulder at me as he passes, he smiles and heads for the house and his afternoon snack. Our neighbors take a keen interest in all this, and look forward to the daily event.

Like my son, some disabled people need encouragement to exercise, until they have their momentum going. Some seem to prefer sitting to walking, but don't let them get away with it! I try to plan our excursions so as not to conflict with Owen's relatively few other enjoyable activities. Your doctor can give you instructions for an ongoing program, but it's up to you to make sure that it takes place on a regular basis. Daily exercises required for orthopedic purposes can burn calories and have beneficial side effects in addition to their primary therapeutic purposes.

The Other Side of the Coin: The Underweight Problem

A developmentally disabled child can be underweight for many reasons. (His ideal weight should be calculated and a doctor consulted before any weight-gain program is initiated.) The youngster may have poor motor coordination, with a resulting excessive spillage of food. The food he eventually does get inside may not meet his nutritional requirements, or he may reject other needed food because of bizarre preferences or behavioral problems. Vomiting, diarrhea, or poor absorption may limit actual net intake, and a high level of activity can burn up energy faster than it's being replaced, as is the case with the involuntary movements characteristic of athetoid cerebral palsy. All you have to do to appreciate what this means is to watch these youngsters for a while as they maneuver about in their daily activities.

Owen is a picky eater with unusual food preferences and is chronically underweight despite ice cream cones. We take advantage of his all-consuming love of applesauce and use it as a reward for the successful conclusion of a meal—its crowning glory. This may seem like bribery. Call it what you will; Mary and I are only human and describe it to friends as "positive reinforcement." In our defense, I say try persuading a 28-year-old man to eat something he would rather not. You can use other strategies to put weight on your youngster. For a child with a poor appetite, snacks combined with a milkshake at bedtime can do wonders, but distribute the snacks throughout the day so as not to interfere with regular meals. You can transform these nutritional necessities into social events, something pleasant during the day both of you can count on and look forward to.

Constipation

Many developmental disabilities can also trigger digestive problems. Constipation—Owen's constant companion for years—can be caused by many factors: lack of mobility, hypotonia (reduced muscle tone), insufficient fluid or fiber in the diet, the use of certain drugs (Valium and Thorazine, for example), and Hirschsprung's disease (dilation of the colon). When we first heard Hirschsprung's disease described we thought, "Eureka! At last we have the answer to at least one of Owen's problems, and we will do something about it, pronto." But our excitement died when testing indicated that this latest possibility proved just one more in a legion of false leads.

Like all food-related problems, constipation doesn't have any easy remedies, particularly for a child who is set in his ways. Plenty of fluids, particularly water and juices, should help, and fruits and vegetables, cooked or fresh, have a high fiber content if their skins are not removed, and should be included in the daily diet. Appropriate regular physical activity is again recommended to encourage natural regularity, but despite our walks Owen's condition is so severe that he must rely on daily laxatives and weekly enemas. Protracted dependence upon such artificial stimulation, however, is not ordinarily recommended, since it tends to curtail normal functioning and become habitual.

Dehydration (or Fluid Imbalance)

Many disabled children are particularly susceptible to rapid dehydration, which, if extreme, can be fatal. Therefore, children with the following conditions should be carefully monitored: those with cerebral palsy, particularly when oral malfunction is involved; slow eaters and ruminators (those who regurgitate and chew previously swallowed food); those with spina bifida, who may also have a susceptibility to urinary tract infection; children taking certain types of medication that might result in nausea or a loss of appetite; youngsters with failure to thrive, who often refuse food or are what I would call "picky eaters"; Down syndrome patients, who may experience difficulty swallowing and have dry mouths; children who drool excessively or who are on certain types of tube feedings; and those with prolonged or high fever or diarrhea.

Some common signs of dehydration are a decrease in urine output, dry mucous membranes (particularly around the mouth), and loss of skin elasticity. Ask your doctor how to judge this. One word of caution: younger children are more susceptible to dehydration and should be watched closely. If you become concerned, get medical advice without delay.

Vitamins

Your doctor may prescribe vitamins or minerals as a dietary supplement. Treat this like any other medical prescription and follow directions carefully. It does not follow that if ten vitamin pills are good, twenty are twice as effective and one hundred will cure everything under the sun. Just the reverse can be the case, and a dosage of vitamins in excess of normal daily requirements should be taken only under a physician's specific directions. For example, under certain circumstances, large doses of vitamin A, vitamin D, and iron have particularly serious adverse effects. From time to time, vitamin-centered programs receive national publicity promising remarkable curative properties, and supporters suggest special diets that supposedly correct such diverse problems as hyperactivity and learning disabilities. (One such approach recommends the elimination of certain food additives and colorings as well as natural salicylates used in some food flavorings and in the production of aspirin.) Consult your doctor before becoming involved in any special dietary or vitamin program, particularly one that seems to be too good to be true—it probably is. His diet is too central to everything your child is or hopes to become to be dramatically adjusted without careful evaluation of possible consequences. Finally, as discussed earlier, remember that if drug use is required as the result of a physician's prescription, find out what effects its use may have on your child's nutritional needs or eating habits.

The Family's Diet

When one family member has unusual eating habits or requires a special diet, everyone in the group is usually affected in one way or another. Here are suggestions drawn from our experience of sitting for cumulative thousands of hours around the dining room table with Owen:

1. Maintain family eating routines whenever possible. Since dinnertime is apt to be busy, prepare some meals in advance and freeze them for more convenient future use. All your children can help out, particularly your special child, who should participate in whatever ways he can to learn skills or to feel he is contributing to the family group. Ask both boys and girls to set the table and to help with food preparation. Too often girls get stuck with the dishes while the boys play football. Mary has a sign above the refrigerator door that proclaims in bold print, "This is an equal opportunity kitchen," and Mary's good about giving everybody an "opportunity." The kids may say they haven't time. Get rid of your TV.

2. Schedule time so that the usual frantic pace slows a bit before the evening meal. This may be asking too much, but how about declaring a half-hour moratorium on ray guns and trench warfare or asking your spouse to read aloud to the kids while you are making final meal preparations?

3. Continue to work on improving your handicapped child's eating habits if they are really "off the wall." It can be a temptation to feed him at a separate time, in isolation, but don't give up without a struggle. He must master basic eating skills if he's going to live independently, although in the interim period, the wear and tear on the family

psyche can become severe. Mary still works on Owen's table manners, which Owen's siblings describe as "gross," and although the situation has improved somewhat, the chair opposite him is still no seat of honor. We usually place a sensitive guest far away—down the table and out of the line of sight. Your doctor or social worker should have suggestions for helpful management and behavior modification techniques, and there are many imaginative mechanical devices designed to help the physically handicapped cope with dinner-table problems, as well as companies that specialize in such equipment (see Resources: Suppliers).

4. During periods of crisis, when good nutrition is particularly important (and Mom may be at the hospital), it's easy for junk food to creep in. Try to continue regular sit-down meals. Involve neighbors or relatives, if necessary, to help out temporarily. Resist the temptation to use healthy food as punishment or unhealthy food as a reward, and bear in mind that, for better or worse, parents will be role models for their children in the way they demonstrate their own food habits around the kitchen table.

5. Food preparation and expense can be problems, but expert advice is available. A dietitian can suggest techniques for buying nutritious food at less cost as well as ways a special diet can be coordinated with other food preparation to save time and money. With careful planning, everyone does not need to be on the same menu. The following organizations often offer nutrition assistance (however, to qualify you may have to meet federal or state income guidelines):

- Your local community action program. It goes under different names but is usually listed in the phone book's Community Services pages under a heading like "Family Services and Counseling."
- Your nearest cooperative extension service, through its EFNP program (Expanded Food and Nutrition Program). This service should be particularly helpful in rural areas and may not require income qualification. The County Extension Agent or your land grant university should be able to help you locate it.
- The Food Stamp program (look in the phone book's Community Services section under "Food").
- Your area's Head Start program. Current law requires that at least 10 percent of Head Start's student population be handicapped, and a consulting nutritionist be available. The local school superintendent should know the location of the nearest program.
- A nearby public residential institution (state or federal), particularly one dealing with handicapped clients. Although it is ordinarily not his responsibility to provide such advisory service, the

staff dietitian may be good-natured and willing to help or to suggest local sources of assistance.
- The Women, Infants and Children (WIC) program, a special supplemental activity that under certain circumstances provides nutritious foods and education and information about health services locally available.

Check with your local community action people or the United Way office for information about the location of the organizations mentioned as well as about descriptive brochures, if they are available.

If none of these organizations provides individual nutritional consultation, professional dietitians are available in most cities, but they charge for their services. If your child is hospitalized, even on an outpatient or intermittent basis, the staff dietitian may be willing to provide information and advice on nutritional matters. One did for us. Don't underestimate the importance that good nutrition and an emotionally upbeat and regulated mealtime environment have on your family. Unfortunately, during times of crisis, good food habits are apt to suffer.

Dental Health

What happens inside the mouth affects an individual, handicapped or not, in many ways. Teeth missing or badly positioned (as is sometimes the case with children with cleft palate) can contribute to unsatisfactory speech patterns. A toothache or a chronically sensitive mouth can affect appetite or food preference, and if the child can't tell you what is wrong, it may be months before you find out for yourself. Unfortunately, many handicapped children are particularly susceptible to the two major diseases of the mouth caused by plaque: gum disease (gingivitis) and dental decay (called "caries" or just plain cavities). As a consequence of poor dental hygiene, gums may become infected and bleed, and an unpleasant odor result, adding one more hurdle to social acceptability. Worst of all, teeth are often lost. (Surprisingly, diseased gums cause more tooth loss in the adult population than do cavities.) Fortunately, dental disease is largely controllable, if you have the tenacity. On the other hand, the availability of adequate dental treatment is a primary concern for those who deal with the disabled population, and our experience with Owen's chronic dental problems indicates that their concern is justified.

Dental health is primarily a case of keeping the mouth and gums clean, although proper diet and fluoride use are also important. That same permissive parent, however, who tolerates obesity in his youngster also encourages dental problems when he offers a candy bar as a bribe or instead of an apple for dessert. And children with multiple food dislikes often prefer trouble-causing sweets (but then, what youngster doesn't?). Problems can even arise when a baby is allowed to take his bottle of juice or milk to bed with him, for if he falls asleep with the nipple in his mouth, a pool of sugary solution may surround his teeth and accelerate tooth decay. Good dental health is a result of parental vigilance and supervision.

Although snack time may be an important ingredient in your child's overall health plan, inappropriate snacking will cause tooth decay. The answer is not to eliminate snacks but to control their content, so as to retain the desired nutritional value and still promote dental health. Foods with high cariogenic (decay-causing) potential, such as raisins and ice cream, are better served at regular mealtime, when the other foods and liquids eaten at the same time will help remove the objectionable material from the teeth. Many foods appropriate for a snack menu taste good, offer required nutrients, and still are compatible with special diets for weight gain or reduction and increased fiber or fluid intake. Among them are juice, hard-boiled eggs, meats, cheese, vegetables, fresh fruits, nuts, plain yogurt, and plain milk. They also can be used as so-called finger foods to help the child gain independent feeding skills.

The same good oral hygiene that you practice with your other children applies to your handicapped child. Be particularly alert with infants and young children, since initiating good habits for the future is vital. Consult your dentist for details of fluoride use. Schedule regular checkups. Brushing after every meal, daily flossing, and control of sugar intake are recommended but sometimes are impossible (they are for us—just the thought of getting Owen to brush after every meal makes me blanch). Do the best you can, but never ignore your child's dental health in the expectation that it will take care of itself. We all have seen too many handicapped folks with unforgivably neglected teeth. The primary tragedy, of course, is the pain and discomfort involved, but a secondary consequence is that it reinforces the sometimes unfortunate stereotype many people still have of the severely disabled person.

A special child's teeth may be normal, but the problems involved in keeping them clean and healthy are not, since many of these youngsters, like Owen, have coordination or behavioral problems that make toothbrushing or flossing a hit-or-miss operation. Mary and I must still do the job if we want it done well. At brushing time Owen approaches his teeth gingerly, but with interest, as though he is inspecting them for the first time and is a bit surprised to find them there at all. As a result, unsupervised, he doesn't do a thorough job and is often subject to bleeding gums and bad breath—a source of embarrassment and dismay to his siblings. Furthermore, some handicapping conditions require special approaches to oral hygiene. Research has been done and material written that may be of help—for example, *Dental Health in Children with Phenylketonuria (PKU)* (see Resources: Nutrition).

We have found that one of the problems with institutional life, even when the staff is conscientious, is that some personal hygiene matters are not always closely monitored. Therefore, parents must check their youngster's teeth and gums on every home visit and stay on top of the situation with the caregivers. Our solution was to ask that a dental hygienist located near the institution clean Owen's teeth every month or so at our expense. We also try to schedule an appointment with our family dentist during Owen's vacation periods for a thorough checkup.

Your dentist may have home-management suggestions and, if he prefers not to treat your child himself, should be able to refer you to a colleague who specializes in children's dentistry (a pedodontist) or the care of the handicapped. If you have trouble, ask other parents in your local support group for suggestions. Another information source is the American Dental Association, which has affiliates in every state, some of which have listings of dentists with wheelchair-accessible offices who serve the specialized needs of handicapped patients. A local dentist or your area hospital should be able to get the name and address of your state association.

Every parent should learn enough of the details of dental hygiene to protect his child from being saddled with one more unnecessary problem. Ignorance is no excuse and is particularly insidious, since by the time symptoms become obvious, serious and irreversible damage may have already been done. Information is available that is clear and specific. One helpful article is "Day to Day Dental Care" (see Resources: Nutrition, Dental Health, and Feeding). If it's not in your local library, ask for a copy through the interlibrary loan program. Another resource is a publication of the National Easter Seal Society: *Helping Persons with Handicaps Clean Their Teeth*, by Arthur J. Nowak, D.M.D. In another booket, *Toothbrushing and Flossing* by Paul Casamassimo, also published by Easter Seals but now out of print, I was surprised to learn that: "Teeth should be cleaned well at least one time per day, preferably right before bedtime. Toothpaste isn't necessary and may in fact hinder efforts to clean teeth due to excessive foaming and salivation. Remember, it is the brush that takes off the plaque, not the toothpaste. A soft brush is less traumatic to the gums and better than a hard-bristled brush at getting to the difficult areas in the mouth. Proper diet and home fluoride therapy can help control plaque. Ask your dentist."

One fact of life evident in both nutritional and dental good health is that parental action—supervision and monitoring—is a prerequisite. Professionals can give you advice and furnish information, but their effectiveness is blunted if you are apathetic. In the final analysis, they aren't going to be able to bail you out. In almost all instances your child's nutritional and dental condition will be as good as you insist it be or as bad as you allow it to become. It will be a reflection not only of your actions and inactions but also of yourself.

14
Safety in the Home

Although handicapped children are vulnerable to the same kinds of accidents as the nonhandicapped, all major disabilities involve limitations that restrict the ability to sense or escape from danger. How safe would you be or feel if you couldn't hear the alarm, read the poison label, smell the smoke, understand evacuation instructions, descend the stairs, call for help, or feel the pain? (Think about this the next time you're impatient with your child if he seems timid or afraid.) These special exposures mean that safety must be a high priority for all of us who are responsible, in any way, for handicapped people. This chapter considers home-related exposures: fire, lost child, safe housekeeping, poison and toxic substances, unsafe playthings, household furnishings, and automobiles. Chapter 21 addresses hazards and risk taking in the outside world.

A Safety Plan

As a first step in developing an accident-prevention program for the home, contact local agencies interested in safety and explain your general situation and concerns. Visit them personally if possible. Request any information they have that deals with safety and ask what resources they offer that might meet your needs. The American Red Cross and your local fire and police departments are natural starting points. Although their information is geared to the general population, you will find that much either is directly applicable or can be adapted to fit your specialized situation. Your visit can be worthwhile for two reasons: it introduces you to people in your community whom you should know—and who should know you—and the resulting conversations may point out safety considerations you might otherwise overlook. With the exception of information on fire safety, I have discovered little material designed specifically for handicapped people, but contact your local department of human services, bureau of mental retardation, or the Association of Retarded Citizens (ARC) to see if anything new is on the market. (Compiling such a manual would make a real contribution to the handicapped population and be a natural project for a parents' support group.)

The U.S. Consumer Product Safety Commission is a useful source of wide-ranging information. For example, it publishes *Buyer's Guide: The Safe Nursery* (a booklet designed to avoid injuries from playroom and nursery furniture and equipment) and a *Home Safety Checklist for Older Consumers*. (In many areas of exposure, safety literature for the elderly is also applicable to the disabled [see Resources: Safety].) Be particularly sensitive to the dangers posed by electrical outlets and wires, stairs, swimming pools, and abandoned refrigerators. The agency also offers a hotline to help answer your questions involving product safety.

Becoming familiar with general safety practices is a beginning, but before these suggestions can be truly helpful, they must be adapted to your own circumstances. Think through, or, better still, record in your notebook the physical and environmental limitations that make your child vulnerable to accident. Such an individualized "safety profile" will help crystallize your thinking and save time later when you meet with resource people to discuss accident prevention. (You may want to include it as part of the profile described in Appendix A.) For example, a nearby lake or river presents a problem to a blind child; fire safety requires another set of precautions for parents of a nonambulatory youngster. When adapting your home for the pleasure and convenience of a handicapped individual, don't forget to make it a safer home. As you speak with experts and study material, begin a list of potential hazards and ways to limit your child's vulnerabilities. You will need it later (see Resources: Adaptive Housing).

Special Vulnerabilities

Traffic Hazards

You need to pay attention to the danger that lies in wait on the highway right outside your front door. Unfortunately, the precautions you can take are limited. Families with children who really can't be expected to look out for themselves or to learn basic concepts of pedestrian highway safety may want to have warning signs posted in both lanes approaching their houses. Yellow signs reading something like "DRIVE SLOW, HANDICAPPED CHILD" can sometimes be installed. Since the responsibility for posting such signs varies from location to location, I suggest you contact the local police for information. They may refer you to a town, county, or state highway department, depending upon who is responsible for the roadway. Other approaches to the problem are to install gates that isolate parts of the house from access to the street, to install locks on outside gates, or even to fence your yard. One of my first chores in every one of our many homes was to install a snow fence enclosure for Owen that was especially designed to confound his remarkable mechanical ability to unlatch even the most ingeniously constructed gate. Show your friends and neighbors how to get in and out, and be sure that they lock up after a visit—if they can figure it out. If your problem is acute, consider discussing the possibility of behavior modification with your doctor.

Around the Home

Poisons and toxic substances pose a special threat to some people with disabilities. Get the number of the nearest poison control center from your local hospital's emergency room and post it. (Ask your doctor about the advisability of having ipecac available in your medical cabinet, to be used, of course, only under medical direction.) Phone and ask for any brochures or checklists dealing with home safety (many are available), and learn what kinds of products are dangerous. You may be surprised, for even such innocent things as plants and flowers can be toxic and have serious consequences if eaten. If you find the idea of a child eating a poinsettia leaf or chips of paint ridiculous, it's just as well you're reading this book; remember that one of the ways a youngster learns about the environment is by popping all kinds of things into his mouth and that pica, a condition that causes a craving for unlikely food, has been blamed for cases of lead poisoning.

Locate all potentially dangerous substances in your house and either safeguard or replace them with nontoxic substitutes. In particular, check areas under sinks and in the cellar and garage, and watch for such products as antifreeze, drain cleaners, and garden sprays. Paint and plaster containing lead can cause brain damage if ingested, and even if your house has been recently painted, old lead paint and plaster underneath can flake off. The local health department can give you advice about lead paint if you are concerned.

Make a tour of your house, looking at everything with safety in mind. Be aware of dangerous objects that can be pulled over on top of a toddler who is reaching up for support—a tablecloth or a hot pan on the stove. Although much can be done to child-proof your home, it all can come to naught if you don't ensure continued and competent supervision. "Who's minding the baby?" is, to me, the most important consideration in safeguarding the disabled child.

Toys and play-related equipment can be dangerous if not properly controlled. Easter Seals has produced an excellent pamphlet dealing with this subject—*Playing It Safe: A Safety Checklist of Children's Toys* (currently out of print). It suggests purchasing fabric products that are flame retardant/flame resistant, stuffed dolls and animals that are labeled "washable/hygienic materials," and only those painted toys that are labeled "nontoxic." It stresses the danger of small toys, pieces of puzzles, or tiny parts that might be swallowed, and warns that ropes or plastic bags can cause strangling or suffocation. This pamphlet makes a real contribution to safety; if enough parents request it, perhaps it will be reprinted. It's too valuable to waste. The *Directory of Living Aids for the Disabled Person* (see Resources: Directories) is another excellent resource that lists devices that assist the handicapped in their daily life and includes the suppliers' names and addresses. For example, one of the many safety items listed is a SAF-T-STRAINT: "Made to hold a person back in an auto seat when a seatbelt is not adequate."

Concern for safety, however, shouldn't be limited to your home or automobile, since your child may spend many hours away from home at day care or a similar activity that involves new exposures—some actually created by your absence. For example, if your child has any condition that might require immediate action on the part of staff, they must know about it. Give them the name of the doctor you want contacted in an emergency as well as your daytime phone number and, if your child's condition warrants such concern, the name of the ambulance service to call. Find out if any staff members have had basic first aid training, including familiarity with the Heimlich maneuver and cardiopulmonary resuscitation. If your child is motor-disabled, you may want to offer teachers guidance about limitations that should be imposed on his activities and interactions with other youngsters, but remember that a certain amount of calculated risk taking may be necessary if your child is going to learn to live in a normal environment.

The Lost Child

Most parents remember that awful sinking feeling that came over them when, in the middle of a crowd, they looked down and found that the child who just a moment ago was by their side has vanished. It's a basic and frightening experience, particularly for handicapped children and their parents. Because Owen is incapable of independent action and unable to communicate in any way, fear that he might get lost is almost an obsession in our family. One of our reactions was to buy a shiny bracelet inscribed, "My name is Owen. I can neither talk nor understand. Please call my parents" (our name and telephone number followed). The message had to be short and snappy because of space limitations, but it got the job done. (If only he wouldn't keep losing the bracelet!) At many pharmacies you can buy bracelets already inscribed with information geared to particular medical conditions, or you can get one uninscribed and have it engraved to your own specifications by a local jeweler. The Medic Alert Foundation (see Resources: Safety), a charitable nonprofit foundation, maintains a central file of vital medical information on all its members. For a modest fee (currently in the $15 to $48 range), each subscriber is provided with a bracelet or necklace engraved with a brief description of his medical problem and file number as well as the telephone number of Medic Alert's information center. Doctors, police, or anyone who may be called upon to provide assistance can obtain vital information immediately over the phone.

Finally, if your child can undo locks and specializes in unauthorized and unsafe nocturnal walks, try attaching one of those buzzers to your door that stores use to indicate approaching or departing customers.

Now that Owen is older and often travels alone by air, we always slip a note in his pocket that explains our son and gives additional critical information. During our many years of experience, the airlines have been compassionately accommodating, and we have encountered no disasters despite our original uneasiness. Actually, Owen loves to fly; it may be the tidal wave of sensation that gets to him. And the staff generally welcome him with open arms. I escort him onto the aircraft ahead of the regular passengers to introduce him to the crew and to make sure, if there is an interim stop, that he doesn't deplane by mistake and get left in Bismarck, North Dakota. On the other hand, he's always the last passenger off and I have to wait alone by the gate, well after everyone else has left except the security guards and their X-ray machines. But once I'm sure he made his connections, the plane has landed safely, and everything is all right, I relax and look forward to seeing him. It's quite a show. Eventually he comes bursting out of the exit gate, always with a broad smile on his face and usually with airline wings and a big identification badge on his lapel. Often he's looking left and right, locked in what appears to be animated conversation—none of which he understands—marching in the middle of the plane's crew with an arm around one of the pilots or, better still, a stewardess. Owen loves to fly.

Sometimes, since Owen always flies home for Christmas, winter travel presents problems. I particularly remember a conversation concerning my homeward-bound son I had one December afternoon with the passenger agent in Cincinnati, Ohio. The weather was awful over much of the country. Owen had just missed the last connecting flight of the day to Maine, and drifting snow was about to close the Cincinnati field. Apparently, as we talked things over, the agent was just beginning to realize what he had on his hands, and desperation began to creep into his voice as the possible alternatives of getting Owen out of Cincinnati were eliminated one by one. I began to notice that the quality of my voice was changing, too. But the story had a happy ending when Owen was finally bundled onto a flight to Boston, and I drove off into the blizzard to pick him up four hours later at Logan Airport, where he sat waiting in the airline baggage room smiling and keeping track of the baggage conveyor as it went round and round.

On the other hand, our relationship with the airlines hasn't been completely one-sided; it has had instructional value for them as well, and I take satisfaction from the fact that, largely because of Owen, almost every flight attendant on Delta Airlines knows the American Sign Language for "When do we eat?" and "Will you please direct me to the men's room quickly."

Fire Safety

The fire-safety precautions you'll have to take depend upon your child's age and handicaps.[1] Certain general approaches, however, can apply to all: First, become familiar with the generally accepted lessons of good fire-safety practice. Next, adapt the general rules to your child's particular limitations and plan the specific steps necessary to reduce risk. Finally, take the steps necessary to put your own plan into action, including acquiring necessary equipment, initiating regular drills, and testing the alarm devices.

To get advice, contact your local fire department and/or your insurance carrier. Because of your circumstances, they ought to be able to make arrangements for an expert (a "safety engineer") to inspect your home, discuss and perhaps meet your handicapped child, and make suggestions. The expert's recommendations may involve specific actions, such as rearranging sleeping arrangements, adding smoke alarms, or making physical changes to the house. Try to get a complete written "safety inventory" from your insurance carrier that evaluates not just fire but all aspects of safety on your premises. If you want additional information, many national organizations will send you materials, usually free of charge. However, practices change with time and are replaced by new techniques. So update information periodically,

---

1. Some of the information in this section was derived from the following magazine articles: "Fire, An Alarming Situation," by Ronny J. Coleman, in *Accent on Living* (Summer 1984); "Fire Safety and Disabled Persons," by Bernard M. Levin and Harold E. Nelson, in *Fire Journal* (September 1981); "Fire Safety Programs for Handicapped Citizens, The Los Angeles Story," by Ed Reed, in *The International Fire Chief* (1980); and "Fire Safety Programs for Handicapped Persons, The Las Vegas Story," by Fred Jameson, in *The International Fire Chief* (June 1980).

and check with your local experts regularly, particularly if you plan to purchase specialized safety equipment.

Developing a specific plan from the advice and information you have gathered should be your next step. Here are several suggestions, covering a wide range of disabilities, ages, and conditions, for you to apply in whatever way is appropriate to your circumstances. We don't follow all these routines in our own family, but we should.

1. If your child has a mobility problem, try to locate him on the ground floor, but wherever he sleeps, draw up a bedroom escape plan that is posted and practiced by the entire family in regular home fire drills at least twice a year. Hold one drill in the dark. But remember that a fire drill is just a test, so don't get carried away and run the risk of hurting someone or catching pneumonia yourself. Unless the bedroom has an exit directly to the outside, alternate escape routes should be identified. Sleeping with bedroom doors shut will retard dangerous hot gases and smoke if there is a fire. Be sure that all house and bedroom doors open outward to make it easier to exit (existing doors can be converted by reversing the hinges). Since power occasionally fails in a fire, a flashlight should be available at each bedside. Mary has always stored a number of short, stubby candles and matches at various strategic locations throughout the house so that the family can function and she can see her way to Owen in the event of a power failure. (Depending upon your child's motor ability and creativeness, matches should be safeguarded.) The passage between your bedroom and your child's room, the stairway, and all exit routes should be kept free of litter and furniture barriers that can cause falls and in the dark might delay escape. A whistle by the bedside of a handicapped older child or adult can attract attention and be heard above a high background noise level.

2. Notify the fire department, describing the limitations of the disabled person, including his room location. Place a special fire rescue sticker, often available from the fire department or the division of public safety, in his bedroom window. If he ever must be left alone, and can operate a phone, locate one by his bed, with the fire or community emergency number attached (written in Braille for the visually impaired). A touch-tone phone or automatic dialer can be helpful. If your child is hearing impaired and has a TTY (teletypewriter), encourage your local fire department to obtain compatible equipment. Ask the area phone company for details.

3. Warning devices that can be "heard" by the handicapped child should be installed in the home in approved locations. Although the normal signal on a conventional smoke alarm is not adequate for many hearing-impaired persons, it's possible to hook two alarms together

and intensify the sound. Emergency warning devices for the sensory impaired are available to augment the usual auditory signal: fire alarms and smoke detectors that activate strobe lights, vibrators (sometimes attached to the bed), and variable-intensity fans or high-intensity flashing lights. (Note that strobe lights that flash more frequently than five times per second have been suspected of triggering seizures in certain susceptible people. Such an episode apparently took place at a dance we attended at Owen's residential school. My only memory is of the seizure victim lying on the gymnasium floor held tight in the arms of a friend while someone went running for the doctor.)

Alarm systems are now being developed that hook directly to the telephone. They are typical of a new technology called ARRAS (Automatic Residential Remote Alarm Systems). Some contain a microprocessor, so that a prerecorded message, triggered by the alarm, can be sent to the fire department, the police, or a health organization in medical emergencies. In some instances, the fire department can record the message for you so that all the information needed is included. An outdoor audiovisual alarm system that warns neighbors of an emergency is also available. For information on such warning equipment, contact the Department of Professional Programs and Services, Alexander Graham Bell Association for the Deaf, Inc. (see Resources: Associations).

4. Mechanical lifesaving devices can be installed to help evacuate the physically disabled person. For the disabled nonambulatory person who must live in a multistoried residence, a tubelike mechanism made of a special elastic material is available. The person escaping can regulate his speed by extending his elbows out against the tube's sides while firefighters at ground level also help control the rate of descent. A much more common installation, the automatic sprinkler system, once almost exclusively limited to public facilities because of prohibitive cost, is now a realistic possibility for private residences, and with the availability of thermoplastic pipe, existing homes can be retrofitted. (For suppliers of safety products, see Resources: Safety; Suppliers and Catalogs.)

5. Designate a safe place outside where all family members are to meet for a roll call. Notify the fire department if someone is still inside, but never go back into a burning building! Instruct all family members on how to report a fire, according to advice from the local fire department, and locate the nearest call box, if one is available in your neighborhood.

6. Smoke and toxic gases may be even more deadly than the flames themselves, so before you open a window, make sure the room's door is closed; otherwise, fumes and intense heat may be sucked into the room. If you can, keep your body low and take short breaths through

your nose. For a nonambulatory person, a small portable oxygen container should be considered, but ask your local safety expert if any special fire precautions need to be taken.

7. Be sure that your babysitter is trained in general child supervision and safety techniques in particular and that he is familiar with your home. It is important that you review fire safety with him, including evacuation procedures. Take nothing for granted; you can't expect an 80-pound teenager to get a 150-pound nonambulatory person out of the house without some training. The National Fire Protection Association (NFPA) publishes an annual catalog of fire-safety products and services (see Resources: Safety). The NFPA also offers fire-safety programs for mentally retarded adults who live in community residential settings. The program may be of interest to you as a model if you are associated in any way with an institution or a group home.

If your child is institutionalized, local and state fire regulations will require that the institution comply with a specific fire code. Discuss safety procedures with staff to learn about their fire-safety program and to see how the code is implemented, particularly in terms of your child's residence. They should respect you for your concern about an important area and be pleased that all their efforts are understood and appreciated.

One concluding note on safety. Translate theory into action by taking your safety list (which I hope you began when we first considered safety and the "lost child" and that has ended now with thoughts about the dangers of fire) and make another survey of your house. Note all the items covered and evaluate your state of readiness—because it's up to you to wage a war against accidents. While you're at it, mark your calendar for a repeat survey next year. On the other hand, keep in mind that despite all your precautions, the very best defense against tragedy is continuing and competent supervision of your child.

15
Financial Resources

Making the Most of Available Financial Resources

Financial concerns will always play an important role in your family life.[1] For many of us, money first becomes a concern when we struggle to pay the first hospital bill and lingers on in varying degrees all our lives. For some it will control their lives. It represents an additional pressure that those not directly involved, including the caregivers, may minimize or overlook—automatically believing that such costs are taken care of by "insurance," the government, the union, or other third-party payers. There is no easy, enduring solution to financial help you may need: everything, from an electric wheelchair from the Muscular Dystrophy Association of America, the salary of your respite worker, or the rent for a supervised apartment, can be expensive if you must foot the bill. Although no one solution can address all financial problems, some general suggestions may help you avoid pitfalls and maximize resources. Pay attention to details, don't be embarrassed to seek help, be a creative initiator, and cast your net far and wide. (Sufficient help rarely is available from one source.)

In the process, as you write letters, hold phone conversations, and attend meetings, you enter the turf of the bureaucrat. Again, I urge you to think through what you plan to say before making contact, using notes if necessary. Confirm all important phone calls with a letter. Speak concisely (recording results of the communication for future reference) and pursue all alternatives, but do so in a courteous, thoughtful fashion. Effective communication is particularly important when seeking resources that may profoundly affect your family's future.

Don't respond in kind if the person on the other end of the phone is abrupt or impolite. Sometimes state agencies have surprising flexibility, and if you are friendly and persuasive, if you can establish a personal

---

1. *The Pocket Guide to Federal Help for Individuals with Disabilities*, Publication No. E-87-22002, produced by the Clearinghouse on Disability Information, Office of Special Education, is an excellent source of information (it has a section on financial assistance), but be sure you get the most recent issue.

relationship, you may convert a negative answer to a "Well, let's see what we can do" response. Finally, don't necessarily accept no as the final answer or take it personally if you're turned down. Policies and people change, and you may have another chance. Don't ruin an economic opportunity for ego satisfaction.

You Are the First Source of Support

In trying to make ends meet, first examine your own financial situation. Is your family prudent about money matters? I am not suggesting that you should live a life of penury, only that it's to your advantage and of importance to those from whom you seek support that you know where you stand and are able to demonstrate that you have made the most of your financial resources (frequently, financial assistance is predicated on *demonstrated* financial need). Some families find it helpful to construct a budget, while others utilize professional counseling assistance (available in most major cities) to get their financial house in order. Once again, *Home Care for the Chronically Ill or Disabled Child*, by Monica Loose Jones (see Resources: Guides), is a first-rate comprehensive manual. Chapters 16 and 17 of that book offer specific advice on the mechanics of getting help and on helping yourself. Also check with your local support group for ways to economize safely on drugs and medical supplies (drugs can be purchased through some national organizations and some dressings can be homemade—ask your doctor).

The Internal Revenue Service

All parents should be familiar with income-tax procedures. Every legitimate exemption taken, and every dollar of income deducted, is money saved to support your child. Learn how to complete both federal and state tax returns, know whether separate filing is necessary for your child and which tax form is best suited to your interests. (If you establish a trust for your child, a "fiduciary" return is required.) Since tax laws change regularly, make no decisions based on hearsay or past experience. Successful filing fits naturally into three stages: collecting information, organizing required records, and filing and submitting the correct form accurately and punctually. Penalties and/or interest charges may be required if you are late or fail to file. Failure to file is frowned on by the IRS.

Information Gathering

The Internal Revenue Service (IRS) provides assistance to disabled citizens and their parents, and a number of helpful pamphlets are currently available, which should be revised and published annually in the future: "Child and Dependent Care Credit, and Employment Taxes for Household Employers" (Publication 503), "Tax Information for Handicapped and Disabled Individuals" (Publication 907), and "Credit for the Elderly or for the Permanently and Totally Disabled" (Publication 524). Brailled instructions are available, and, for a nongovernmental perspective, *Exceptional Parent* publishes an "Annual Income Tax Guide." IRS Publication 907 of November 1986 says:

> This publication covers the federal income tax rules of particular interest to handicapped and disabled people and to taxpayers with disabled dependents. These rules, for example, allow taxpayers to claim a credit if they are permanently and totally disabled, to deduct medical expenses, and to claim a credit for disabled dependent care expenses. The publication also gives general information on what income is taxable and on certain deductions and credits. . . . In most instances the Internal Revenue Service will mail you either Form 1040 or Form 1040A and Form 1040EZ with related instructions.
>
> If you have not received a form in the mail, or wish a form other than the one received, you may be able to get it at your local bank, post office, or public library. Or, you can order it from the Internal Revenue Service Forms Distribution Center for your state. . . . If you need information on a subject that is not covered in this publication, you should check our other free publications or call the toll free telephone number for your area listed in the instructions for the tax forms.

To obtain these government publications and to get information you need to get going, contact your local IRS office, which is listed in the phone book under Internal Revenue Service or U.S. Government, IRS. (Telephone help for the deaf is available for those with access to TV/Telephone-TTY equipment.)

When you contact the IRS, ask if any additional material of interest to handicapped citizens is available. Ask how appointments with an IRS representative are made, what arrangements are required if you wish the IRS to help you complete your return, and whom to contact locally for information on filing your state income tax return. Later, phone or write that office to find what services they offer disabled taxpayers and to ask them to send you any descriptive materials available.

Once you receive the federal material, read it carefully, examine the returns, and clarify any questions with the IRS representative or by using the 800 number listed on the return. Here are some things you should know: who must file a return; what kind of income must be declared (Are payments in kind, such as rent subsidies and food stamps, exempt?); under what circumstances you can claim your child as a dependent (if you do, he can't file a separate return of his own); what deductions you can take; how costs of residential programs, medically related transportation and child and disabled care are treated; what schedules you will need (a schedule is an addition to the basic form that provides for entering explanatory information or claiming deductions).

Accurate record keeping is critical. Although the IRS doesn't, in general, require submission of substantiating material with the return, your return may be audited. At that time you must back up your submitted figures, particularly expenses claimed, including dates, receipted invoices, or canceled checks, as well as a description of services provided. Currently an audit may be ordered up to three years after your filing date, and under some circumstances records can be inspected up to seven years after original filing. Our Owen-related expenses were audited on several occasions, but the meetings were friendly, the auditor polite and fair—and I escaped unscathed. I was pleased to be able to go into the conference armed with well-kept and complete substantiating data. Keep good records. You'll sleep better. A friend of mine files a letter from a doctor who knows his son with his tax return along with copies of bills and canceled checks for unusual expenses for which he has taken a deduction. The doctor's letter, updated regularly, describes the nature of the boy's disability and the fact that he is unable to feed, bathe, or clothe himself, etc. Such detail is not required, but my friend's returns have never been audited. Maybe there's a connection. File your return between January 1 and April 15, and retain copies of returns from the seven most recent years.

Completing the Form

You have three options: prepare your own return, get help from the IRS, or seek private professional advice. If considerable money is involved or the form is complex, I suggest you contact a tax consultant, but be sure he's knowledgeable about this specialized area of tax preparation. Ask your local support group, association (the ARC is good in this area), or social service representative and find out about billing practices before you become committed. I was badly burned by a professional who charged by the hour and educated himself on the fine points of handicap tax law at my expense. My advice is not to agree to an hourly arrangement unless you have had satisfactory experience with the consultant or know those who have. (Costs involved in tax preparation have, in the past, been deductible items.)

Private Medical Insurance

What Kind of Coverage Do You Need?

In my opinion, every parent should carry health insurance for his family unless total medical needs are covered by a public agency. The challenge is to obtain a policy you can afford that covers the areas most important to you. The goal is maximal coverage for minimal premium, but the coverage must be the right coverage. Special parents, particularly, must protect themselves against catastrophic medical expenses that, if not covered, would bankrupt their family, and they should be alert to the fact that some insurance coverage excludes pre-existing physical conditions. Overlooking this fine print could jeopardize coverage for your child.

To choose wisely, a basic understanding of health insurance is a necessity. (Many issues raised in Chapter 27, under life insurance, also apply here.) Health insurance is generally divided into two categories: basic and major medical (often called extended coverage), although some insurance companies use other terms. Basic coverage is defined in the individual policy, which you should carefully read and understand. Basic insurance often includes hospitalization costs up to a certain maximal number of days, certain surgical practices as well as stipulated emergency outpatient care, and, depending upon the policy, specified diagnostic work and medical procedures in the doctor's office. Be sure allowances for surgical procedures are realistic in terms of local practice. (Some policies stipulate the maximal daily rate allowed for a hospital room. I prefer a policy that guarantees coverage for a semiprivate room without any dollar limitation.)

Major medical coverage goes into effect when "major" medical costs exceed certain limits, but coverage usually applies to only a portion of these expenses. Eighty percent coverage is common, with the patient being responsible for the rest, but if excessive expenses are incurred in one year, insurance companies will sometimes assume the additional 20 percent. This feature is commonly called a "stop loss" clause; however, some major medical policies contain another clause that sets a lifetime limit on expenses the company will pay the insured. Read the fine print!

A feature of many policies is the stipulation that the insured (that's you) must pay a specified amount of expenses (called a "deductible") after the basic coverage has been exhausted and before the major medical coverage becomes effective. Find out how much this deductible is. (Under certain policies the insured must pay part of the expenses incurred on individual items—a "co-payment.") Insurance can be purchased both for the individual and for the entire family. I recommend you get family coverage; sometimes it's the only way you can obtain insurance for your child.

Some critical points to clear up when you consider a particular policy are: Does it cover treatment for emotional or psychological problems? Does it exclude from coverage any pre-existing medical conditions or require a waiting period before coverage begins? (This could be a disaster and unacceptable for a special family.) Can the policy be terminated by the company without your consent? And, are all dependents included? Be sure your handicapped child can be continued in family coverage after age nineteen. Owen, at twenty-nine, is still included in our policy, at an additional premium, although I had to file a doctor's statement certifying the severity of his disability.

Some parents have changed jobs or chosen one job over another because of the employee health-insurance plans they were offered. On the other hand, changing jobs can endanger coverage, and you should evaluate the implications of even a temporary lapse of protection before you make a move. If you have any choice in the matter, don't leave your family uncovered during the move, and do your best to convert to a new plan offering at least as good coverage as you currently enjoy. I can't emphasize too strongly the importance of maintaining medical insurance coverage and to avoid a gap at all costs. Insurance companies are never overjoyed at the prospect of having to deal with the heavy expenses that can, from time to time, be associated with individuals who have disabilities. Get maximal coverage, and once you have it, hang on to it. See what your group plan says about converting coverage if you change employment, and be particularly sensitive to exclusions, waiting periods, and increased premiums. If your child can look forward to working in the outside world, the law requires that, if he wishes to participate, he must be included in any group plans offered by his employer.

What Kind of Plan Is Best for You?

Insurance is available through group and nongroup plans and health maintenance organizations (HMOs). Group plans ordinarily are sponsored by companies for their employees, and by associations and nonprofit organizations for their members. The ARC, for example, offers life insurance and in-hospital income coverage. A nongroup plan offers coverage for someone who isn't working, is self-employed, or is employed by a company that doesn't offer a group plan. (*How to Provide for Their Future* [see Resources: Law] gives excellent information on insurance and government benefits.)

Generally a group plan is less expensive, is not subject to cancellation as long as employment continues, and is not apt to include exemptions or waiting periods. But check to see what rules govern your child's continued inclusion after age nineteen and find out when you can enroll in or make changes to the plan. In some companies this can be done only at the time of initial employment or during a designated period each year. Insurance companies' coverage of newborns with birth defects or congenital problems when family coverage was in effect before their birth is now required in all states for both group and nongroup coverage.

One disadvantage of group plans is that since they provide uniform coverage for a large number of participants, normally no provision is made for policy individualization to meet particular family needs. Nongroup plans, on the other hand, because they are *not* standardized, can be tailored to meet your needs, but they may, unless you are alert, contain provisions that work to your family's disadvantage. Again, examine the policy carefully. Whatever your coverage, it's important to receive assurance that your child is immediately covered or, if he isn't covered, to know under what conditions such coverage can be arranged.

The HMO system, also called "prepaid medical insurance," is a relatively new approach to health insurance in that it not only provides protection once your child is sick or injured and in need of medical attention but also emphasizes good health practices, preventive medicine, and health education so he will stay well. One possible disadvantage of such a plan is that you must utilize the doctors retained by the HMO (unless you wish to pay out of your own pocket), and services are rendered only at facilities specified by the HMO. On the brighter side, all procedures, medicines, and treatment prescribed by these doctors are generally covered, with the exception of some elective procedures, prescriptions, and treatment of mental or nervous problems, when partial payment by the insured (co-payment) may be required. HMOs are available in most major urban centers and usually offer both group and nongroup plans. Since this is a fairly new approach to health care and practices vary, contact the individual HMO you're considering to see how it handles the sticky problems I have been discussing, particularly consultation with specialists outside the HMO. (Some HMOs may resist covering special families.)

Record Keeping Is Important

Whether or not your child's medical expenses are large, keeping track of claims can be time consuming. The family financial advisor, mentioned earlier, usually can suggest procedures to reduce the process to a system—ways you can coordinate your payment of bills with filing of claims so as to place the least strain on your budget. The ideal arrangement, of course, is for the doctor or supplier to bill the insurance company directly. I find it helps if you deal with one insurance claims representative all the time, and sometimes your doctor will help by deferring billing until you are reimbursed by the company. If your finances are tight, ask him what arrangements can be made.

Accurate, uniform record keeping is vital for both reimbursement and tax purposes. Find out what information is required and complete the claim forms completely and accurately. Considerable time is lost and your money is still tied up while forms are returned and redone. Details are important. For example, our son's full name is Peter Owen Callanan. The fact that we always refer to him as Owen has inadvertently caused misunderstandings and delays in the past, particularly when dealing with large, computerized companies.

Here are a few observations about health insurance in general that you should know:

- Private insurance providers will not reimburse for medical services covered by a federal or state compensation act or similar legislation.
- Every state has a commission controlling insurance practices within that state. Contact them for general information. Your state senator, state representative, or any large local insurance agency should be able to furnish their address.
- Some group plans offer a choice of coverage. If your child has problems, it is usually better to select the largest amount of health coverage available.

Prudent budgeting of family resources, alert income-tax management, and an informed approach to insurance coverage are important but often not enough to sustain a family that contends with the additional fiscal drain that caring for a special child entails. Often another source of help must be tapped.

Government-controlled Assistance

Probably the most important financial assistance to disabled citizens, in terms of total dollars expended, comes from three general sources. First, there are those programs operating under the umbrella of Social Security: Supplemental Security Income (SSI), Medicaid, Medicare, and Social Security itself. Next comes the Crippled Children's Services. Finally, there are those state-operated programs assisting developmentally disabled citizens. Many books are written each year describing these programs, and almost every year major changes are made and new books are written describing these changes. Little is to be gained and perhaps some disadvantage lies in describing them in detail when it is easier for parents to contact the agency involved at the time help is needed. Some general observations are in order, however, to point out the nature and future benefits to your child of the services these programs provide.

Supplemental Security Income provides income (currently $340 per month) to disabled individuals of modest means, but until a youngster is eighteen, the entire family income is considered in the formula used to determine program eligibility. The problem involved in meeting financial requirements is discussed in Chapter 27, but one lesson is clear: parents should not give significant property to a handicapped child without first checking current federal regulations to see how increasing his net worth will affect eligibility for governmental support, either at that time or in the future. The intent of the regulation is that governmental aid should not be given to someone who has adequate means to support himself.

Medicaid is a medical assistance program, and, as with SSI, only low-income citizens qualify for benefits. Criteria vary from state to state, but ownership of property as well as income are involved in the formula. In many states the financial and medical qualification requirements for SSI and Medicaid are identical, although even individuals who don't meet financial guidelines may sometimes qualify for assistance by being "medically needy" if their medical expenses are extraordinarily high. If your child (under age twenty-one) qualifies for Medicaid, he also is eligible for a special health program called Early and Periodic Screening, Diagnosis and Treatment (EPSDT). Ask about it when you contact the Social Security office.

Medicare is medical insurance available to all who qualify for benefits under Social Security, irrespective of their personal financial status. If someone who qualifies for Social Security dies or retires—and if he has a handicapped child—that child may qualify to receive benefits until he is eighteen. The size of the benefits will depend upon the size of the parents' total contribution to Social Security. After he reaches age eighteen, the child will continue to receive such payments as long as he is unable to perform gainful work. If the child's income is sufficiently low, he may receive both SSI benefits and Aid to Families with Dependent Children (AFDC).

Crippled Children's Services are state-operated but federally subsidized organizations providing diagnostic and medical services for many kinds of handicapping conditions, including chronic diseases, birth defects, and accidental disabilities. This program's title is a misnomer, since services are not limited to orthopedically crippling conditions. Some services are provided free to all children, while other services may require a partial payment from the parent, depending upon his financial situation. This program can be particularly helpful in that it not only provides parents with medical and financial planning advice but also often assumes part or all of the costs involved. It's important to know the details of how the program operates in your state, since some services are not covered without prior approval.

Another particularly helpful organization available in every state goes under different names but is often called the Developmental Disabilities or simply D.D. Council (federally funded under the Developmental Disabilities and Bill of Rights Act, Public Law 98-527). Although their services vary, councils often promote planning, advocacy, and research and act as actual funding sources for services to developmentally disabled people with neurological problems, both motor and mental. Your council should be helpful in identifying local resources. It also may help you determine if your child qualifies for public assistance and, if so, where such assistance is obtained. Help need not be limited to the strictly medical, but can include other services, particularly those that make it possible for an individual to remain at home or live relatively independently under his own control and escape institutionalization. (Changes in the law in 1984 also required state councils to support projects in employment-related services.) Although disability services can be closely associated with some state agency, they also may be contracted out to private or not-for-profit organizations.

Help from the Private Sector

Another source of individual support, often overlooked, is not-for-profit associations and foundations. Operating on both national and local levels, they are dominated nationally by such large organizations as the National Easter Seal Society, the Spina Bifida Association of America, the Epilepsy Foundation of America, the American Foundation for the Blind, and the Association for Retarded Citizens. Many of these groups offer a broad range of assistance by sponsoring research, respite facilities, and hospitals. Some of this help is specific, in that it deals exclusively with one kind of disability or disease, while other help is more general, such as the cost benefits of volume buying in group health insurance plans and discount prescription services.

Even less obvious is the individual support sometimes available on a state or local level, which, although usually limited and specific in nature, is worth exploring, particularly if other sources are unavailable. Sometimes this help takes the form of funds available through local hospitals dedicated to specific populations or foundations that concentrate in areas of interest to disabled people. The hospital social worker or your contact person in the department of human services or special education department may know if such local resources exist. Occasionally, statewide directories are published that describe foundations and the areas in which they concentrate. Ask your reference librarian.

How to Start Your Search for Help

You may already have established your entry into the financial support network long ago, at the hospital when the business office referred you to a social service organization for help in meeting your first medical bills. On the other hand, you may have managed to get by on your own resources till that one day when it finally became obvious that some form of outside help was necessary. A natural first step in your efforts to locate financial resources is to seek advice from someone in your school system or a medical professional with whom you have established a close relationship. An alternative is to begin the search by contacting your nearest Social Security office (listed in the phone book under Social Security Administration or U.S. Government, Social Security). You will probably end up in that office eventually anyway.

In addition to giving you information about whether any of Social Security's programs can provide assistance, "the people in the Social Security office will help disabled or blind people get in touch with community organizations that may provide assistance. For example, the local health department can help meet some health needs. The public assistance office may provide extra financial help or other services." (U.S. Department of Health and Human Services, Social Security Administration Publication No. 05-11000, January 1987. Get it at your Social Security Office. It's free.)

After you have asked the switchboard operator at the Social Security office to connect you with someone who is familiar with disability benefits for a disabled child under SSI, your phone conversation might go something like this: "I'm the parent of a mentally retarded, twenty-year-old son. He has no personal financial means and is incapable of supporting himself. Can you help me find out if he qualifies for *any* form of U.S. government assistance and, in addition, can you suggest organizations here in the state that will counsel me about local resources available?"

Don't waste time. Publication No. 05-11000 says, "You should apply for SSI *right away* if you think you can get SSI or if you have a child who can. This is because SSI payments can start only with the day you apply or the date you are eligible, whichever is later. You can apply for

SSI at any Social Security office. You can call, write, or visit the office. You may apply for someone else who might be eligible for SSI if the person is not able to apply."

The information that such a meeting might furnish you includes:

- If your child's request for assistance is rejected, you have the right to appeal the decision. (Get the free leaflet "Your right to question the decision made on your SSI claim" at your SS office.)
- It is sometimes possible to arrange interviews at home.
- SSI can change its mind, so don't consider its decisions irrevocable.
- Everyone who applies for disability benefits, irrespective of whether he receives them, will be "referred to the state vocational rehabilitation agency for consideration of possible services. Such services include counseling, medical services, training in the use of prostheses, teaching of new employment skills and job placement."

You'll probably eventually need more resources than the Social Security office has to offer, and your contact with them probably will be only the beginning of your quest. But you will be making a beginning by dealing with people whose job it is to provide help and who are armed with the most recent and accurate information. Finally, since money matters are discussed in many places in this book, I suggest you refer to "Finances" in the index for additional information.

Dos and Don'ts
from Birth to Age Five

1. *When in doubt, find out.* If you become seriously worried about your child's development, learn the pattern of normal human development, and consult a doctor if your child is falling significantly behind.

If your doctor's response doesn't satisfy you, request a second opinion. Don't shop around seeking the opinion you want to hear, but be sure the testing process has examined all aspects of your child—physical, emotional, and mental.

Don't be reluctant to seek this kind of information because of concern over costs or the availability of services. There are people in your state whose job it is to help you. Determine, with their guidance, the most appropriate methods of taking care of any charges that may be involved. But get the services!

2. *Government help.* Know what rights you and your child have under laws pertaining to the handicapped. Under Public Law 94-142, all states provide educational services to handicapped children (discussed at length in Part Four). Identifying and providing diagnostic services to youngsters who need special services is one of the state's responsibilities. Contact your local school system for details.

3. *Take maximal advantage of your professionals.* Select all key care providers carefully; a physical therapist can be as critical to your child's health as the most specialized physician. Insist there be one coordinator who knows the whole picture and won't pass the buck.

Don't be intimidated by specialists. You have much to contribute that is available from no one else. Maintain high expectations and be realistically demanding of those who work with your child. But be courteous and understanding. Professionals are human beings, too.

Be "professional" yourself: prepare for appointments, be prompt, think through the questions you would like to have answered. Become familiar with the technical language used; listen carefully, particularly to directions or prescriptions in which you are involved (take notes if that helps). Let it be known if you don't understand something or can't handle an assignment.

Change professionals if you're sure it's warranted, but only after careful consideration. Changing is preferable to continuing an unsatisfactory relationship, since your child's progress is affected by your family's attitude toward the professional team.

4. *Establish a home safety net.* Learn the nature of any reactions, symptoms, or susceptibilities characteristic of your child's condition so you can take steps to protect him. Know what constitutes an emergency and whom to call.

Understand the side effects of the medication and drugs prescribed and the details of how medication is to be obtained, administered, stored, and replenished.

Adapt your home to meet your child's needs. Contact local and national safety experts and follow safety guidelines.

5. *Begin intervention and stimulation "early."* The clinic's interdisciplinary team, or your pediatrician, should develop a specific plan indicating all actions recommended to improve your child's condition. Generally, during the first two years of life intervention is best carried out at home. After that, children often prosper by moving out into the mainstream of the community to center-based programs. Investigate the early intervention programs available and see that your child takes maximal advantage of them. Find out the services your state provides and get cracking!

Don't be passive or immobilized. If your child's diagnosis is unclear and/or your pediatrician feels "things will work out" but you're still worried, there are things you can do to help that require no doctor's prescription: Play with your youngster, and see to it that he receives all the physical manifestations of love and affection that you would lavish on a nonhandicapped child.

If you live in a rural area, locating resources may be difficult; however, with help you should be able to accomplish more things with and for your child than you thought possible.

Learn enough about the details of your child's handicap to understand treatment alternatives and to evaluate both progress and performance of attending professionals. Develop a basic library of resource materials that will make you a more effective advocate.

6. *See that your family—including the handicapped member—remains healthy.* Don't isolate your child. To shelter him unnecessarily will increase his limitations and "differentness." Don't become so preoccupied with disabilities that abilities are overlooked. The goal is to maximize his potential and possibility of eventual independence. A newborn requires extraordinary assistance, but as he grows older, help should be

kept to a minimum. Develop a toughness that allows you to do what is necessary. A sense of humor will help, too, and can provide a refreshing interlude of laughter.

Don't shortchange the rest of the family. Try to maintain regularity in all things—medical and dental checkups, immunizations, exercise, and bed- and mealtimes. In your concern with one child's special diet, don't neglect the balanced nutritional requirements of the rest of the family.

When signs of excessive strain appear, seek help. It's normal for everyone to suffer feelings of frustration and guilt, but if stress gets out of hand it can cause serious problems and make a bad situation worse. For many, it's difficult to admit that help is needed, and one trick in being a successful parent is the willingness to accept help.

There are moments when it's best for everyone to take a break, even from one another. Respite homes and special resources are available to care for children while families unwind or attend to necessary business. Seek out someone reliable to take over for you. It just might make your day—and your youngster's, as well.

Beware of expensive, unorthodox remedies that seem too good to be true. Thoughtfully examine all alternatives, but guard against something that seems to be too good to be true—perhaps it is.

7. *Generalities won't solve financial problems.* (Read Chapter 15 and immerse yourself in the details.)

8. *Finally, always assume there's an answer to your problem.* In most instances Mary and I eventually found a solution to even the most perplexing problem. Never take no for an answer unless you have checked, rechecked, and explored all alternatives. Keep your perspective and your sense of humor, and nurture hope.

PART FOUR

We educate one another; and we cannot
do this if half of us consider the
other half not good enough to talk to.

GEORGE BERNARD SHAW

The Promise of
Education for All
Disabled Children

Prologue

In the late 1960s college students shouted anitwar slogans while senators in Washington just shouted. No one understood what anyone else was saying, and no one cared. In Baltimore, Owen was six, the age most kids begin first grade. He wasn't interested in communicating either. By now we had uprooted our family twice to seek medical help, but Owen remained a mystery and we knew we were in trouble.

One day we heard that a technique called "operant conditioning"—practiced at a large and reputable local institution—was achieving remarkable success with patients whose problems sounded just like Owie's. Simply put, the theory suggests if a person is rewarded with something he particularly likes immediately after he has performed some desired action, he will be inclined to repeat that action, seeking further reward. By means of a complex system of rewards and withdrawal of rewards, he could be led into a pattern of approved behavior. It sounded great! Our hearts began to beat faster, and Mary and I quickly arranged an appointment.

At our initial interview, as we explained Owen's unusual problems, the attending specialist leaned forward in his chair, rapidly taking notes, obviously excited by the challenge. At the conclusion of the meeting, while we stood in the hall shaking hands and pulling on overcoats, the doctor urged us not to worry, saying that in two months he would have our son talking—not only talking but doing so in complete sentences. This sounded awfully good (Mary and I were young then), and after we read up on the subject and checked things out with both the family doctor and our bank balance, we said, "Okay, let's give it a try." We enrolled Owen in the program.

Visiting wasn't permitted, but after a week or so we were allowed to observe a work session through a one-way mirror. This arrangement has always made me feel awkward—like a divorce lawyer or a Peeping Tom—but our first observation was worth waiting for. It was delightful, and even today the memory of it makes us smile. There was Owen seated at a table in one of those antiseptic cubicles, working on a complex jigsaw puzzle. Across from him in a wrinkled white coat sat a balding resident physician with a large pile of multicolored M&M candies in front of him and a small plywood board with an electric light bulb and an activating toggle switch by his right hand. He was following Owen's progress closely and rewarded every correct solution with a piece of candy and a bright flash of his light. Right from the start, Owen apparently saw a humorous side to the whole business, because as he began work he was smiling almost imperceptibly to himself.

Everything went well for a while, with Owen popping his M&M rewards into his mouth and the light flashing on and off, but gradually his correct responses began to accelerate. The resident had trouble keeping up, and in his haste occasionally scattered candies into his lap and onto the floor. What he apparently didn't know was that Owen, despite his many limitations, has remarkable abilities in certain fields, puzzle solving being one. He can polish off a 2,500-piece representation of the Battle of Gettysburg before the average person can get the cellophane off the box. But Mary and I had seen this many times before and had just gotten up to leave when the reward light began to malfunction. Interested, we sat down again.

Owen's therapy continued, except that now the light no longer responded regularly to the toggle-switch pressure, and Owen would stop, often with his hand arrested in midair, waiting for the flash and looking expectantly at the resident, who in turn would whack the light board on the table and glance over his shoulder at the one-way mirror. Once he inadvertently hit his index finger on the table and winced. Perspiration began to form on his forehead. Our son was now assembling the puzzle about as quickly as I have ever seen him go, and it was obvious the resident was outclassed. Finally, with a concluding blue flash, the light gave out entirely. By then Owen had moved the pile of M&Ms over to where he could reach them more efficiently and was rewarding himself as he continued the puzzle. The resident had apparently lost interest and was sitting quietly, rubbing his finger, which looked red and inflamed. Mary and I got up and left. It hadn't been such a bad day after all.

As you can guess, Owen didn't learn to talk in two months, but I think he had a wonderful time, and we have no regrets. Research must continue and new techniques and approaches must be explored if progress is to be made. And parents, as important participants in the process, must be thoughtfully supportive. Operant conditioning has apparently proven helpful for many; it just didn't work for Owen. It was a serious professional attempt by dedicated people supported by a recognized institution. Mary and I did our homework, too, by investigating the program and conscientiously following instructions.

The moral isn't that one should avoid new approaches or even unorthodox therapy that is supported by competent practitioners. Quite the contrary. Mary and I learned by this and other experiences that to be an effective advocate you must constantly press for your child's welfare, examining all available resources. You are bound to encounter disappointments, even disasters! But the answer is not to abandon all action. Those of our friends who have succeeded continued trying despite setbacks. They picked themselves up after each defeat and kept their sense of perspective and humor. No cure is yet known for what ails Owen, but someday one will be found, and I'm as sure as I can be that when it is, it will come as the result of efforts of the people like the man in the wrinkled white coat. Meanwhile, he will have to get a new light bulb—and more candy.

16

Your Child's Right
to an Appropriate Education

In the beginning was the Word.

In Part Three, I concentrate on that first transition period when parents begin to assume their new responsibilities as leaders of a special family. One of their problems is coordinating everything and everybody involved in the diagnostic phase and the resulting medical plan. Often this is an involved process, and it becomes even more involved as the child grows older. The focus of attention, which initially is concerned almost exclusively with physical health and the medical profession, must expand to include the child's mental and intellectual health and the people involved in its development.

Acknowledging the necessary interrelationship of intellectual and physical growth—where neglect of one will adversely affect the other —is nothing new. Two thousand years ago, Juvenal, the Roman poet, described the ideal human condition as "a sound mind in a sound body," and even today his well-worn quotation stands high on the list of educators' favorites. But unlike so many educational cliches, it is one to take seriously. Working toward a healthy developmental balance is important for all parents but should be a priority for mothers and fathers of handicapped children. They must help their youngsters take advantage of everything the kids have going for them if they are to grow up to be as sound as possible. It's easy to become so preoccupied with a physical handicap that it monopolizes your waking hours and distorts your perspective. Although this single-mindedness can make you feel noble, resist it; it usually is a disservice to everyone, and a bore to a few.

Maximizing intellectual development is easier said than done, since it requires coordinating an entirely new cast of characters—the educational establishment—with the medical profession, some of whom may be unaccustomed to being coordinated. But unlike the preschool years, when many of us received little or no coordinated help at all, the years when your child becomes legally of school age and enters the educational cycle are—glory be—the focus of a national program that guarantees handicapped children certain fundamental educational rights. On that wonderful day when your child reaches the age at which the law in your state applies to him, and indirectly to you, you inherit a powerful partner. Now the government, on all levels, is obligated to stand by your side through your child's years of mandated free instruction and to work with you to see that he is offered what the law describes as a "free appropriate education." Rarely have three words meant so much to so many.

Your local school system, the partner with whom you will now deal most directly, will henceforth be called the local education agency, or LEA. The state education agency (SEA)—where you live, it may be called the State Board of Education—is also a partner, seeing to it that your local agency meets its responsibilities to both you and your child. It's important for parents to realize that the LEA has a *legal* obligation to serve as advocate for the children under its care and that the youngsters really have three protectors: you (as parents), the federal government, and the LEA. Remember this if you have a disagreement with representatives of the school system. They are probably acting in what they believe are your child's best interests. That doesn't mean that they are always right. Children who live in a state that offers special educational services beginning at birth qualify for this support from infancy. Others must wait for varying periods of time, but all states have educational responsibility toward handicapped children during the same years that free public instruction is provided to nonhandicapped children.

Part Four deals with all aspects of the special education system you now enter: its organization, its people, and its language. (Lists of facts are dull but these can be important.) This section touches upon the rights and responsibilities of both parent and school. It discusses what to look for in a good school system, how to seek out and evaluate educational services, and what to do if the results are disappointing. This section concentrates on the actions you can take, since the quality of your child's education will be influenced by your ability to do three things at least reasonably well: first, learn and stay up to date on applicable federal and state laws and make maximal use of the educational rights they guarantee; next, work with your school system in a spirit of cooperation that is courteous yet demanding; and finally, develop the skills (many of them bureaucratic) and strength of character (not necessarily a bureaucratic trait) required to function effectively in a field dominated by professionals and cluttered with red tape. This chapter deals specifically with the legal underpinnings of special education and the specific rights they guarantee. I make the assumption that you are in favor of or at least have no objection to your child's receiving appropriate special educational services. Although much that is required of you may be difficult, stick with it; special education can be the difference between your child's making it in life and being left forever behind.

The Legislation

Special education for handicapped children has developed from a wide-ranging complex of interlocking laws. For our purposes I will consider four laws that have had a significant impact, paying particular attention to eight basic rights that the laws guarantee:

- Equal access
- Confidentiality and access to educational records
- Nondiscriminatory admission
- Least restrictive environment
- Individualized education program
- Nondiscriminatory testing
- Parental participation
- Due process

All laws we discuss have been amended down through the years, so when you refer to them, get the most recent amendment.

These rights are "basic" in that, together, they make possible one of the most fundamental rights of all—the right to a free appropriate education—and they establish the guidelines that govern your relationship with your local school system. They are also of particular importance because they're not limited to the educational experience but spill over to affect your child later, in other areas of his adult life.

One word about rights. At the beginning of our life with Owen, I found my role as his advocate embarrassing; sometimes I failed to be assertive enough, believing that I was defending rights for Owen that others didn't enjoy. With time I realized what should have been obvious: the laws' intent is to give handicapped children not an unfair advantage, but an *even* break to help them enjoy rights that others enjoy automatically just because they're healthy.

You should know that the term *Public Law*—often shortened to P.L.—means legislation that has been passed by Congress, is the law of the land, and, therefore, applies to all of us. (Individual states may expand coverage and rights provided under federal law but *may not* reduce or limit them.) The numbers that follow the P.L. provide further identification; for example, 93-112 indicates the 112th law passed by the Ninety-third Congress.

Since much legislation is amended from time to time, be sure, whenever consulting federal or state laws, to obtain the most recent amendments. Out-of-date information can be worse than no information. The Office of Special Education and Rehabilitative Services, U.S. Department of Education (see Resources: Federal Agencies), is a source of ongoing updates. Write and ask to be placed on the mailing list for their publication *OSERS News in Print*, which in the past, in addition to other useful material, has included a "Summary of Selected Legislation Relating to Handicapped Individuals." If you've put together the ABC library described in Part Three, you should already have available for quick reference copies of much of the legislation and other key materials that will be referred to in the following chapters. For further reading I particularly recommend *Negotiating the Special Education Maze: A Guide for Parents and Teachers* (see Resources: Education). It has been helpful to me in the preparation of this book and goes into much greater detail than I have found practical here.

Section 504

The first piece of legislation to examine is the Rehabilitation Act of 1973, but I will particularly refer here to its Section 504, since it's that part of the law in which we are specifically interested. (Sections 501 and 503 will be discussed later.) This bellwether legislation, the first federal civil rights law specifically protecting the rights of handicapped citizens, says:

> No otherwise qualified handicapped individual in the United States
> . . . shall solely by reason of . . . handicap, be excluded from the par-
> ticipation in, be denied the benefits of, or otherwise be subject to
> discrimination under any program or activity which receives or benefits
> from Federal financial assistance. And these activities must take steps to
> make [it] possible for handicapped people . . . to learn, work and com-
> pete on a fair and equal basis [with nonhandicapped citizens].

Section 504 will prove equally important later, when you help your youngster with other transitions, from the formal learning cycle to postsecondary education, then possibly to employment, housing, recreation, and all the other aspects of independent living.

This law's key provision affords handicapped people the right to equal access, an "access" to life that nonhandicapped persons often take for granted. The provision makes it discriminatory for an LEA to allow barriers of any kind to interfere with a handicapped child's right to learn, and it applies not only to schools but also to colleges, hospitals, and all health, welfare, and social service organizations receiving federal assistance. If science labs are located on the third floor of a school, ways must be found for the orthopedically impaired student to have access to them—for example, an elevator or stairlift can be in-stalled, or the class can be rescheduled to the first floor. Partly because of Section 504, all new school construction must be accessible (usable) by all handicapped students. If a child is blind, Braille or taped mate-rials (or readers) must be provided. One morning I sat, spellbound, in an elementary school classroom and watched as a special education teacher signed the day's lesson to her client. The signer, with her back to the front of the room, sitting directly in front of her small, deaf student, was apparently oblivious of the classroom teacher, who paced back and forth behind her. The signer's eyes were locked on those of her student, and her hands "spoke" in a fluid, graceful monologue. For everyone else in the class it was just another routine day; for me it was a demon-stration of equal access in action. Have you ever seen a good signer when she's really rolling? It's a sight to behold and does your heart good—even when she's "talking" about quotients and the lowest com-mon denominator.

Although the results of federal intervention will probably please you, you may wonder what place the government has in the education business in the first place. Isn't education a state, not a federal, func-tion? The answer lies in the Fourteenth Amendment and to a certain extent in the Fifth. These amendments forbid the states to deprive any person of life, liberty, or property without due process, and further guarantee equal protection for *everyone* under the law. These wide-ranging principles have been interpreted by the courts to apply spe-cifically to public instruction wherever it takes place. In effect, they guarantee handicapped students the same educational opportunities afforded the nonhandicapped and protect them from any discrimina-tion limiting these opportunities.

Copies of Section 504 regulations can be obtained from the U.S. Department of Education, Office for Civil Rights, Washington, D.C., or from your congressional delegation, an excellent source of informa-tion involving governmental operations and regulations. I have often looked to my representatives for help, with good results. They have a vested interest in satisfying their constituents.

The Developmental Disabilities Assistance and Bill of Rights Act

The second significant law, for short we'll call it the Develop-mental Disabilities Act, is concerned with a wide range of planning, coordinating, and advocacy services for the developmentally disabled individual and also is not exclusively concerned with education. More-over, one of its provisions dramatically improves the prospects of handicapped children's receiving all the benefits that the various education laws now guarantee but sometimes don't deliver. It accomplishes this by providing funding for each state to establish a "protection and Advocacy System," an independent professional corps of advisers (advocates) to look out for all the interests of disabled citizens, not just their educational interests. Your state has such an organization, whose job it is to provide you information on your child's individual educational rights in understandable language and to assist or represent you if it appears his rights have been violated. To insulate the advocacy system and keep it independent, it is required to be autonomous and without ties to any other organization, state or federal. (For information on how to utilize the advocacy system, see Chapter 24.)

Other goals of the Developmental Disabilities Program are improvement of services for handicapped citizens, coordination of existing resources, and development of programs to fill gaps where critical services aren't currently available, including the transition from school to the adult world (a noble aspiration dear to the hearts of all of us who have fallen into one of those gaps).

Every state has an agency designated to administer the overall program, and since the specific services offered to individual clients will vary from location to location, I suggest you contact your own state agency for a description of its offerings. (Your NICHCY State Resource Sheet lists the responsible agency and its address.) Get acquainted with the people running the program. They should be keenly interested in your input.

To be eligible for services, individuals must be "developmentally disabled," as defined in the most recently amended legislation. This definition has changed significantly over the years and may continue to change, so check it out—it is not identical with the requirements of other federal programs.

Many parents find that establishing their child's eligibility is one of the most frustrating and time-consuming problems they face. Keeping accurate records and getting acquainted with knowledgeable resource people—even before you need their help—make this road easier. Although our son has the mental age of a three-year-old, because of an inexplicable twist in the definition contained in the law, in his late teens he did not qualify for certain services reserved for the mentally retarded. I would love to have the lawmakers responsible spend one 24-hour day with Owie. It might sharpen their thinking.

Confidentiality and Access

The Buckley Amendment

The third critical piece of legislation is the Buckley Amendment to the Family Education Rights and Privacy Act. The act applies to all citizens but is particularly meaningful to handicapped people, since the Buckley Amendment assures them the right to confidentiality and access to educational records. This protection can both save those who are "different" from humiliating embarrassment and ensure that they obtain critical information. It guarantees to *all* parents, legal guardians of students under eighteen, and students over eighteen that the LEA will be open and aboveboard in its relationship with them, that it will protect a youngster's privacy and anonymity, and that it will, in a timely fashion, make school records available for inspection—and correction if they are in error. The confidentiality of such information is specifically guaranteed, particularly against its release to unauthorized persons or to the public without appropriate consent. In short, the LEA is the custodian, in trust, of privileged material concerning your child, which it must administer in a controlled and responsible fashion.

The Buckley Amendment requires all public schools to establish written policies—*available for you to inspect*—describing the specific way student records will be handled. (All LEAs receiving any federal money from the Department of Education must comply; for all practical purposes, this includes every public system, but private or parochial schools that receive no federal support are exempt.) Some requirements of the law are:

1. All "records, files, documents and other materials, discipline folders, health files, grade reports, and other records which contain information directly relating to a student," irrespective of where they are kept, fall under this act. Included is such routine information as students' and parents' names and addresses, phone numbers, whom to notify in case of accident, and attendance records. This so-called general Directory Information applicable to all students may be released under certain conditions, but only if parents are given the opportunity to refuse their consent. Other not-so-routine information covered by the law includes standardized test results, teachers' notes, individualized education programs, and evaluation results.

2. Although the school must make information covered by the amendment available to you as parent in a "timely" (reasonable) fashion, the staff is not required to drop everything to dig it out immediately, although it often will in an emergency. The law gives the LEA 45 days to comply, though most LEAs usually act more quickly. Check your local regulations for specifics.

3. A school can refuse to show you certain student records: for example, a teacher's or counselor's personal notes that are not part of a student's cumulative records or shown to anyone else except a substitute teacher; personnel records of school employees, which may mention the student; or records of school security police, which must be kept separate from the rest of the school's files. Although there are other exceptions, they are complicated and rarely apply. If you are concerned about this point, ask your local superintendent if there is any information about your child you can't see and if so, why it is unavailable.

4. Once you have asked to see a particular record, the LEA may not destroy anything in the folder. Each school system's record policy must contain procedures on the length of time particular types of records will be kept and under what conditions they will be disposed of; P.L. 94-142 (legislation discussed later) requires that LEAs maintain records either till the student is twenty-one or receives a high-school diploma, and it stipulates that records concerning his special education *must* be destroyed (after notifying the student) five years after the special services are no longer needed. One state's policy says, "A permanent record of a student's name, address and phone number, grades, attendance record, classes attended, grade level completed and year completed may be maintained without time limitation. [The ability to recapture this information can be important, since in future years you may need to supply it for many reasons—in an application for Social Security benefits for your youngster, for example.] Any other information that is part of the confidential [student] file must be destroyed within five years after the data is no longer needed to provide educational service to the child. Parents and student shall be informed prior to the destruction and may request a copy of all or portions of the data."[1]

5. You have the right both to have information in the file explained to you and to have someone of your choosing accompany you when you inspect the file, although you may be asked to give written authorization for this exception to the confidentiality rule.

6. Before records may be released to anyone outside the school (a doctor, an insurance company, the SSI, a private school), you must sign a consent form, which usually contains such information as the name of the individual requesting the records, what particular records are required, and the reason for the request. This release of information may be important to you. (In addition, the school must keep a list of every-

1. "Handicapped Children, Their Right to an Education, Information For Parents," Nebraska Department of Education, Special Education Branch, 1981, p. 5.

one who requests or receives information about your child.) However, the school can release records without prior parental consent to other school officials or to officials in another system in which the student plans to enroll. This is understandable. It would be difficult for school administrators to conduct their daily business if they didn't have such flexibility.

7. You can have copies of certain records made by the system. Although you may be charged for the service, the law allows only the material cost of reproduction to be recovered; no clerical time may be billed. Some LEAs send copies of records by mail, but ordinarily they require a signed release-of-information form.

8. If you believe any information in the file is misleading or incorrect, you are guaranteed a specific procedure to help straighten things out. You can:

- Bring your concern to the attention of the principal. If he corrects the error, the issue is settled.
- If the principal disagrees, you may send a written request for a hearing to him or to the person designated in the school policy to handle such matters. The principal must inform you of your right to a hearing, which, if requested, has to be held without unreasonable delay.
- The school must have established a procedure for a hearing administered by an impartial committee or an individual, known as a "hearing officer," who has no direct interest in the hearing's outcome. The purpose is to allow each side to present its point of view. If you wish, you may bring someone with you, such as a lawyer, a doctor, a psychologist, or another parent or friend.
- The decision of the hearing officer is final; however, you have the right to enter a written statement into the file describing your objections to the material or to write a letter of complaint to the organization responsible for enforcing the Buckley Amendment (Family Education Rights and Privacy Act Office (FERPA), Department of Health and Human Services, 200 Independence Avenue SW, Washington, DC 20201). In some states you may sue the school system in a civil court. I would not recommend such action unless you consider the information involved to be absolutely crucial. It can be expensive and time-consuming to sue.

In short, your child enjoys the right to privacy in his career in school and only the professionals working directly with him may see his records.

It's critical that your youngster's records be accurate and complete. Record keeping—both yours and the school system's—is a necessary tool that can be a godsend. Check your child's files periodically and make copies of important documents for your notebook. If your family moves, find out what records the new school will require and notify your old LEA far enough in advance that they have time to send on needed information. (Remember that the efficiency of many schools is reduced in the summer.)

P.L. 94-142

The last, and perhaps most important legislation, is Public Law 94-142, the Education for All Handicapped Children's Act of 1975 and all its many amendments. I will refer to it as either the Education of the Handicapped Act (EHA) or simply P.L. 94-142. In contrast to Section 504, which is involved in many areas, P.L. 94-142 is strictly an education law, overseen by the Office of Special Education of the U.S. Department of Education and concerned with handicapped children from age three to twenty-one (or graduation from high school). Although both laws contain many similar provisions—Section 504 actually has a more liberal definition of those who qualify for coverage—P.L. 94-142 as amended is referred to as the foundation for education of the handicapped, and you should be most familiar with this legislation. It not only sets forth certain educational rights that handicapped children enjoy but also establishes guidelines (procedures) to be observed by everyone involved in the public education of handicapped youngsters. Like Section 504, P.L. 94-142 ensures compliance with its provisions by providing for the withholding of federal funding from any institution in violation. There's nothing like the prospect of losing federal money to motivate people.

The goal of P.L. 94-142 is to assure handicapped youngsters "a free appropriate public education which emphasizes a special education and related services designed to meet their unique needs." The director of a developmental center in Maryland, describing her program, got at the heart of what this bureaucratic language means when she said, "What we try to do here is to provide specially designed experiences for each one of our handicapped kids that will make his later adult life as meaningful and productive as possible." In its own special language, the law goes on to explain:

> "Special education" means specially designed instruction, at no cost to the parent, to meet the unique needs of a handicapped child, including classroom instruction, instruction in physical education, home instruction, and instruction in hospitals and institutions (94-142, 300.14).

Related Services

The earlier emphasis upon "related services" implies that coverage isn't limited to what goes on in the classroom, and the law goes out of its way to describe several basically noneducational services that must be made available if the learning meant to take place in the classroom is actually going to. The law says:

> "Related services" means transportation and such developmental, corrective, and other supportive services as are required to assist a handicapped child to benefit from special education, and includes speech pathology and audiology, psychological services, physical and occupational therapy, recreation, early identification and assessment of disabilities in children, counseling services, and medical services for diagnostic or evaluation purposes. The term also includes school health services, social work services in schools, and parent counseling and training (94-142, 300.13).

In short, P.L. 94-142 includes as its province all areas that affect the quality of the education offered. And even though Medicaid currently will not reimburse for medical services provided at a school location, this fact represents a rare exception to the position taken on July 5, 1984, by the Supreme Court when it ruled unanimously that neither costs, staff liability, nor medical needs should be allowed to limit a handicapped child's school attendance. In other words, nothing having to do with your child's handicap should be allowed to stand in his way educationally, and if he has medical needs that must be attended to at school, it is the school system's responsibility to help you solve the problem (but not, at the moment, to pay for it). In 1979, even though his dental abnormality might have been a factor in Owen's speech problems, our LEA refused financial assistance, saying in a letter, "In reference to orthodontia, this is medical treatment and not an allowable cost. The parents should be contacted for any dental work that Owen needs." I did not contest this position then, but I would if I had it to do over again.

The legislation makes coverage even more comprehensive by stipulating that "special" education need not be limited to the public school setting, but can involve any education-related activity carried out in such places as a hospital, an individual's home, or a special state or private institution if (and this is an important "if") adequate services are not available in the local school system.

Owen was a teenager when P.L. 94-142 was passed, and in the five years that he qualified for services, we—our school system, Mary, and I—repeatedly moved the poor kid from one institution to another. In all, we entered him in five different "schools," always optimistically, in an attempt to find the special "best place" that we knew was out there somewhere. Owen is an alumnus of a large institution in Pennsylvania, a small group home, two sheltered workshops, and a school for the deaf in Maine, but he never got a varsity letter. Even though our LEA covered all tuition, the search demanded a price of another kind, and each change of school had its own collection of bittersweet memories (a little child can look small in the halls of a big institution).

Although Owen has never developed intellectually, it wasn't for lack of trying on the part of a lot of people and the humane support of our home school system. Some staff members obviously shared in victories and in defeats. P.L. 94-142 made it possible for us to give Owen every opportunity available at the time, irrespective of cost. Doing everything we could was, and is, important to us and how we feel about ourselves.

Nondiscriminatory Admission

Another key concept in the opening passage of P.L. 94-142 quoted earlier is contained in the word *available*. The law goes to great lengths to see that the education described will be available in the most extensive sense of the word. P.L. 94-142 was enacted partly as the consequence of a Senate committee report highly critical of the country's educational system. The report estimated that of all handicapped children in the country at that time, "two-thirds were either completely barred from the public schools or 'sitting idly in regular classrooms awaiting the time when they were old enough to drop out.'"[2]

The guarantee of availability—the insistence that handicapped children should no longer be barred from school—is the most important of the basic rights upon which the philosophy of special education rests. Educators call it *the* right to nondiscriminatory admission (or "zero reject" if they're in a hurry). In general, zero reject stipulates that no child can be excluded from public education because of a handicap. It says it's not good enough merely to allow a handicapped student to attend school if he is in *any way* excluded from participation in activities regularly available to his nonhandicapped classmates; to be allowed to be in attendance "physically"—to be admitted but not in-

2. *Summary of Existing Legislation Affecting Persons with Disabilities* (U.S. Department of Education, Office of Special Education and Rehabilitative Services, Office for Handicapped Individuals, Washington, DC, Publication No. E-88-22014, August 1988, p. 14), prepared by Robert M. Gettings, Executive Director, and Ruth E. Katz, Assistant Executive Director, of the National Association of State Mental Retardation Program Directors, Inc.

cluded—is educationally unsatisfactory and discriminatory in the eyes of the law.

To guarantee full educational availability, P.L. 94-142 makes it clear that its regulations apply to all aspects of school life, not just the purely academic. It says your handicapped child must have equal access to such normal activities as "counseling services, athletics, transportation, health services, recreational activities, [and] special interest groups or clubs sponsored by the public agency" (300.306 [b])—the whole works! And in today's world of the two-wage-earner family, don't forget early-morning and after-school day-care programs. Everything the other kids have available to them, your child should have, too.

The law also says this education shall be "free." Note that "free" does not mean you will have no costs at all, only that the special educational services part of school life will be free. You are responsible for the charges, fees, and dues that other parents have and that would apply were your child not handicapped. Note, too, that if the LEA does not supply transportation for any of its nonhandicapped population, it is not required to provide it for its disabled students unless parents can show why it is necessary—usually a note from a doctor is sufficient. Freedom from additional expense is central to the law, since services for a handicapped youngster often are expensive, and the parent who is unable to educate his child properly because of financial demands over which he has little if any control is discriminated against.

The Least Restrictive Environment

Another basic right upon which much of P.L. 94-142 rests and which has upset prior practice is the guarantee that the handicapped student will receive his education in the least restrictive environment. This means your child enjoys the right to go to school—and to be involved in everything that school means—in a setting as free of artificial limitations, as representative of the normal world, and having as few restrictions on personal freedom as possible. Such "normalcy" is essential if your child is to learn the skills that will be required of him later as a participant in adult society.

Ideally, your child will attend the neighborhood school he would go to were he not handicapped and wherever appropriate he will be assigned to a classroom *with* and participate in activities *with* non-handicapped students. The law says, "removal of handicapped children from the regular education environment [can be allowed to take place only if and when] . . . the nature or severity of the handicap is such that education in regular classes, with the use of supplementary aids and services, cannot be achieved satisfactorily" (300.550). The burden is upon the school system to see that this requirement is met. When a handicapped child is integrated into school life, he is said, in nontechnical language, to be *mainstreamed*; however, it's important to realize that nowhere in the laws is the term mainstream used, nor is it anywhere required that *all* handicapped children must be educated in regular classrooms. The only stipulation is that integration be the maximum consistent with meeting individual educational needs.

Seeing that their child is mainstreamed is, for many parents, the first skirmish in a battle that will continue until their child is no longer a child. The struggle to be treated like a human being may begin in the elementary classroom, move from there to postsecondary education, and then extend to adult life, with all its complex questions about how much mainstreaming is either possible or desirable in housing, transportation, sexuality, employment, recreation, travel, and on and on and on. This first attempt to reverse the debilitating isolation of differentness is the original link in a chain that you hope will lead toward the maximal independence of which your child is capable.

I am now convinced the interests of most people with handicaps can best be served by including them in noninstitutional environments. However, everyone involved in the integration process must be primed and ready if mainstreaming is to be successful: the handicapped student making the move, the school administrator arranging it, the teachers who are receiving and accommodating the student, and, finally, the nonhandicapped classmates who will be accepting or unfortunately perhaps rejecting their new classmate. One of your jobs as a parent is to encourage programs that promote student understanding of differentness and to insist that the school be thoughtful and thorough in its preparation.

Whatever you do, don't demand a short-order miracle. Even under ideal conditions, mainstreaming is not best, nor is it possible, for everyone. Owen, because of his many disabilities, was, is, and, in my judgment, always will be, unable to function in a completely nonrestrictive environment; it must be restrictive to some degree. Thus in his case a "restrictive" setting is a supportive necessity. Unfortunately, there are many Owens in this world; for them institutional life, or some type of protective environment, remains the most humane answer and is, even with its custodial characteristics, their own "least restrictive environment."

Individualized Education

The intent of P.L. 94-142 is to ensure that your child has an individually tailored education, one that helps him make the most of life. Educators call this desirable state "reaching one's maximal potential." Toward this end, the law requires that every special education student receive, and continue to receive as long as he is in the program, what is known as an IEP, an individualized education program. In educational jargon, both the written program (often called a "plan") that describes the program and the program itself are referred to as the IEP. The law is specific about what constitutes an acceptable IEP: It must specify in writing exactly which special education and related services are needed and how they will be provided. (The IEP is, of course, primarily concerned with the special services required *in addition* to the regular school program, but to meet least restrictive environment requirements, it should give an indication of the amount or percentage of the student's time to be spent in the regular school program.) Since it is often impossible for the school to do everything that needs to be done—and that you desperately want done—all at the same time, the IEP will determine educational priorities by deciding what must be scheduled first. The plan must describe the stage of educational development your child has achieved at the moment (his current performance level), as well as the degree to which he will be able to function in the regular school instructional programs; it must state what you hope he will be able to accomplish in both the short and long terms. Finally, the IEP must state when the program will start, how long it is expected the various services will be continued, and how the program's success is to be evaluated. (Your right as a parent to approve or disapprove of the educational placement that evolves from the IEP as well as your role in the design of the IEP itself is discussed in later chapters.)

This individualization is nothing new. Good teachers have done it since teaching began; it's one of the characteristics that makes a teacher good in the first place. What is new is that now it's required by law, and rather than just one teacher, a team of interested people is involved in the process. In a way, an IEP is an agreement between your child (with you as his representative) and the appropriate educational agency, usually the LEA. The implication underlying the law is that the regular curriculum will be changed to fit the child, and not the other way around. The IEP is, in effect, a road map describing the route your youngster will follow on his educational journey.

Three Other Important Rights

In addition to the guarantees already mentioned, three other critical rights were written into the legislation to see that it functions as intended: the rights of nondiscriminatory testing, parental participation, and due process.

Testing

The right to nondiscriminatory testing, the right to be tested in a fair, unbiased manner, guarantees that your child be given no tests that place him at a disadvantage because of his handicap. Never underestimate the importance of test results! They will influence decisions concerning eligibility, IEP development, class placement, advancement, and, for some, even graduation. They must never be misleading! Although testing is a complex business, a general understanding of the fundamentals, particularly what constitutes a good and useful test, is important for parents in their role as advocates and decision makers. Much material on testing is available; *Parents Can Understand Testing* (see Resources: Testing) provides an excellent overview, written in understandable language. Mary and I have been frustrated by our dependence upon the testing process and the conclusions that others draw from test results, since Owen has never been able to give us feedback of any kind except a primitive body language vocabulary of likes and dislikes (he's particularly good at dislikes). Down through the years, when his testing was unreliable, as it frequently was, and decisions were made on the basis of those results, we were in deep trouble and often never even knew it until it was too late. If feasible, tests should be given in your youngster's native language (no matter how much biology you know, you won't do well on a biology test if the questions are written in Russian and you can't read Russian). If your child is visually impaired, questions should be read to him. As a general principle, not just in educational testing but throughout your child's life, whenever important decisions of any kind are made affecting his future, all federally supported organizations involved in the decision-making process must see to it that he or those representing him are not disadvantaged because of communication problems. Although testing discrimination can often be caused by inadequate communication, many other factors can unfairly influence results.

An orthopedically impaired child whose mental processes are unaffected may need an extension of time to record his answers on tests measuring cognitive, and not motor, ability. And it's not realistic or fair to expect that a youngster who has spent his life in an institution will understand some concepts and relationships important in many intelligence tests; "home," "share," and "private," for example, may, unfortunately, be alien to him.

Parental Participation

The guarantee that parents will be allowed to join the professionals as equal partners places an obligation on parents to play active and constructive roles in the decision-making process. It is a responsibility for which many are unprepared. (Federal law *requires* parent participation only after the child has been found eligible for special services.) To be invited into the territory of the expert is an opportunity too good to turn down. Don't be hesitant; LEAs are directed by P.L. 94-142 to encourage, not just tolerate, parental participation. To ensure most effective participation, the law requires that LEAs notify parents of the time, place, and purpose of the IEP meeting as well as of the names of all others who will attend. This notification must be early enough so parents can make necessary preparations; every effort should be made to schedule the meeting at a mutually convenient time and place, and the LEA must furnish parents with a copy of the resulting educational plan upon request. Our LEA always made every effort to see that meetings were held at times convenient for us and that we were well informed and treated as equal participants.

If parents are unable or refuse to be on hand, their participation can sometimes be obtained by using other means of communication, such as conference telephone calls. The intent of the law is that IEP meetings be conducted without parental involvement *only* when parents have refused all efforts by the agency to involve them. Don't let this happen. It can dramatically reduce your advocacy position. It's difficult to criticize a decision in which you have refused to participate.

The educator's continuing responsibility to be clear and to see that parents understand is similar to the doctor's responsibility to his patient. It's difficult to participate if you don't understand what it is you're participating in. On the other hand, it's your responsibility as a parent to let the educator know if you're not on the same wavelength.

Parents can participate in other, more indirect ways. Although sometimes it's human to become so immersed in your child's problems that you lose sight of the forest for the trees, it often is helpful to extend your interest outward into the larger community. Fortunately, the law encourages you to do so on both the local and state levels. The state education agency (SEA) is required to conduct public hearings as it develops plans for providing special education and related services. Local agencies are also expected to offer parents the opportunity to participate in the development of the annual application for P.L. 94-142 funds. If you're interested, get in touch with your special education contact person or superintendent of schools and ask for more information— who knows, you may end up on a committee. Here is a direct way you can influence policy, change things you don't like, and encourage things you do.

Due Process

The right to equal treatment and due process, the last major principle, has its origins in the Fourteenth Amendment and guarantees that
neither you nor your child can be taken advantage of in the "process" of
seeking an educational fair deal. Due process ensures that decisions
made and actions taken affecting a handicapped child in the areas of
identification, evaluation, and educational placement—anything having to do with his acquiring a free appropriate education—are fair to
the child and those responsible for his welfare. It's as simple as that! But
remember that this right protects not only the parents but also the
school system, which is also entitled to a fair deal. Such protection is
sometimes called "procedural guarantees." Again the law is specific in
what it requires.

Several provisions were briefly touched upon earlier in connection
with other guarantees, for example, parental access to student records,
the timely notification of parents before meetings and other important
events, and the obligation of the LEA to make sure parents and/or students understand critical communications, particularly those involving
procedures that require their consent. Due process means that parents
must be "fully informed of all information relevant to the activity for
which consent is sought"; for example, they should understand their
rights and options, when and how certain decisions will be made, why
a certain action is suggested, what result is desired, what other options
may have been considered, and what consequences may result if they
refuse to consent.

Federal law, through its procedural guarantees, ensures that your
child's special education is neither interrupted nor delayed by excessive
bureaucratic delays. If there are disagreements between the LEA and
the parents, a child may not be removed from his current educational
program without mutual consent nor can he be refused initial admission to public school while disagreements are being worked out. The
law ensures that the special education process will be conducted in a
timely fashion (a phrase used to indicate reasonable promptness) by
requiring that certain actions take place within specified time limits.
For example, there should be no unreasonable delay between the time
parents have consented to an evaluation and the actual date their child
is tested, and re-evaluation must take place at least every three years.
The meeting to develop the IEP must be held within thirty days of the
evaluation, and the program agreed upon must begin immediately after
parental consent and reviewed at least annually.

Generally speaking, due process requirements influence the manner in which five general areas are handled. You should be well enough informed about your state's regulations to know if you are being treated correctly in these areas:

- Notification and informed consent
- Participation in decision making
- Treatment of privileged educational information and student records
- The right to an independent evaluation and information about where one may be obtained locally
- The opportunity to offer any complaints to your LEA regarding the conduct of the student's educational program

If you make a complaint and are dissatisfied with the results, you are entitled to have your grievance heard in a structured way, called a "due process hearing," and adjudicated, or settled. You may obtain the advice of a lawyer or some expert, and an impartial third party, acting under specific guidelines, judges whether your rights have been violated and if so what remedy must be taken. Even in this process you are guaranteed additional procedural rights. For example, you have the right to a public hearing, to reject any evidence not disclosed at least five days before the hearing, to bring your child to the hearing, to receive an exact record of the proceedings and decision (written or electronic), to face, question, and require the attendance of witnesses, and to receive what is called "timely and specific" notice of the time and location of the hearing. Finally, if you're dissatisfied with the findings and decision of the hearing officer, you have the right to appeal and ultimately to go to the civil courts. Fortunately, Mary and I never had to go that far, and I urge you if possible to work things out in a less formal and usually far more satisfactory fashion, as described in more detail in Chapter 18.

In conclusion, it's important to know and safeguard your legal rights. It can be a mistake, however, to misuse them or to view your relationship with professional educators as one-way, in which they give and you take. Remember that the school system, too, can invoke due process if staff feel the interests of the student or of the system as a whole have been violated. Although P.L. 94-142 sets forth the general outlines of due process, it leaves the details of implementing them to the various states, and there is a great deal of variation throughout the country. Consult your school's parents' manual and state and local laws and regulations to learn the details that apply to you. Positive participation on your part will further your child's education much more effectively than a series of avoidable confrontations. When you're work-

ing for your child, leave your need for ego enhancement at home. Much
mischief is caused when parents get too personally involved and view
the relationship as a contest. You may win some battles and your child
will still lose the war.

17

The Law in Operation

The Special Education Cycle

Chapter 16 looked at the laws that *should* enable a qualifying handicapped child to receive an appropriate education. It also examined the rights safeguarding the quality of this education. Does your child need special services? This chapter deals with your child's entry into the program and the contribution you as a parent can make to guarantee that this education becomes a reality.

Although the details of each state's special education plan vary slightly, the basic process follows a similar pattern nationwide and consists of a series of steps, each building logically on the one that preceded it. Although sometimes the steps may be combined, all must take place in sequence. The progression is as follows:

Step 1. **Referral**—Your child is referred for an evaluation by a qualified person who feels the youngster needs special services. These services may be requested at any time during the regular school years, and all provisions of P.L. 94-142 apply, not only to preschool children but also to older school-age youngsters. It's easy to be confused by the similarity between the terms *assessment* and *evaluation*. Although, in education, they are sometimes incorrectly used interchangeably, I use *assessment* to mean the general process of getting every bit of information possible from the widest variety of sources to provide a youngster with the best education. The term *evaluation* is more specific and refers to the process through which, in a legally prescribed manner, information is gathered to assist in determining the nature of a child's handicap, whether he qualifies for special educational services, and the development of an appropriate educational plan.

Step 2. **Evaluation**—Your child is thoroughly examined to determine his strengths, weaknesses, and individual needs.

Step 3. **Recommendation**—On the basis of the evaluation, a decision is reached about whether your child is "eligible," that is, has a handicapping condition that interferes with his ability to learn in the school's current education program and, therefore, requires special attention.

Step 4. **Program Development**—If your child is found to be eligible, an individualized education program (IEP) is drawn up.

Step 5. **Program Implementation**—Specific arrangements are made to put the program into action. In some states short-term objectives and the methods to be used to evaluate the program are decided during a second, separate phase of this step.

Step 6. **Program Review**—The IEP is re-examined and updated at least annually.

Step 7. **Triennial Evaluation**—Your child is evaluated again, at least once every three years.

There is no one time, common to all circumstances, when parents begin to consider special help for their children. Not all handicapping conditions are obvious at birth or are diagnosed during the early childhood years. Many develop or become apparent later, after a child has begun "regular" school. On the other hand, many children who have trouble in school are not really handicapped at all and end up graduating with honors. Some late bloomers even grow up to become lawyers or college presidents (although this doesn't make my point). So if one of your kids begins to experience academic or behavioral problems, don't assume the worst and immediately request a formal evaluation. An extreme reaction on your part can be counterproductive. As we have seen, each child develops at his own special rate, and there are many ways within most school systems' regular curriculum that parents and school, working together, can help a child over the natural rough spots that sometimes occur as children grow up. (As ridiculous as it may seem, perhaps even you, now a parent, had some minor trouble in school.)

Two of our children stayed back a year in school, and two required intensive, special tutoring, but all later did well in college. Shepherding six kids through their school years involved the kinds of traumatic experiences most parents have lived through but would like to forget. One of our most perplexing problems during those years was deciding which problems were serious and worthy of attention and which were just normal stages. This process became more difficult after Owen's birth, when, having seen what can happen when things go wrong, we began to run scared and, I'm afraid, have given our last daughter fits.

Mary and I did our best not to overreact, but sometimes we did. We erred once when we had one child tested for a possible learning disability and involved a friend who, coincidentally, happened to be a psychiatrist. Probably our biggest mistake was overlooking the fact that in those days many people—not just children—didn't want anything to do with psychiatrists, even friendly ones. Our daughter did not like being singled out and tested; teenagers don't like being different. The episode, which in our eyes was a conscientious precautionary action, was for her an unnecessary and unfortunate experience. Fortunately she didn't have a learning disability after all, and she eventually graduated magna cum laude from professional school. I was a headmaster at the time and supposedly a sensitive professional educator. So much for adult or expert infallibility.

One way to sort out potentially serious problems from normal developmental fits and starts is to establish close communication with the school. If you are worried and losing sleep, set up an appointment and have an informal chat with your child's teacher. Make her aware of both your concerns and your insights. A parent who is already involved in school activities—the PTA, classroom volunteering, the school board —will be more knowledgeable about academic life and routines and find interaction with administrators and teachers easier. As a consequence of normal supportive routines, your child's teacher may involve other school personnel in an attempt to find solutions, so don't be concerned if new faces appear; they're professionals, and confidentiality is part of their job. Often adjustments can be made in your child's regular school activities, such as a minor change of his schedule or class section, some tutorial help during study hall, or informal conversations with the guidance counselor or teacher with whom he enjoys a special relationship. Just knowing about your concerns and your child's out-of-school behavior may help teachers individualize his regular classroom instruction more responsively.

Keep track of these early efforts, including copies of any letters. This documentation may be helpful later if you request an evaluation and become involved in the IEP process. If your child's handicapping condition is only now becoming obvious, start keeping a notebook with a section that includes all school-related matters (see Appendix A). Particularly important will be diagnostic test results, a copy of the referral, minutes of IEP meetings, professional reports, and a notation of such important dates as when you consented to your child's evaluation. If you have a significant telephone conversation, follow it with a confirming letter and keep a copy. Everything should be dated. Undated information loses much of its value. Time and again I recall some professional looking over his glasses and asking, "And how old was Owen when that happened?"

Often as a result of school–home cooperation, solutions are found, and if you are a worrier, you can move on and concentrate your worrying on something you can get your teeth into. However, if your child continues to experience difficulties and you think he needs more attention and possibly different services from those the normal school curriculum provides, you may wish to have him included in the system's special education program. Your state education regulations set forth specific ways that such a request should be made. Many LEAs offer a brochure describing their procedures. Ask for it!

The Referral Process

The Referral (Evaluation Request)

In addition to the state's federally mandated child-find network (involved mostly with preschool children), there are ways a child can become a candidate for special services after he's enrolled in the regular school program. The process of entry into the special education program differs somewhat from state to state. Sometimes the school itself becomes concerned because of a student's performance and sets up a screening committee to consider whether the youngster's problem warrants the individualized testing of a formal evaluation. But since at this stage no special testing is involved (and legally can't be without your permission), the guarantees of P.L. 94-142 do not yet apply and the LEA is under no federal obligation to notify you that such a group is meeting. The first you may learn of the committee's existence is when you're notified that the school system recommends your child be evaluated and requests your permission for a formal evaluation. Don't rant and rave and get everybody excited. The LEA may have kept you in the dark temporarily only to spare you anxiety in the event that they decided there was no cause for concern and, therefore, no need for an evaluation. Note that federal law requires that parents *consent* to an evaluation but does not require that states allow them to *participate* in either the evaluation or the resulting eligibility decision.

On the other hand, several states on their own initiative stipulate that once a formal referral is made, the LEA must conduct an evaluation—if the parent gives consent—irrespective of whether there has been any prior screening committee action. Some states require parental notification, even participation, in the preliminary screening stage. Practice varies. Where it is allowed, I strongly recommend you participate.

Who Can Request an Evaluation?

Many people can make a referral; some are legally required to under certain circumstances. Your state regulations specify who is so authorized. However, as we have seen, federal law stipulates that parents always enjoy this right. You may ask for an evaluation, perhaps as an outgrowth of conversations with your child's teachers, when you feel attempts to correct the situation using regular school resources have proven inadequate. The school personnel involved should help you make the referral as well as explain the details of what is involved, even though they may disagree with your decision. Even if your child is not in school and you have questions about referral, contact the superintendent's office and ask for help. One of his responsibilities is to comply with federal law and to see that you are informed of and understand critical features of the education regulations. If he isn't available, his secretary should be able to clear up the matter or refer you to someone who can.

Ordinarily, all a parent needs to do is to submit a letter (it can be handwritten) containing the following points:

Superintendent's Name in full   Date
LEA Name   Your Name
LEA Address   Your Address

Dear Mr. (Mrs., Ms., Dr., etc.) _____,

I am the parent of (child's full name and age), who is a student in Grade___ at (school's name). I believe my child has special needs that can't be met by the regular school program and request that as soon as possible he/she be evaluated so that an appropriate program can be provided. [The following paragraph is optional and not a necessary part of your formal request:]

I make this request for the following reasons: (In your own words briefly describe your child's condition, explain why you feel the existing program is unsatisfactory, and what services you believe are required.)

Please let me know when this evaluation will take place.

Sincerely,

(Your Name)

cc [copy to]: Director of Special Education [if there is one]

Your state may require that you describe the handicap and how it does, or would, interfere with your child's learning. I suggest you include this information even if it's not mandatory. Don't worry; just describe the problem in your own words or ask someone at school or your doctor to help you. It will soon be important for you to learn to describe your youngster in more professional terms, and you can start here.

In states where special services are mandated for eligible students *before* the regular school years and your youngster is preschool age, call or write the superintendent, requesting an evaluation. Give the name, age, and address of your child, your reasons for concern, and whether you have had any contact with the LEA. In most instances it's a good idea to informally consult someone in the system before you write and to follow the normal child-find procedures outlined in your state's regulations. The superintendent is probably required by state law to respond to your referral letter within a certain time. Find out what that limit is, and if you don't hear from him by the time it expires, inquire about it.

It is an interesting point that, legally, even if the parent makes the referral in the first place, the LEA still must have written parental consent before the evaluation can take place. So don't get edgy if it seems that the LEA is insisting you grant permission for something you, yourself, have requested. Under the law, for consent (which is often spoken of as "advised consent") to be binding, the school system must see to it that the person being asked to give consent understands all that is involved, including possible consequences. The LEA's Request-for-Consent Form is often accompanied by a letter including such information as who referred your child, what professionals will make the evaluation, a listing of all tests to be done, and an explanation of your options. The 1985 New York State cover letter accompanying the form concluded by saying: "I [chairperson of the evaluating committee] have also attached a description of your legal rights. The description is very informative and I urge you to read it carefully. I will gladly provide you with more information if you are interested." If your request for evaluation is turned down, you must be notified in writing of the reasons for the rejection and given a full explanation of the rights you as a parent have to appeal the decision.

In the rare event that the LEA initially recommends evaluation and you refuse to consent, your child's right to go to school is in no way affected by the disagreement. However, the LEA has the right to appeal your decision, just as you have a right to challenge theirs, through due process. I strongly urge you not to challenge an evaluation request coming from your LEA. Even if you are doubtful of the advantages a special program has to offer, agreeing to an evaluation does not irrevocably commit you, for even if your child is eventually judged eligible for services and a program is recommended, you must still give permission before the first IEP can go into effect, and your ability to reject unsatisfactory educational programs is in no way diminished. In addition, many states schedule additional services to meet a child's needs even if he has been judged ineligible for special educational services. Several states forward the test results of children not currently enrolled in the LEA to those providing that child's current education program so that they can adapt their regular curriculum to reflect lessons learned through the evaluation cycle. Your child has little to lose and much to gain by an evaluation.

In an attempt to achieve wide coverage and to ensure that no handicapped child slips through the cracks and is missed, various states allow others besides the parent and the school to make a referral—for example, a doctor, a nurse, a social worker, the student himself, or perhaps any staff person in the school system. One state not only allows but also requires that "any certified (licensed) personnel working in the public school system shall (or must) refer a child if they suspect or have reason to believe that a child has an exceptional education need."[1] Other LEAs require that all new students take screening tests, the results of which may cause the school to suggest an evaluation. Many people are involved in seeing that your child has a chance at getting an even break before the decision to evaluate is finally reached. Suggestions are given later in this chapter to help you prepare for and participate in the meetings involved in the evaluation cycle.

Evaluation

What is a pre-entry or preplacement evaluation? The primary purpose of an evaluation is to determine whether your child needs to receive services. To be eligible, he must be diagnosed as having one of the handicapping conditions set forth in the law, and the impairment must be severe enough to interfere with his education. P.L. 94-142 is specific about the handicapping conditions that qualify. This attempt to make qualification requirements specific and nonsubjective is understandable and not just bureaucratic mumbo jumbo. It is easy for us, with our vested interests, to forget how others may view the hundreds of thousands of taxpayers' dollars that can be involved in one child's special educational career and the impact such expenditure may have on a school system's tight budget. According to P.L. 94-142, eligible children are those who are: "mentally retarded, hard of hearing, deaf, speech impaired, visually handicapped, seriously emotionally disturbed, orthopedically impaired, other health impaired, deaf-blind, multi-handicapped, or [have been diagnosed] as having specific learning disabilities, who because of those impairments need special education and related services" (300.5).

Complete descriptions of the qualifying handicaps are too extensive to quote here in their entirety, and will change with time as the law is amended. However, it's in your self-interest to become familiar with

1. *The EEN Triangle of Support—A Guide for Parents,* Wisconsin Department of Public Instruction, Bulletin 4294, revised Feb. 1984, p. 5.

the technicalities involved in the referral and evaluation process, since it's your child being evaluated.

The law describes the "evaluation" as those "procedures used to determine whether a child is handicapped and the nature and extent of the special education and related services that the child needs." Specifically, the term means "procedures used selectively with an individual child and does not include basic tests administered to or procedures used with all children in a school grade or class" (300.500 [c]). The school staff may conduct subsequent evaluations more frequently than every three years if they think it is necessary, and your consent is not required after the initial placement, although you must be notified (I believe it's highly unlikely they would act in opposition to your desires).

In a formal evaluation, more than one test must be used to develop an educational plan or placement, and the evaluation must be made by a group of professionals who include at least one teacher or specialist in the area of suspected disability. All tests, sometimes called "instruments" or "procedures," should be selected to reflect true aptitude or achievement in one specific area and not to be discriminatory—influenced by a handicap in another area. One final requirement is that the evaluation must consider the child "in *all* areas related to the suspected disability, including, where appropriate, health, vision, hearing, social and emotional status, general intelligence, academic performance, communicative status, and motor abilities" (300.532[f]). This is consistent with the approach of looking at the total child.

An often overlooked evaluation goal is to determine the factors that are affecting the child's school performance; sometimes other forces unrelated to the handicapping condition are found to be involved and may be corrected. Even if special services are not authorized, the evaluation can be of real value, since information gained can help a youngster's current classroom teachers modify or adjust his regular program to better meet his needs.

We all have probably heard some variation of the story about the "profoundly retarded" child who after years of institutionalization was discovered to be hearing impaired and not retarded at all. That's the stuff from which nightmares are made; unfortunately, mistakes do happen, and in my life as an educator I have been personally involved in a few of them. We never realized our own son had little tactile sensation until he was almost six. This lack of sensitivity explains his need for extreme and sometimes bizarre stimulation in other areas. Today a complete examination should pick up this type of condition much earlier.

The law stresses the importance of incorporating a child's strengths in the development of his special education, and there's a lesson to be learned here by all who work with handicapped children. It's easy to overlook a child's strong points and to become preoccupied with his deficits, thereby missing the opportunity to build his future on the things he *can* do. Never sell your child short. Owen's fine-motor coordination is excellent and has made some sheltered workshop activity possible that otherwise would have been out of the question (such work activities, discussed in Chapter 22, can be—but unfortunately seldom are—an escape hatch to the normal world). Owen's sense of humor and wonderful disposition (real strengths) have pulled all of us through difficult moments and made him a welcome member in every community in which he's lived.

Eligibility

The Eligibility Decision

Federal law does not specify the exact procedures that states must use to determine if a child is to receive special educational services. Procedures used must follow the law's protective guidelines (previously discussed) and result in a fair decision. (Due process protects you and your child if you feel your rights have been violated.) In most instances the eligibility decision is made by a committee, which follows guidelines set forth by state regulations and makes the decision primarily on the basis of the child's evaluation. In some states the committee consists of the same people who conducted the original evaluation.

The decision-making group goes under different names in various states. Some, logically enough, are called "eligibility committees," and I use this designation. Since parental participation depends on state regulations, you cannot necessarily insist on being included. In some SEAs parents can attend the entire meeting and present their views, and in others they are barred from the final decision-making session. Irrespective of your state's regulations, I suggest you ask permission to attend, to provide your input into the discussion. But remember, you're a guest of the committee and have everything to gain by being courteous and positive. If you can't attend, you almost certainly can submit a written statement outlining your position.

The eligibility committee addresses three critical issues: (1) Does your child qualify for special education? (2) What is his handicapping condition? (3) What special education and related services are needed to provide him with an appropriate education?

If the eligibility committee decides that your child's condition is not serious enough to warrant special education or even if it agrees that he is eligible but names a handicapping condition that differs from your understanding, you can appeal. For example, the state may identify the primary problem as mental retardation, while you are convinced that it is an obvious case of learning disability. You may say, "What does it matter what handicap the committee arrives at, just as long as it gets your child into the program?" *It* can make a profound difference. Correct identification is essential, since the IEP evolves directly from the identification and legally no service can be provided for a handicap not identified. Occasionally the committee has difficulty deciding which of a number of conditions is the primary educational problem. In such a case the committee has the option of ruling that the child's eligibility is based on the multihandicap category, thus giving the program maximal flexibility. I urge you to campaign for this option if it is at all possible.

Once the committee has decided which handicapping condition is to be the one "of record," I suggest you ask for a concise definition in lay language. This articulation may not only help clarify the situation in your own mind but also give you some indication of how clearly the evaluators themselves see the picture.

How the Committee Determines Eligibility

In theory the work of the eligibility committee is quite straightforward. In practice it can be exquisitely complicated. It sounds easy. All the committee has to do is examine the evaluation and any information included in your child's school file, determine whether he has one of the qualifying handicaps, and, if so, judge whether it adversely affects his educational performance. But any veteran parent knows the pitfalls between even a well-intentioned committee judgment and a straightforward, definitive answer. (Remember the joke that a camel is a horse designed by a committee?)

If your child's handicap is severe and has textbook symptoms, you can feel safe. However, in situations in which the diagnosis is complex or borderline, as is the case with Owie, parental monitoring during all stages of the process is absolutely essential, since an inappropriate diagnosis can have unfortunate educational consequences. In the case of diagnostic ambiguity, the committee should be even more inclined to welcome parental participation. In some instances involving a rare syndrome, Mom and Dad may actually know more about the condition than the committee's professionals, and parental input can and often should be decisive.

Involvement in the eligibility process offers you the opportunity to gain another perspective and to see your child through the eyes of the school staff responsible for his education. Don't be so anxious to change their opinions that you miss the chance to expand your own understanding. If you are eventually forced to negotiate differences between your views of what is best for your child and theirs, it's vital that you see the existing conflicts as clearly and objectively as possible.

Once the evaluation has been completed, many LEAs hold a conference with you to explain the results; this may be unnecessary if you attended the proceedings, although you may have further questions. Now is the time to be sure you understand what is to come! Due process grants you the right to receive a copy of the evaluation report if you want. Study it. An understanding of both the evaluation's findings and the conclusions drawn from them is important if you are to make an informed decision whether to accept the evaluation or to ask for an independent evaluation and if you are to participate effectively when your child's IEP and subsequent educational placement are drawn up.

If you disagree with the committee's eligibility ruling, you have three alternatives:

First, even if the committee decides your child does not qualify for special education services, it may suggest how the regular curriculum can be adapted to meet his needs, and this may satisfy you—at least for the moment. You may find that because of the attention that has been focused on your child's situation, he will continue to receive unofficial special attention.

Second, you can work informally with the LEA, hoping for a reversal. Ask them to add new material to the file as it becomes available after the meeting or to eliminate material that you find unacceptable or inaccurate but that you didn't challenge at the time. It's possible that once you have discussed the decision with school officials, their answers will satisfy your objections. Or they could eventually reverse themselves.

The third option is to seek an independent evaluation. P.L. 94-142 allows a parent to obtain a second evaluation, at public expense (under certain conditions), from a "qualified examiner who is not employed by the public school responsible" (300.503 [a]). Under some circumstances you might exercise this option before the eligibility decision. The LEA, on its part, can object through a due process hearing if it feels an additional evaluation is unnecessary. If "the final decision [of the hearing] is that the [original] evaluation is appropriate, the parent still has the right to an independent educational evaluation but not at public expense" (300.503 [b]).

The decision to ask for a second opinion at either public or your own expense is not simple. Your state regulations outline the steps required, and I recommend that you ask for an explanation of all the details, particularly the question of how the evaluator is to be selected. You have to form your own judgment whether he is sympathetic to your point of view and, what can be more important, whether school officials will be favorably influenced by the results or antagonized by what they see as an attempt to go over their heads. Might an adversarial feeling cause them to disregard the results of the new evaluation, no matter how favorable it is to your cause? Since the results of a publicly funded evaluation are made part of your child's formal evaluation with or without your approval, it might make more sense to pay for the evaluation yourself if you can. You may then select the evaluators yourself and decide whether to make the results available to the school. There are so many unknowns in this option that I suggest you request financial assistance only if you have particular confidence in your case.

It is entirely possible that the committee will decide your child is not to receive special education services even though the evaluation is competent and irrespective of whether it is privately or publicly conducted. If so, you may appeal the eligibility decision itself through due process appeal procedures. The mechanics of doing this are discussed in Chapter 18.

If you are able to participate, you can take certain steps to prepare for and to be effective at the various meetings, where you may be the star witness. (Many of these recommendations are general and apply to all group meetings that you are involved in, so refer to this list when other types of meetings are discussed in later chapters.) Since so much of your success in working with other people depends upon common sense and courtesy, several of these points have already been made in discussing meetings with individual professionals. However, preparing for group decision making with a committee involves many additional and fundamentally different relationships. Here, then, are general observations and recommendations Mary and I have found helpful. Down through the years some of them have saved us from bouts of insecurity the night before the meeting, when, after the other kids were put to bed, we sat together and talked about the next day. Since circumstances vary, you may find some points helpful and will certainly discard others as being inappropriate to the situation or just not your style. Fine, use what makes sense to you.

First, a few observations about general approach: *Listen* and let others have their say. I have found two productive ways to present questions and concerns. One is to mention them to the group (always in a positive way) at the beginning by saying something to the effect that your personal goal for the meeting is to be able to end up at adjournment time with the answers to the following questions that are important to you, your child, and your family—and then spell them out. Another approach, the one that has worked for me, is to write our concerns down the evening before. Be sure you or your partner checks them off during the session as they are covered. Find out from the chairman how long he expects the meeting to last. Then, pace yourself and before adjournment bring up any topics not covered.

I favor seeking maximal informality consistent with protecting your child's interests, believing that it's counterproductive to arrive at the meeting armed with a tape recorder, a professional consultant, a list of demands, and an aggressive attitude that will certainly impress the school people—but not necessarily in the right way. I have experienced better results with a quiet, positive approach that attempts to cover all questions of importance, that encourages the making, and recording, of critical decisions, and a free, honest, and complete exchange of information.

No matter what your approach, differences of opinion can and often do arise. If that happens, try to keep yourself below the boiling point by remembering that if a member of either side loses his "cool," your child, who spends more waking hours at school than at home, will probably be the one to suffer the consequences. If, despite your best intentions, you are afraid you may lose your cool, request a temporary recess or request that the meeting be adjourned and rescheduled. I have never found this rather unusual step necessary, nor do I expect you will, but people *are* human, and it's easier to tell someone not to lose his cool than it is to keep your own.

How you respond to the environment of a relatively formal meeting will depend upon your experience and temperament. Many find it a positive challenge, an opportunity to meet new people, to participate in a different world. A meeting can be interesting and fun. On the other hand, you may find it difficult to function well in a setting where you feel overpowered or intimidated. Some parents find it helpful to have an informal get-together with the chairperson before the formal meeting or to have someone on the IEP team whom they know. If there is a staff member at school or a therapist out of school, for instance, whom you feel knows both you and your child, ask the chairperson if that individual could be included in the meeting. You, of course, can and should have someone there to support you—your spouse or, if you are a single parent, a friend, but a friend who is familiar with your child.

Several parents' groups publish materials providing tips to make you more effective at crucial meetings. Some suggest that parents become more professional themselves by attending assertiveness-training sessions, or that they take several deep breaths before beginning to speak (I find this advice has amusing potential, particularly if everyone sitting around the conference table were to practice it simultaneously). In no way do I underestimate the importance of being assertive. It's critical that you be a persistent advocate for your child and stick to your guns on his behalf when you feel you are right, and there are ways in which this can be done that are effective and yet upbeat and courteous. Little is gained by being confrontational. I have found most school people are almost as interested in your child's welfare as you are, and welcome a cooperative attitude.

Now that we have considered general approaches, let's look at more specific things you can do to become an effective meeting participant, no matter what the topic:

1. Prepare yourself. Get a special education parents' handbook from your LEA or SEA if available. Find out if the state advocate or a local parents' association publishes material specifically designed to help parents prepare for the subject you're concerned with at that particular meeting. Publications of this kind abound and go under such names as "Checklists," "Parent Fact Sheets," "Action Charts," and "Organizers." You should be able to locate one. Use it to augment the suggestions contained in this book. I recommend you digest the material in a checklist-type brochure before the meeting, however. I found that trying to keep track of where I was while checking off multiple columns of "do this but never do that" variety distracted my attention from the important issues of the meeting.

2. Contact the chairperson before the meeting date and double-check on its time and location (you should have received a notice). Find out who will attend, including descriptions of their school duties and meeting responsibilities. Another approach to help you keep track of who is who is to ask if you can pass around a sign-up sheet; it should be of assistance in matching up faces with names. The chairperson may make introductions as part of his first order of business, at which time you can introduce your guest(s), if any. In the event you're introduced, you may want to comment on how you look forward to working with the team. Some parents find tape recording helpful (clear this with the chairperson); I don't.

If an agenda has not been sent out, ask the chairperson what subjects will be discussed, what decisions will be made, and whether minutes will be kept and distributed. Tell the chairperson if you wish to distribute material and ask how and when he prefers it be done. Mention any particular topics *you* would like discussed so they can be included in his agenda.

3. Ask if a body of rules governs the conduct of the meeting, so you will know what to expect and how to act: for instance, how will decisions be made—by vote or by consensus? Will there be a specific adjournment time? If you have any official requests to make—perhaps you want a meeting date postponed because of an emergency in the

family—be sure to go through the chairperson and not "step on toes" by speaking informally with a friend on the faculty. Protocol can be important to some people.

4. Discuss the meeting with both your partner and, if appropriate, your child, covering the important issues involved and your reactions to them. Try to work out any important intrafamily differences before the meeting to present a united front.

5. Attend *every* meeting that affects your child, and be prompt. Don't arrive late, breathless, and disorganized; it can get things off to a bad start. If you can, arrive early. This way you'll have a chance to break the ice, to meet those you don't know, informally, and to introduce your guest personally. If possible, mother and father should go together. Parents can provide mutual support and divvy up duties so that when one is speaking, the other can take notes (dual attendance will also be an indication to the committee of your seriousness).

6. Although this point may be controversial, I suggest you dress as though you were going to the bank to apply for a mortgage. A single-parent friend insists that committees, which are usually dressed in professional attire, respond more receptively to her when she wears a nice dress than when she appears in jeans and T-shirt. I realize appearances shouldn't affect attitudes, but sometimes they do.

7. Unless it's obviously inappropriate, take your youngster with you. After all, he's the one you're all talking about; and if he's over eighteen and he's competent, he has a legal right to be there. Some suggest taking a child only if he can understand what's going on and is mature enough to participate in a meaningful manner. This is a judgment call on your part. I believe that a handicapped child, even a silent one like Owie, can be his own best spokesperson. If his attendance is impossible, make sure every member of the evaluation team, including administrators, meets him. Owen almost always went along despite the fact he couldn't participate. I'm convinced it was helpful for the committee to see him in person; I'm also convinced it would have been difficult at the first meeting for them to have found him ineligible after having had personal contact. On the other hand, certainly don't bring him along if it might upset or embarrass him. Owie loves crowds and doesn't often get embarrassed.

8. Always come prepared, with your "homework" done. Know both the general background and the specific facts concerning the matters to be discussed; this will require some effort. At *every* meeting you should be as up to date as possible on your child's situation, which in most instances involves reviewing the in-depth inventory you prepared for the evaluation stage. You may feel more comfortable if you

have your notebook along to refer to if necessary; however, it's probably more effective to make brief notes of vital facts you have organized
and want to remember and take them along instead.

9. Make sure the committee understands the impact that the
handicap has on your entire family. The total involvement of all family
members can easily be overlooked or underestimated.

10. Bear in mind the purposes of the meeting and your objectives,
and do what you can, tactfully, to keep the meeting from adjourning
before the necessary decisions have been reached and your questions
answered.

11. Finally, find out when the next meeting will be and, if appropriate, thank the committee.

The Evaluation: Preparing for a Specific Meeting—an Extension of These Eleven Recommendations

Most meetings are called for a certain purpose, or at least will have
one agenda item of primary significance. At sessions involving the
screening/evaluation cycle, you need to know the answers to certain
basic questions: Who asked for the evaluation, and why? What procedures will be used, what timetable followed, what tests given? (As we
have seen, the LEA is required by P.L. 94-142 to explain the nature of
the evaluation to you, *including all tests to be given,* when asking you to
sign the consent form. Often an explanation is part of the form itself.)
You have a responsibility to supply information, and at this particular
meeting you will make a real contribution by ensuring the information
describing your child is accurate and complete.

Information usually comes from three sources: you, the parent; the
perceptions of school staff, whether drawn from the records or their
own experiences with your child; and school records, including test results and former evaluations, if any. Since much information may be
available only through you, and since incorrect material currently in
school files may also be identified and corrected only through you, your
testimony is crucial. Your preparation for these meetings, therefore,
should center more on collecting and corroborating this material than
on running through a checklist of things to do and points to cover. At
many future meetings you will need to repeat or update the background
information gathered at this time, but it will be more easily accomplished then if the job you do *now* is comprehensive and correct.

Your efforts in preparation for this meeting will pay dividends
when you help draw up the resulting IEP or at the due process hearing if
your referral is rejected and you decide to appeal. The time you have
available and your built-in record-keeping tolerance will determine
your own particular approach. There is no best way for everyone, but

leaving a lifetime of dates and experiences to spontaneous recall is al-most sure to be ineffectual, particularly during the excitement of the meeting. Playing something by ear often means playing it poorly.

Help the Committee Understand Your Child

If you have little free time, the least-involved preparation is to write down randomly the characteristics of your youngster that you feel are important: things your youngster does, doesn't do, or does poorly that give you serious concern or that please you. Organize and reinforce your points with specific examples from his past. Educators call them "anecdotal records." (The profile described in Appendix A is one way to keep such information for the future.)

A second approach, a bit more time-consuming, is to contact the evaluation chairperson or your friend on the committee. Ask what types of information are of particular interest to the committee (for in-stance, examples of how your child interacts with his peers); write down his suggestions and then, referring to your notebook, try to re-capture both facts and memories that fill in the gaps between the writ-ten record the committee has available and your personal experiences. If you can translate these cold facts into a picture of the warm child you know—who is more than a collection of dates, test results, and evalua-tions—you will, in my opinion, have done your job.

A third and much more involved approach is to observe your child for measured periods of time under controlled conditions. Record what you see, covering such areas as communication, interaction with others, and mental or physical development, including hearing, eyesight, and senses of smell, touch, and taste.

You may have insights into his self-concept, how he feels about himself. His teacher, guidance counselor, or school psychologist should be able to provide help in this area. Observe his agility, thinking skills, and learning style. Does he learn about something most easily by read-ing about it, by having it explained, by looking at a picture of it? Does he appear most comfortable and learn best in a group, by himself, with the radio blaring, or when it's completely quiet? Does he seem to be most responsive when he moves about the room or when he sits motionless?

Many LEAs ask parents to complete a questionnaire before the screening/evaluation meeting; it's sometimes called a "Case History Form." If one is used in your system, look it over. It can give you ideas about what the committee feels is important and the kinds of informa-tion you should brush up on. These observations require thought, orga-nization, and discipline, in addition to considerable time. I wouldn't suggest attempting such a program without some professional guidance or, at the very least, the use of reference materials. The book *Negotiating the Special Education Maze* (see Resources: Education) includes an extensive section on observing your child that will be helpful to anyone wishing to do a more comprehensive job and looking for a structure in which to do it. (This approach would be too difficult for me to handle successfully.)

Learn from Others Who Know Your Child

Another way to update yourself is to communicate. Sit down and talk with your child; although this is often not possible, sometimes parents give up too soon. His school is another obvious and effective source of information. Speak with your child's teachers or other staff members who know your youngster, such as the school nurse, social worker, and guidance counselor. In all your academic dealings, now and in the future, be familiar with the routines expected of *all* parents and, except in emergencies, observe them scrupulously. Your LEA's parents' manual probably contains visiting procedures. There is no surer way to get off on the wrong foot than to wander unannounced around school halls with your notebook under one arm and state regulations under the other, grabbing unwary teachers as they hurry by on the way to class. On the other hand, don't be apologetic; most teachers understand and will be receptive if you're considerate.

Speak in Ways the Educators Can Understand

Make sure you'll have an opportunity to describe your child to the committee. I'm sure you'll find committee members genuinely interested in what you have to say, but you will be much more effective if you communicate in language they find useful. Educators, being professionals, are accustomed to and in most cases are required to deal in facts and controlled observation, not impressions or incomplete recollections. The conclusions they reach concerning your youngster—whether he should be evaluated, the nature of the evaluation, whether he will receive special educational services—must be based as much as possible on specifics, because their reports must be written in specifics. Avoid such comments as, "My Johnny didn't turn over till he was almost one-and-a-half—or was it two? Let me think. Of course I had to help him a little bit to get him started rolling. But now that I think about it, it might have been Tom who had the turning-over problem and not Johnny at all."

One way I found to communicate effectively with professionals is to report your personal comments or observations in concrete terms, addressing the traditional questions of what, where, when, how, who, and why. For example, Owie's bizarre mannerisms are a cause for concern to us. At an evaluation meeting Mary or I might describe them to professionals in this way:

QUESTION: What is it that bothers you about your child?

ANSWER: Owie's crazy way of jumping around. Our son will bend slightly over toward his right side, raise both arms in the air and flap one or both hands with his fingers rigid and extended. He'll bend his knees slightly, tense his entire body, screw up his face, and thrust out his jaw. Then he'll open his mouth as wide as possible, skewing it dramatically to one side, and make an intermittent, high-pitched noise.

QUESTION: Where is this behavior apt to take place?

ANSWER: Almost anywhere he encounters excessive stimulation from light or sound.

QUESTION: When is it most apt to happen?

ANSWER: He's been subject to this stylized mannerism from early childhood—beginning as well as I can remember around age two. Although I haven't been able to detect any pattern, he is definitely more susceptible at some times than at others.

QUESTION: How does he conduct this rather unusual performance?

ANSWER: Owen always carries on this performance with complete absorption and apparent delight.

QUESTION: Who is involved?

ANSWER: Obviously Owen, either by himself or in the company of any interested onlookers who happen to be passing by. But I'm convinced he doesn't do it to draw a response from onlookers.

QUESTION: Why does he do it?

ANSWER: That's what I would like to know.

Looking at Your Child's Record

Take advantage of the guarantees of the Buckley Amendment (described in detail in Chapter 16) and inspect all your child's records to see that they are complete and accurate. Check them against your notebook information and ask to see your LEA's policy on record keeping so that you will know how to look at all the applicable material on file. You will be particularly interested in finding out:

- What kind of information is kept on your child and where it is filed
- What you must do to see your child's records and how you can make copies
- What you can do if you believe there are inaccuracies
- Who has access to this material
- If there is any information that is not available to you
- How long records will be kept

Make an appointment in advance to examine records, don't just show up, unannounced, at the superintendent's office. Since many records are stored in locked, confidential files, a secretary will probably have to be taken from her regular duties to see that your needs are met.

You may want to find out if the committee plans to consider any material not currently in school files. If so, ask to see what is to be added, and, of course, check it for completeness and accuracy. I never found this to be necessary and would not advise it unless you have experienced problems in the past. On the other hand, if you have information you feel is pertinent, including professional reports or records of which the school is unaware, be sure to ask that these items be considered at the meeting and offer the committee a chance to look them over beforehand.

This can be an important point, since it's not at all uncommon for parents to have received evaluations, many of them done before the school years by nonschool sources, which might shed light on a child's condition. If the LEA refuses to admit such material, which is unlikely, ask for a letter explaining the reasons for that decision. Later, if the committee eventually decides your child is ineligible and you decide to appeal, the letter will be useful. Remember that the purpose of the due process provision is not to offer you the opportunity to be an obstructionist but to ensure that the screening/evaluation process is conducted fairly and expeditiously.

In conclusion, the evaluation cycle can, one way or another, have positive implications for your child. Even if he is found to be ineligible, he is still entitled to all the benefits of a regular public school education, and much of value to you and your child should have been learned by this interplay of experts. I'm confident that the system works; if everything realistically possible has been done to ensure your child's best interests, he will be admitted to the special education program. Then the important work of drawing up his IEP begins.

18

The Individualized Education Program

I'll learn him or kill him.—Mark Twain
(He was probably trying to explain a federal law to someone.)

If, at the conclusion of the evaluation, your child is ruled to be eligible for special educational services, the next step is the construction of a program to meet his needs. To be effective this program must have its roots in, and grow out of, the initial evaluation. The job of ensuring its effectiveness is the responsibility of a special team of which you are a member. The team goes by different names in various states: special education evaluation/placement team, pupil evaluation team (PET), child study evaluation team, school-based admissions and release team, admissions and release team, M (multidisciplinary) team, and so on. For consistency, I'll call it the IEP team.

Federal law is specific about the IEP team's membership, which as a minimum consists of the following:

- Your youngster's teacher (if there's more than one, the state may specify who will participate).
- One or both parents.
- The child himself, if appropriate (you have to be the judge—if there's a question, include him).
- Someone from the school (in addition to the child's teacher) with authority to see that the services agreed upon are provided.
- Other individuals (guests) at the discretion of the parents and/or school system; if this is your youngster's first placement, a member of the evaluation team or some staff member familiar with the results of the eligibility evaluation and procedures used. Guests are just that—guests—and, in effect, are included through the courtesy of the regular membership (having too many guests can be counterproductive). They are in no way official committee members.

As a normal administrative routine, the LEA will appoint the chairperson of the IEP team (often the administrator on the team; for us, frequently, it was the principal). Find out the chairperson's name, his position, and how he can be contacted.

Previous chapters briefly described the IEP process as required by federal law. Now let's examine it in more detail. Many lessons you have already learned regarding preparation for meetings with professionals are applicable here. Since each state enjoys some leeway in its procedures to meet federal requirements, familiarize yourself with what is mandated in your school district. Refer to the descriptive and checklist materials mentioned in the chapter on evaluation. So armed, and with the help of this book—you should be ready to get to work.

In addition to furnishing crucial background information, you will be a central figure in the committee's deliberations in another way. Before its educational plan can be put into action, you must consent by signing what is sometimes called a "placement permission form," a written indication that the IEP meets with your approval. This authority, which gives you a kind of veto power over team decisions, is a wonderful safeguard; it is also a heavy responsibility, for such power, if exercised without careful thought, can adversely affect many people. Committee members may be chagrined, but *they* can forget it by suppertime. The damage it may do your child can last much longer.

As a member of the team you will help design your child's final plan. If the program proves to be a poor one or you unreasonably withhold consent to approve a good one, you bear partial responsibility. Some states are flexible and provide for a preliminary period during which a new program is tried out. Even if such an option doesn't exist in your state, you always have the right to withdraw your youngster from special education services later, if you think it is in his best interests, so you really are completely protected.

To prepare intelligently, think through the purpose of the first IEP meeting and the details of what should—and legally must—be included. The meeting is held to discuss the evaluation report and from it and other available materials to develop a plan. This is the first of what probably will be many IEPs, which, if properly done, will result in a constantly evolving, flexible program that changes as both your child and circumstances change.

If the IEP is to be successful, you and your new colleagues must:

- Give each team member an opportunity to become familiar with your child's strengths and weaknesses and with the general recommendations of the evaluation committee.
- Examine and give priority to his total educational needs.
- Set preliminary short-term objectives and general goals.

- Consider the most effective ways to teach your youngster, and set forth *all* the services needed to provide this instruction.
- Examine all the instructional and placement possibilities and arrive at recommendations for an overall IEP. (In some instances, setting specific objectives and making final program design and placement recommendations require a second meeting, and the special education program may not begin until the complete IEP is drawn up.)

Chapter 17 described in detail the seven minimal ingredients of an acceptable IEP (state law may add to this list). In brief, it must contain the educational and support services necessary to provide a special and individualized program based upon short-term objectives and long-term goals, integrated as much as possible into the mainstream of school life and designed to provide for continuing program evaluation. (That's a mouthful!) To function effectively as a team member, you should understand the implications of these requirements and their effect on your expectations *for* and participation *in* the IEP.

How You Can Influence Details of the Plan

The IEP Must Be Individualized

When the law says the IEP must be "special," it means the program differs from, and to some degree is outside of, the regular school curriculum. For example, a student who must walk with braces because of an orthopedic problem might be included in regular (nonspecial) school activities for most of his school day and need an IEP and its special attention only for adaptive physical education.

When the law says the IEP must be individualized, it means the plan considers and prescribes for each student separately and individually, apart from any group program. Such individualization is required not only in academics but also in other areas: perhaps in social adjustment, vocational training, health education, and adaptive behavior (how successfully your child is able to adjust to different circumstances). Don't expect that individualization guarantees one-on-one instruction—it doesn't. But do keep in mind that the focus of the IEP meeting is on your child as a worthwhile "somebody" who is significantly different from all the other "somebodies." Your job is to insist he's viewed not as a collection of disabilities but as an individual with a personality and many normal needs and desires.

The IEP Must Be as Nonrestrictive (Normal) as Possible

In apparent contrast to the insistence upon *specialness* that sets special education apart from the normal school curriculum, the IEP must meet the special needs of the student within an environment that has as few restrictions as are appropriate—in other words, an environment as normal as possible. Toward this end the program must contain a statement describing how much the student will be able to participate in regular activities with his nonhandicapped peers, both in the classroom and in nonacademic activities. Your job is to remind the committee that, if possible, your child should not be perpetually surrounded by handicapped people, staff that minister to only the disabled, and equipment that is peculiar to the disabled. Remind them that if the committee has "tunnel-vision" and is afraid to let your child take a chance and spread his wings, the eventual effect on his physical development and self-image will be predictably destructive. One of the committee's many jobs is to see that along with the appropriate education, large breaths of fresh air from the outside world are allowed to come into your child's life.

The potential destructiveness of segregation is what the framers of P.L. 94-142 feared when they stressed the least restrictive environment. At every stage of program development you should push for as much normalcy as is consistent with your child's ability to cope. In IEP meetings see that priority is given to scheduling normal student experiences into your child's program, including both academic and extracurricular activities. During the primary-school years integration is more naturally oriented around classroom-centered activities, and a great deal of its success will depend upon the initiative and originality of the teachers. Ask the teacher representative on the IEP team how he feels integration opportunities can best be offered at your child's age and level of functioning. As your child grows older, or if he is entering special education at a later stage in school life and this is his first IEP, ask such critical questions as Will he be able to go to the cafeteria? (Join a club? Work in the shop? Attend an athletic contest? Go to a dance?) It should be your job to see that at the appropriate time your child's IEP takes into consideration his prevocational and vocational education needs. If possible, his program should work progressively toward the time when he will move on from school into the "outside world." Often too little of this necessary preparation is done. The skill development required for this transition—described in Part Five—can and should be anticipated in your child's curriculum at an appropriate time. In short, the IEP should be optimistic and wherever possible plan for a more normal tomorrow—a least restrictive environment.

The IEP Must Determine Your Child's Current Level of Functioning

The program must include a description of present levels of functioning. To set goals for your child or even to begin to think about evaluating program or student progress is impossible unless a starting point, a frame of reference, is determined. To develop plans for your child's future, you must know where he started. This determination serves the same function as pretesting does in the normal academic program. And the description of present levels of *total educational performance* must be based on evaluations in all areas and be more than just a listing of test results.

The committee determines your child's current status by studying the recently completed evaluation and any other earlier individualized testing that might have been done; by questioning, in detail, the committee member present who participated in the initial evaluation; by taking advantage of your observations as a parent; and, finally, by examining school records. As discussed in earlier chapters, the ways that you can gather information describing your child and effectively present it to the committee are applicable here.

The IEP Must Set Goals and Evaluate the Program

P.L. 94-142 requires that the IEP contain a listing of annual goals —statements describing what your youngster can realistically be expected to accomplish within the year in his special education program. To decide on the areas needing particular attention and/or remediation, the committee must examine the student's strengths and weaknesses and assign priorities to those skills it feels most urgently need attention.

Goals are general, and often between five and ten are involved in a typical IEP, although the number required is affected by the severity of the handicap. A typical goal might be: "By next June we hope Owen will be able to assume complete responsibility for his personal appearance and hygiene; the criteria for goal completion will be 80 percent." This means that the goal can be considered to have been met when at least 80 percent of the intermediary steps required to reach that goal have been satisfactorily accomplished.

Goals are ordinarily set for twelve-month periods that coincide with the annual evaluation cycle. Sometimes this is as far into the future as parents and staff are able to look (particularly with a young child), although as later chapters point out, general and far longer-term goalsetting related to the child's transition to the outside world *must* eventually be part of the committee's thinking as it plans future IEPs. Many handicapped students are unprepared because goals were set too late.

Mary and I learned the hard way that exquisite care must be taken when you attempt to look into the future, especially when prediction of ultimate placement in society is involved. For most handicapped children some kind of independent functioning is both realistic and a natural outgrowth of a succession of least restrictive environments, and it should be aggressively planned for. If that avenue is not open, however, and ultimate independence of any kind is out of the question, don't live on unrealistic expectations. Instead, bend your energies to building the best sheltered life possible for your child, and don't spend a lifetime feeling guilty or frustrated. One of the most difficult decisions required of a parent is determining what future is realistically possible for his child and establishing the long-term goals resulting from that decision. Set your goals high, but temper enthusiasm with realism.

Besides being at the very heart of the process to build an effective educational program, establishing realistic goals is also the key to evaluating both the effectiveness of that program and whether the placement and services originally written into the IEP were and still are appropriate. To evaluate program effectiveness, you must answer two additional questions. The committee must know not only where your youngster is functioning at the moment but also whether he is headed in the right direction to reach his overall goal and whether he's making satisfactory progress toward that goal. For example (exaggerating to make a point), if at the end of a year *not one* of the many goals in your child's IEP has been met, you could not escape the conclusion that something has gone dramatically wrong either in program planning or in execution and that immediate changes are in order. The LEA should and probably will use sophisticated evaluative techniques to examine your child's rate of goal completion and translate what it learns into appropriate adjustments in the program. Ask your special education contact person to explain how the evaluation process works.

The intermediate steps required to reach the IEP's annual goals, called short-term instructional objectives, are specific statements describing the timelines (schedule) and the progress, or changes in behavior, you hope your child will make in the short term—often in the next two to three months. For each goal, one or more objectives should be listed in the IEP. Since objectives form the basis for day-to-day program evaluation and will be constantly referred to later, it's important they be clearly stated and commonly understood by all IEP members. In working toward our hypothetical goal of complete hygienic independence for Owen, the objectives would be something like this:

- Owen will remember to button or zip up his pants before he leaves the bathroom (failure to meet this criterion has embarrassed me and disconcerted passers-by, but left Owen unconcerned).

- He will learn to tie his shoes in the morning without assistance.
- He will be able to take a shower and master the following skills: control the cold/hot water faucets, wash himself (covering most areas of his body), rinse off, refrain from dropping the soap on the bottom of the shower stall and leaving it there, hang up his towel after drying off, and put on his clothes before leaving the shower area.

These skills are, of course, nonacademic and apply to a residential school program, but they are typical of basic life skills that are of deep concern to parents. For many handicapped children, survival or living skills are just as important as academic skills—and often must be mastered before the academic skills can or should be attempted. Your job is to help the educators develop objectives that are realistic in terms of your child's abilities and future needs *and* to help the professionals by reinforcing these skills when your child is with you at home. Often the parent's role as a partner and reinforcer of the child's school activities is overlooked or poorly handled. Be sure that the school realizes the extent of your ability to help out when your child is not at school and takes advantage of this potential without overloading you.

It's also your job to help the IEP team evaluate program success by providing out-of-school observations about how your youngster is progressing toward his intermediary objectives and general goals. Make an effort to provide this information to the IEP committee in the specific and objective terms, discussed previously, which are so important in parent–professional dialogue.

The timelines for objectives must be set forth in the IEP. They say, in effect, "This is the skill our son should be able to learn and *this* is when he should be able to have it satisfactorily mastered." Timelines may be included both in the IEP as objectives are set forth, and later when program evaluation is discussed. For example, "Owen will learn to handle his toothbrush by January 15th, will be able to hang up his shower towel by the end of March, and will master his clothes-buttoning skills by April 1st."

The IEP Must List Specific Special Education and Related Services

It's especially important to anticipate and include all special services involved, since an LEA is obligated neither to provide nor to fund anything not set forth in the plan (unless it is part of the regular school program). Services left out of the IEP may, from a budgetary point of view, be difficult or impossible for the system to provide later. (Have you ever seen what school committees go through to add to their budget once it has been approved?) Join with the professionals in seeing that the plan is all-inclusive. Don't forget such important considerations as special transportation arrangements and, particularly, summer camp or tutorial help if necessary. In September it's easy to forget the problems that may arise in July and August.

Although P.L. 94-142 doesn't specifically require a twelve-month program, your LEA may consider including summer educational services in the IEP if a child's special education will suffer significantly because of the break in continuity caused by prolonged vacations. States vary in their response to this question. Such factors as the type and severity of the handicap, concern that the student might harm himself or others if left unsupervised, and, of course, the costs involved can enter into the decision.

My advice is that you request that such continuing special coverage be included if you believe it would benefit your youngster, but try to get substantiating professional opinions and carefully document your case. Our school system granted our request and paid for Owen's summer tuition on the basis that he would lose too much of the advantage he had gained during the regular school year if skills learned weren't continuously reinforced. It was a lifesaver for both him and our family.

The description of included services *must* be specific and in such detail as to allow for no misunderstanding. Unnecessary vagueness can be cause for future friction. Now is the time to hammer out the details. For example, here is one way to avoid misunderstandings:

Each week at school Owen will receive:

- Five 20-minute sessions of speech therapy.
- Instruction in math, language arts, and living skills in the resource room (60 percent of classroom time).
- Three 40-minute periods of special adaptive physical education. *(Never underestimate the value of proper exercise for your child. It can dramatically improve his functioning and overall health.)*
- Instruction in music and art in the regular classroom (15 percent of classroom time).
- Special transportation providing pickup and return every regular school day.
- Three 40-minute sessions of physical therapy. (Your LEA may require that certain related services, such as various therapies, be incorporated into the IEP only on the basis of professional recommendation. To avoid problems and possible delays, ask that a physical therapy "consultation" be written into the plan if that is the service needed. If the therapist, after examination, thinks such therapy service is warranted, it can then be incorporated into the IEP. At the initial meeting find out what, if any, services fall into this category in your district.)

Federal law requires that the dates when services are to begin and their expected duration be included in the IEP and, although perhaps not available at the first meeting, be included before placement can be made. For instance, the IEP might say, "Both physical and speech therapy will begin September 20th and last until the end of the first semester; all other activities will start at the beginning of the school year and, unless the committee is reconvened and the LEA changed, will continue until the end of the school year."

Now is a good time, when you have a complete listing of all the services your child will receive, to stand back for a minute and look at the program as a whole. See if it makes sense with all the pieces put together. Does it satisfy all the concerns raised in the preceding pages? Take some time. At the meeting don't be embarrassed to ask the chairperson for "just a few minutes to review the overall picture." He shouldn't object. Probably other committee members can use these few moments to equally good advantage. Your child's daily schedule, with details like the names of teachers and classroom location, may not be available at this time and is not required as a part of the IEP. However, ask that this information be sent to you as soon as it's available.

The Placement Decision

The most critical decisions you make during your child's school years will involve placement—the nature and location of the program in which he will be "placed." This decision should be based on his educational, physical, and behavioral needs, satisfied in the least restrictive environment. I suggest that your attitude during this critical initial IEP meeting be that the lack of available services within an LEA must in no way limit the IEP. It's quite the contrary, according to the law. The services needed to provide an appropriate education must be arrived at first, and only later are ways found to furnish these services. If they are not available locally, they must be acquired somehow, somewhere— perhaps through an out-of-district arrangement. Locating the appropriate services is the responsibility of the LEA. Owen was covered by special education until he was twenty-one, and never once was it possible to place him within his local system.

Educational placement should come as a natural outgrowth of goals set and services needed. Although the IEP is *not* in any sense a detailed lesson plan, teachers should build their daily classroom activities as a normal outgrowth of the IEP's goals and objectives and resulting placement, since both an IEP and a lesson plan are reflections of student needs. If this natural relationship doesn't evolve, something is fundamentally wrong and should become quickly evident when you compare goals with program implementation.

In many instances, your child's needs will be met at the same public school he normally would have attended on the basis of your home's location. There, depending upon the severity of his problem, he may be scheduled in a variety of classroom settings. In general, if his handicap is not severe, he is apt to attend a homeroom along with his nonhandicapped peers, participate in the regular school curriculum, and receive appropriate supportive services on an individually scheduled basis—perhaps in what is called a resource room. To qualify for resource-room placement, however, students must spend more than half the academic day in normal school activities. If a child's disability is extreme, his placement may be with other handicapped youngsters in a classroom (they come in infinite variety, depending upon the LEA's approach) where he spends all or a significant part of the day receiving instruction specialized to meet the needs of handicapped youngsters who have a common level of functioning. (In addition, your child may be pulled out of class for the individualized services prescribed in his IEP, such as speech therapy.) This classroom is often described as "self-contained" since most of its needed resources are contained in the classroom and integration into the regular school curriculum is limited.

If the school nearest home is unable to offer these services, or if other circumstances warrant, your child can be placed, with your permission, in one of the following: a regular or special public school within your LEA that is better able to provide special services; a program offered by another LEA or a consortium of LEAs for which services your system has paid tuition; an appropriate private day or residential school; a special hospital program or a state residential program offering the sought-after educational curricula.

If it becomes necessary for a student to be sent outside the local educational authority, the ultimate responsibility for developing and supervising his education program remains with his home system. And the home system must see to it that a representative of the outside institution participates in the IEP meeting when it first decides on such outside placement, either by being present at the meeting or through telephone or some other kind of communication.

Once a child is placed in such a program, representatives of the new institution may initiate and conduct meetings to review or revise the IEP—a reasonable provision, since the program and its staff may be located at a considerable distance from the local area. The meeting, however, is held at the discretion of the LEA, since it retains the responsibility for seeing that the parents and one of its own representatives attend. In short, although there is flexibility in the practical day-to-day administration of a student's education program in outside placement, the LEA cannot be absolved from the ultimate responsibility for a handicapped child's appropriate education and compliance with the law, no matter where his education takes place, as long as it is at public expense.

Preparing for the IEP Meeting Where Placement Is Decided

Now that we've seen what must be accomplished by the IEP meeting, let's look at ways to make your participation effective. In preparing for the IEP cycle it is helpful to break the process down into two interrelated categories: first, the general approaches and attitudes that affect the whole business, and second, the specific, almost mechanical things you can do to ensure thoroughness (that is, the necessary details to check on, the points to remember, the questions to ask).

The first, or general, category can be summarized in a few short words: be thorough in preparation, flexible of mind, specific in approach, and cooperative in attitude. It's vital that you go into this meeting knowing the territory. Be thorough! This book and the material you collected in the preliminary evaluative stage should give you all the information you need to help you describe your child to the committee and to understand both the process and the rights you enjoy in the planning process. Mastering the material should be only a matter of review.

If you have not yet committed such background material to memory, begin to do so now by reviewing a number of materials: the complete material on your child that you prepared during the evaluation stage, the final evaluation report, the report of the eligibility committee, and the form your state uses to write up the IEP. This review should give you an overview and help you understand what options are available, what decisions must be made, and what information you need to supply.

I'm convinced you accomplish more if you can acquire the flexibility that comes from exposure to other interpretations and opinions. I know Mary and I tended to be the most rigid and least effective when we were most uncertain or frightened. Before the meeting, speak informally with someone in the school system about the IEP process as it is practiced in your LEA and as it pertains to your child in particular. Ideally it should be someone who will participate in the IEP process and with whom you have already established contact and a comfortable relationship. Much of practical value may be gained by such a meeting. You can get an indication of the kinds of decisions that will be made at the meeting and see them presented through another's eyes, and you won't be taken by surprise at the meeting.

Since your child's placement may have far-reaching implications and affect others, you'll want to talk over the oncoming meeting with your entire family or with a close friend if you are a single parent or guardian. If your child can communicate, find out what particular things concern him, what he likes to do, and what he finds difficult. Listen to what he says. It's important to know how he feels about school, his teacher, his friends, you, and the family.

It is particularly important that you do as much intrafamilial collective thinking *before* the meeting as possible. Some subjects you will face may be controversial "hot topics"—the possibility of institutionalizing your youngster, for example, can really stir things up. It is preferable, although not always possible, for a father and mother to iron out their disagreements beforehand rather than to show signs of family discord at the meeting. If you are taken by surprise at the meeting, the chairperson will probably allow you to excuse yourselves for a brief time to speak confidentially with each other. This can, however, be awkward, and I suggest you ask for such a courtesy only in unusual circumstances.

Most issues you will encounter at the IEP meeting can be anticipated, and careful planning should protect you from having to make quick decisions. Here are some things to think about as you do this planning.

Some Pre-IEP-Meeting Suggestions

1. Discuss with the chairperson of the IEP meeting any preparations for the meeting that would involve school visitation or discussions with staff or with other parents of children currently in the school.

2. Find out, through either the chairperson or a friend on the committee, possible placements for your youngster and what kinds of information concerning your child the committee might find of interest. The contribution you can make to the committee's understanding of your child will probably involve much the same preparation as was the case during the evaluation cycle.

3. Visit possible placements to see them in action. Walk through the physical plant. See if there are any real or potential problems involving access to necessary facilities, any barriers you should discuss with the IEP committee. Your youngster has had enough problems without adding access problems to the list. Remember Section 504?

4. If you have any concerns, make an appointment to discuss evaluation results with the chairperson of the evaluation committee, particularly if you have concerns about the committee's decision about the classification of your child's handicap and its implication for placement and programming.

5. Since this is such an important meeting, you should consider having a kind of dress rehearsal the night before with your spouse or guest at which you discuss the various issues that may arise and your response to them. Review this chapter to refresh your memory on the points that must be covered.

6. Think through the critical points about which you should have specific ideas, for example: What are the skills you feel your child needs now or will need in the future? What do you feel your youngster is currently missing in the school curriculum? How do you feel about mainstreaming—do you want as much or as little as possible? Are there specific goals or placements you find particularly acceptable or unacceptable?

7. Since transportation can present problems, be sure you understand how it is handled in your LEA, paying particular attention to accessibility of vehicles, other children involved, total time committed, and arrangements for the return trip. Little things are important. Does the driver make sure the parent is at home before dropping off the severely handicapped child? Talk with the system's transportation coordinator, and maybe even take a look at, or ride on, the equipment involved. (If it's appropriate and possible, arrange some of your own transportation to allow your child to participate in after-school activities if school transportation is unsatisfactory. This may require coordination with other special parents.)

Seven Suggestions for the IEP Meeting Itself

1. When services are listed, be sure you understand the answers to the six "W" questions: *Who* will provide the service, *what* will the service consist of, *where* will it be provided, *when* will it be provided, *why* will it be provided, and *what* are the hoped-for results? You may be particularly interested in the way the program or school handles such things as behavior problems and rewards and punishments. If you are dissatisfied with any of the answers, speak up, particularly if you think the skills to be worked on are unrealistic or inappropriate. With Owen the educators occasionally became so preoccupied with the strictly academic component that they overlooked the necessary living skills that make a least restrictive environment possible.

2. Be sure you understand in exact detail how you and your spouse can work at home with your youngster, but don't take on too much, and be prepared to adjust the home activities to reflect your experience and endurance. It does no one any good if you overdo and the entire family suffers as a consequence.

3. Inquire if special equipment or materials will be used, and, if so, ask that they be described.

4. Establish your communication network with the school. Find out who will be your contact person and when you can expect follow-up communications about your child's progress. Discuss how that contact will be made: by letter, phone call, or personal conference at school? Would a home visit be necessary?

5. Find out who on the committee will take care of any loose ends that must be seen to before the next meeting, particularly the things that might interfere with the initiation of the IEP.

6. Before the meeting adjourns, find out when the IEP will be reviewed and if a copy of the IEP and minutes of the meeting will be sent you (if so, keep both for your records). At a later meeting, you may feel the IEP can benefit from a re-examination, even if it is informal, before the annual review required by law. Remember that you, as a parent, can call an IEP meeting if you think it is necessary.

7. Under no circumstances should you sign a placement consent form (or any consent form) that you don't understand or feel comfortable with. Don't feel pressured; the LEA must give you time to think over the decision carefully. The exact amount of time will probably be contained in your state regulations. The LEA should be flexible and not stand on formality. Again, your child can't be deprived of his program because of a delay of any kind and must be allowed to continue his current placement until a new IEP is drawn up and accepted.

Five Post-IEP-Meeting Suggestions

1. Ask to have selected samples of your child's work sent home so you can follow his progress and better coordinate your own supportive efforts.

2. Take the initiative. If your child's teacher hasn't contacted you after a reasonable period, call him and begin the communications process that must be ongoing. Keep the teacher advised of significant events at home that may affect your child's classroom behavior. If the IEP is for a next-year placement, see if your child can meet his new teacher before school begins.

3. If you feel your child is not making progress in the schoolwork that you are reinforcing at home or in the life skills that the classroom is concentrating on and that you have the opportunity to observe in the home setting, notify your child's teacher. Give him specific examples.

4. If you have time, become a classroom volunteer. You could be particularly helpful because of your experience with special youngsters. Ask if the LEA has a volunteer coordinator.

5. Join the parent–teacher organization. Consider forming a sub-group of parents with exceptional children; however, you could be more effective by remaining a part of the regular group and offering them your insights and perspectives.

Due Process: What to Do If You Can't Work Things Out

No matter how well-intentioned or reasonable parents or school systems are, occasionally differences arise. Usually such problems, like most honest disagreements, can be worked out informally, and this is invariably the best way. However, when the two sides are unable to reach an agreement, federal law on due process provides general rules, and many states offer specific regulations, for how these disagreements are to be settled. However, the law does not cover all possible causes of conflict—only those rights and responsibilities that are specifically identified in federal and state law as being central to a handicapped child's guaranteed right to a free appropriate education. The other complaints not covered must be worked out by parents of the handicapped as best they can with school administrators—just as other parents in the general school population must do.

Some conflicts due process does *not* cover, many of which are considered to be the legitimate decision-making province of the LEA, are listed below.

- You have a personality clash with a teacher and want your child moved to another class, but the school won't agree to the change.
- You ask that a particular textbook be used for your child, but the school insists on using another manual, which, although you don't like it, is accepted by many professionals.
- You wish to speed up the special education process so it fits in better with your vacation plans, but the LEA will not accelerate its procedures to shorter periods than the maximal limits required by law.
- You don't like the director of special education who attends your child's IEP meeting as an official LEA representative, but the school refuses to replace him.
- You want to attend your youngster's eligibility meeting, but the LEA says, "No, neither state nor federal laws require it and this is not the way we do things." (You can, however, ask for a hearing if you disagree with the decision reached at that meeting.)

Although P.L. 94-142 sets forth the general outlines of due process, it leaves the details of implementing them to the states, and there is variation from location to location. Consult your local parents' manuals and state and local laws and regulations to learn the details that apply to you.

Alternative Ways to Settle Problems

Due process can be expensive, time-consuming, and frustrating. Luckily some states offer alternatives when parents and school have reached an apparent impasse. If your state sanctions any alternative to the formal appeal process, it should be described in the regulations.

One approach sometimes offered by state regulation is a "conciliatory conference" or "administrative review." It is a process in which other people (third parties) not involved in the disagreement are brought in to listen to the dispute and try to settle it voluntarily, although some states stipulate that the decision be binding on the LEA. Sometimes the third party can be a school department employee, and occasionally local regulations offer or prescribe a review by the superintendent of schools and then, if that fails, a hearing by the local school board.

Some states have built a "mediation" process into their regulations. Mediation is similar to the conciliatory conference in that an impartial third party, often professionally trained, brings together the two disagreeing parties and, by placing the conflict in a new perspective and perhaps a more objective framework, attempts to promote compromise, new understanding, and agreement. The suggestions of a mediator are, by definition, nonbinding; he is a conciliator and not a dictator. The state may also ask for mediation but mediation may not be used to deny or delay a parent's rights. *A Guide to Mediation of Special Education Problems,* by Judith Raskin (see Resources: Advocacy), is a helpful book on this subject published by a first-rate parents' organization, the Parent Information Center of Concord, New Hampshire.

In some states in which mediation is not required and the alternative problem-solving procedures are not prescribed, independent organizations offer services. When it looks like tempers might flare, ask your LEA what conciliatory services are available. Your state advocate should be your best source of information and support in this area. He should be able to get you a brochure describing alternatives. (See Chapter 24 on advocacy.)

I recommend mediation or any nonlegalistic process that brings people together and keeps them talking. As soon as the formal courtroom-type setting is introduced, a new dimension is bound to creep into the picture, and alternatives that avoid seeking legal advice are much cheaper. On the other hand, mediation, being noncompulsory, is apt to work better when both sides have some flexibility left and have not worked themselves into an intractable lather. For this reason, don't wait until you are as mad as a wet hen before considering mediation. It's difficult to mediate if everyone is shouting!

The Due Process Hearing

When all informal efforts have failed and progress has ground to a halt, a parent may ask in writing for an impartial due process hearing. (The school has the same right of appeal as you, but if it does appeal, you must be informed of its action. The school can appeal your decision not to allow the evaluation of your child, your request for a free evaluation, or your refusal to accept an educational placement.) The entire appeal process, the outcome of which is based primarily on facts, is one more reason why you should keep good records in a well-maintained notebook.

If you reach the point at which you're convinced that formal appeal is the only solution, your letter requesting a due process hearing can be modeled on the following letter (but changed to reflect the nature of your complaint):

(date)   (your name)
                                          (your address)
                                          (your phone number)

Mr./Ms. _____ (person in charge of special education)
(LEA's name and address)

Dear _____ :
    I am the parent of _____ , age _____ , who is currently a student in the __th grade at _____ School.
    The special education staff and I have discussed my child's proposed placement and have been unable to reach an agreement. As a result, I am requesting that a hearing be scheduled before an impartial hearing officer so that I can present my point of view and request a decision on _____'s placement.

Sincerely,
(Your name)
(copy to the superintendent of schools)

Once parents are engaged in a formal appeal, they have a number of procedural guarantees:
    1. Your LEA must inform you of any free or low-cost legal services locally available.

2. The hearing cannot be conducted by an employee of the school system or anyone else who has a conflict of interest. Usually a number of specially qualified impartial professionals are identified in each state to serve as hearing officers; check your local regulation.

3. You may "be accompanied and advised by a lawyer or by individuals with special knowledge or training with respect to the problems of handicapped children."

4. You may "present evidence and confront, cross-examine, and compel the attendance of witnesses."

5. The introduction of any evidence at the hearing that has not been discussed with you at least five days before the hearing will not be allowed.

6. You may obtain a written or electronic verbatim record of the hearing.

7. You may have your child present and request that the hearing be open to the public.

8. You will receive findings of fact and the decisions reached by the hearing officer no later than forty-five days after you made your original request for a hearing. Basically, the decision will either uphold the action that was taken or that is proposed to be taken, or direct that certain specific changes be made to bring the action at issue into line with the law.

9. If you are dissatisfied with the results, you may appeal the decision to the state education agency. Check with your state's regulations about procedures, but beware: the law will undoubtedly stipulate a time limit after which, if no appeal is made, the decision becomes final.

The state agency, as a result of your appeal, will conduct a due process review, examine the record, see that the previous procedures were consistent with the requirements of due process, seek additional evidence if necessary, "afford the parties an opportunity for oral or written argument or both at the discretion of the reviewing official," and reach an independent decision on completion of the review thirty days after you have appealed unless an extension is granted. You will receive a copy of that decision, which is final unless you bring civil action against the LEA in either state or federal district court. In addition to the rights granted you under P.L. 94-142, Section 504 of the Rehabilitation Act of 1973 allows educational decisions to be appealed to the Office for Civil Rights of the U.S. Department of Education. Consult your state advocate's office or the American Civil Liberties Union if you want additional information.

In summation, whether you resort to due process is a very personal decision with many persuasive arguments on both sides. The advantages are that:

- You are assured of a fair hearing.
- A definite decision will eventually be reached.
- Your grievances, as you see them, will be aired in public if you so desire.
- If you are satisfied with the current placement of your child, he will remain there until the final and last appeal is answered.

The disadvantages are that:

- Much time and, almost certainly, money will be spent. Although you will not be responsible for the direct costs of the hearing, you may incur travel and legal expenses.
- If your child has been found eligible for special education but you are appealing a school decision concerning the nature of your youngster's qualifying handicap, or his placement, your child will be forced to remain in his current placement during the appeal process. If this is an unsatisfactory placement, the delay could negatively affect his education.
- Your relationship with the LEA may become strained and could make future working arrangements difficult.

Although it's always good to know what to do if worst comes to worst, if you're like the great majority of parents, you will never have need for due process, and you and your new partner, the LEA, will together design a first-rate education plan for your child.

19

The Special Education System

How Special Educational Services Are Provided

A public educational system exists to serve everybody, and everybody seems to complain about it at one time or another. Everybody who has a child is an expert; quite a few who don't have children are, too. At every town meeting around tax time in my part of New England, you can hear those who tell you in great detail why the educational system isn't worth the money or why special education, in particular, isn't worth the money. Parents of handicapped children know better; they should attend more town meetings, or if they don't have town meetings in their part of the country, at least they should fire off an occasional, thoughtful letter, explaining why education in a democracy has got to be an education that meets the needs of *all* the citizens. As your youngster begins his formal education, you should become familiar with how the local system works so it can work well for you.

The Structure

Your state will have its own details of operation and will vigorously defend its right to be different, but, in general every state has an organization responsible for educating its children, often called the State Education Department, with a commissioner in charge and a section responsible for special education. The states' legislative bodies, usually called legislatures, decide in general how the schools shall be run: how many school days are required per year, at what ages students are required to attend school, how teachers are certified, and so on. These regulations, sometimes called school law, are supervised and enforced by the State Department of Education under the general direction of a State Board of Education, appointed by either the governor or the legislature. To carry out the day-to-day work of educating students, each state is divided into divisions—the local educational agencies (LEAs)—which are locally controlled by school committees or boards of education.

Different states form their LEAs differently, some by combining them with city or county geographic subdivisions already established, others by establishing new subdivisions drawn up solely for LEAs. They go by many names: school districts, systems, administrative districts, and so on. If you are a newcomer to an area, find out what district you are in by asking your neighbor or by contacting your reference librarian, municipal office, or nearby public school. All LEAs have one person in charge, usually called the superintendent of schools. His office is the natural starting point when you make your first educational contact, since he or his secretary should be able to answer questions or to direct you to people who can.

Although the details of how your education system is organized may not seem important, you should know certain facts: the name and phone number of your local LEA and its superintendent, the person in charge of special education, the chairperson and members of your school committee, and the phone number of the Special Education Division of the State Department of Education. Administrators' decisions are not absolute but in the final analysis are controlled by the citizens of the state through their local boards of control or the state legislature. In some important matters, as we have seen, you can appeal a decision to a higher authority.

The Educators

The superintendent of the LEA in which you reside, whether you rent or own your home, usually identifies one person in charge of special education, often called the special education director. In large systems, special education may be an assistant superintendent's sole responsibility. In small LEAs the responsibility could fall to a resource-room teacher or some other staff member. Sometimes a school principal is assigned the role. Still, your local superintendent of schools must bear ultimate local responsibility, just as the commissioner of the State Department of Education can't avoid overall responsibility for all special education in his state.

Find out who the special ed director is in your school. Under his direction, staff members will help design your child's IEP and put it into action. Some of the specialists involved may be familiar to you from your child's preschool years, such as the physical and occupational therapist, the speech clinician or pathologist, the psychological examiner, the psychologist, the audiologist, and the social worker. Added to these old friends may now be teachers who have training in special areas. Their titles vary from state to state; their specialty areas include: special education, the educable mentally retarded (EMR), learning disabilities, the emotionally handicapped, the trainable mentally retarded (TMR), resource room, and services to exceptional children. Large systems employ these people as full-time staff members, and smaller LEAs sometimes retain them on a part-time basis. Special education specialists may work only in one building or travel around the system, in which case they are called "itinerant" teachers; they may even make hospital or home calls.

As a safeguard to guarantee minimal competency, all states require some kind of special education certification, indicating that certain minimal requirements of training and experience have been met. Become familiar with the certification requirements for those who are involved with your child. Since in many states special education teachers are scarce or too expensive for tight budgets, it's possible some uncertified instructors may be used to "fill in temporarily." Inquire in a courteous fashion about the educational background of your youngster's teachers. Certification does not guarantee that a teacher will be good, but a good teacher who is certified, too, is just that much better.

One person who frequently occupies a key role for parents is rarely mentioned in official publications. This is the secretary to the Special Education Department. Get on his good side as quickly as possible. He sets up appointments, makes schedules, and usually has the rare gift of being able to explain things so that you can understand them. He remembers names, and generally knows more about what is going on than anybody else. He seems to know things first and forget them last.

Instructional Approaches

To be a key mover in your child's IEP planning, you must be familiar with the basic educational approaches and terminology currently used. Although practices vary across our country, and names for similar practices may differ from one location to the next, here are a few techniques you may encounter in your travels.[1]

The Self-Contained Classroom

This approach generally represents a most restrictive school environment, where students with similar levels of functioning share the same segregated classroom, usually for more than 50 percent of the school day. In this program, even if your child is severely handicapped with no apparent hope of any kind of eventual independent living, see that as many of his activities as possible, regular and extracurricular, are integrated into the school's mainstream. So that this program is not completely isolated within the school, many LEAs include shop, home

---

1. For some of the information in this section I have drawn upon *Programming for Secondary Age Handicapped Students*, Division of Special Education, Department of Education and Cultural Services, State of Maine, November 1981.

economics, art, and other basic courses from the regular curriculum in the handicapped students' basic courses.

One fringe benefit of involving handicapped youngsters in the regular curriculum is that faculty and administrators not normally involved with handicapped students are drawn into the picture, thus adding diversity and new role models to the students' program while widening teachers' horizons. Although, today, Owen can't function independently, he still derives pleasure and relief from boredom by frequent forays into the world, which wouldn't be possible if it hadn't been for earlier efforts at school to familiarize him with that world.

If your child is in a self-contained classroom, be sure the performance levels of his classmates are similar enough to make it possible for the teacher to develop an educational plan that has relevance for the entire class and does not neglect children on both ends of the ability scale. (No matter how good the teacher, he can't give individualized instruction to a classroom of children with widely diverse needs.) The best way to see if the class is appropriate is to visit before your child is placed.

The Resource Room

This facility, familiar to us from the elementary years, can be particularly effective in secondary transition education because of its flexibility. It should be a room where a whole variety of resources are coordinated. Community experiences, speakers, trips, and projects can be an integral part of its daily activities. Students can operate in the integrated environment of a regular homeroom and use the resource room only for the special services the IEP calls for. It can function as a center for guidance counseling, special classes (such as crisis solving), special tutoring, team teaching, and sex education. Finally, the resource room can act as a halfway house between the school and community-based programs, where practical living skills can be tried out as students move back and forth between the school and the outside world.

Consulting Teacher Programs

In these programs, special education students attend a regular classroom on an ongoing basis while receiving minimal special assistance from their regular teachers, who in turn receive support from specialists, sometimes called "consulting teachers." This is one of the least restrictive alternatives available to special education students. For this program to be successful, however, the consulting teacher must be accepted by other teachers as a knowledgeable, competent source of advice. The classroom teacher involved must be willing to entertain suggestions and to adapt his own classroom programs. Finally, school administrators must be sufficiently committed to the program to provide teachers with planning time and the materials required, so that individualized programs can actually be put into effect.

Alternative Learning Programs

The term *alternative education* often refers to any program apart from and significantly different from the regular curriculum. This flexible approach is best suited to students whose handicap is relatively mild or behavioral in nature, and inappropriate attitudes stand in the way of achievement. The concept behind this approach, which stresses close student–teacher relationships, is to change the student's attitudes and behavior, promote his feelings of self-worth, and develop both social and academic skills. Close counseling must be maintained and joint teacher/student—and even parent—participation is encouraged in the goal-setting process. Although the program is alternative, it is structured, and progress should be evaluated regularly, as in any other program. The success of the program is *particularly* dependent on the support of school staff, parents, and the taxpaying public, who may feel, because the program is nontraditional, that it is somehow less effective and rigorous than the regular classroom instruction we all remember. The support of the general public is especially critical, since separately allocated funding may require citizen support at school budget time, and participating students will often be involved in very visible out-of-school locations as part of their alternative programs.

In view of the lack of success of traditional programs, creative approaches that offer new ways of solving old problems should be welcome. Just be sure you have confidence in the teacher, understand what the school is attempting to accomplish, and find out how and when progress will be evaluated. The program should be located in some space set apart from the traditional classroom setting. (Owen once followed a farmer around his barns and helped him feed the animals as part of his alternative program. He got dirty, smelled bad, and enjoyed his most successful "academic" experience ever.) Teachers must be flexible and highly motivated to spend the time necessary to meet the unique and often demanding needs of the students.

Curriculum and Materials

Providing a program of studies for handicapped students—that is, deciding the kinds of things students are expected to learn, the times they are supposed to learn them, and the materials and teaching devices and methods to be used—presents problems not encountered in the regular program of studies, which is usually geared to a group of students with relatively common needs and abilities. Instruction for the disabled student, on the other hand, must grow out of the IEP, which emphasizes not group instruction but specially designed plans for each individual child. Handicapped students are often unique, and what is good and appropriate for your child at a particular time frequently is not suitable for others. How does a school prepare to meet the needs of thousands of IEPs as yet unwritten?

The challenge of special education is to build a flexible network of available services within a school system, a kind of arsenal from which any particular IEP can be drawn to put together an acceptable overall plan. This service network often consists of the use of a combination of the following approaches:

1. Regular school classes and materials, if possible (the more, the better, if they meet the child's educational needs, since this approach offers the potential for eventual integration in the least restrictive environment).

2. The regular curriculum *adapted* by a special education teacher to meet the needs of a particular child or other handicapped children, who individually or as a group could benefit from this instruction and would eventually be able to enter the mainstream curriculum from which the course was adapted. Insist that attention be paid to sex education in whatever fashion and at whatever age is individually appropriate. This part of the curriculum has often been overlooked (see Chapter 25).

3. Special courses in no way related to the regular school curriculum, designed for special students who as a group or individually need to learn certain skills or attitudes. (Part Five considers curricula dealing specifically with the transition to the adult world.)

4. The various therapies required to remove physical and emotional barriers to learning. The physical or occupational therapist, the psychologist, and other specialists utilize their professional skills to meet the child's individual needs on a one-to-one basis.

Many school systems have written their own programs, sometimes called syllabuses, for groups of handicapped children with similar needs. Often their goal is to help the student build skills needed to become self-sufficient in personal care or to enter the job market. A few words of caution: Be sure, if it is suggested that your child be placed in a homogeneous class of handicapped children, particularly if the class has a label, such as TMR (trainable mentally retarded) or EMR (educable mentally retarded), that you find out all the details about that class —its goals, its techniques—before you agree. Visit a class, talk to parents, and be sure the program furthers your child's goals. Insist that your IEP, even at the elementary-school level, has long-term goals somewhere in view and that the self-contained class is a step toward that goal.

In the past, some special education curricula have been seen as ends in themselves and resulted in a holding pattern; the description of the program sounded great but the youngsters never made any real progress. To be specific, don't let your child's program remain exclusively academic. Owen worked on letters and numbers for ten years, and a whole succession of teachers, with obvious satisfaction, showed us how our son could now multiply 2 times 2 or copy the letters O-W-E-N. Our enthusiasm, however, was dampened early on, when it became apparent that Owen hadn't the foggiest idea what the symbols meant and couldn't care less.

In contrast, take a clear fall morning. Give Owen some nails to drive into a pine plank, and an 18' × 20' shed to build. Pull a cloth cap sporting a yellow Caterpillar Tractor emblem on his head. Tie a carpenter's belt around his waist and he's in seventh heaven. Forget that the hat's too big and falls down over his eyes or that he doesn't always hit the nail with the hammer (neither do I). He's doing something he likes to do and that he can do, and each time he does it, he seems to get a little better and, maybe, a tiny bit better coordinated.

Special educators would nod in apparent agreement when I asked that Owen be given more work-type experiences so he could learn to do something he enjoyed doing in the outside world, but the next time we came to parents' night we would be shown the same old "2 times 2" worksheets. I believe we made a serious mistake in being too nice and not eventually saying, in effect, "You professionals have had your turn to plan my son's curriculum. Now it's my turn, and I would like—no, I insist—that he receive some practical prevocational experience." The IEP process gives you the leverage to see that this happens.

Some national publishing houses have produced special education curricula, and you should be familiar with these materials if they are to be used with your child. You may be able to help with lessons at home. It is equally important for you to become familiar with the techniques of instruction recommended for use in your child's area of disability, whether or not that technique is used locally. If Mary and I had been more aware of the curriculum for deaf children, we would have known that certain options in sign language existed that, if attempted earlier, might have made it possible for Owen to communicate with some minimal effectiveness. We didn't begin learning the technical side of special curricula until late in the game. (See *The Silent Garden* in Resources: Disability; Hearing.) We had left such decisions exclusively to the experts, which, in retrospect, was a mistake. Our reluctance to get more involved in Owen's curriculum probably sprang more from our feelings of inadequacy and awe of the professional than from any laziness.

Special Services Offered away from Your School

Many systems can't furnish the broad range of services required to meet all possible needs. As a result, students—with parents' approval —can be sent ("tuitioned out"), on a full-day or part-time basis, to a program run by some other organization, public or private. It may be a special developmental kindergarten or a program for autistic children, a state school for hearing disabled children, or a cerebral palsy or muscular dystrophy center. Our family struggled through Owie's early education years before P.L. 94-142 was a reality. As a consequence of having no LEA to help out and arrange for programing (not to mention financing), we moved our family from state to state and from city to city, rather than moving Owie. Even when the education laws came into being, our son's needs were so unusual that his curriculum became a potpourri of programs. His evaluation's statement of needs was enough to ruin the day of all but the most intrepid special education director.

Sometimes, often in a rural area, a group of school systems band together into what is called a consortium. Together, they offer special programs with specialized staff and equipment housed at a central location—programs that one system would find economically unfeasible on its own. And in many high schools students leave the classroom to go into the community and participate in various volunteer or work programs to gain experience in the outside world (see Chapter 21). All of these out-of-school activities should involve no expense to the parent, including transportation, provided each one is included in the child's IEP.

The advantages of moving your child to a more specialized facility are obvious, and usually the move is in his best interests. However, you should be aware of the disadvantages of some programs. Think them over and discuss them at your IEP meeting if you feel they are a problem. For instance, will the placement constitute a more restrictive environment, grouping your child with other handicapped children? If so, do other opportunities for him to mix with nonhandicapped kids back at the "sending" school compensate? (This was never a concern with us, for Owen really couldn't cope with a normal peer group. When he was younger, other kids his age would ignore him as soon as they learned he wouldn't respond and play their games. Later, his contemporaries proved too much of a challenge to him, and except within the family group, he would withdraw and watch quietly from a distance or turn his back and gaze off into space at something we have never been able to identify.)

If long-distance commuting is necessary, it's important to know if bus transportation is arranged that puts the least strain on your child and that is efficiently scheduled so as to save time for other, less specialized activities back at the regular "sending" school, such as art, music, and dance. If the program is a full-day activity, take maximal advantage of opportunities available at home during nonschool hours to expose your youngster to his nonhandicapped peer group through church youth groups, Scouts, camp, and so forth. More and more, on the elementary-school level, teachers have developed techniques for involving special students in the mainstream of classroom life, and these approaches are even taught at some colleges and universities. For instance, friends can be assigned and games played that stress interaction between youngsters rather than individual, parallel play or competition.

In unusual circumstances, a residential placement may be decided upon. Such action, often a last resort, is usually arrived at reluctantly by both school and parents. It is expensive, works counter to the concept of least restrictive environment, and, at least for the moment, breaks up the family. Be sure to find out beforehand whether the school system will pay for both direct educational charges *and* residential fees, or only the educational charges. For Owie, the 24-hour supervision and the structured living of residential life are a necessary part of his educational experience without which his education suffers. This interdependence between classroom and living arrangements is true of many youngsters who are forced to live in institutions, and many parents can argue convincingly for complete coverage of charges. (For us it was a bitter, wrenching moment when we had to acknowledge that all our family sacrifices to avoid separation had come to naught.) P.L. 94-142 basically concerns itself with public education. However, when appropriate services are not available to meet the needs of a child's IEP in a public school, the LEA may expend public funds for services at a private or church-supported institution where the services are available. Individual parents are free, of course, without IEP sanction, to take advantage of such a program at their own expense if the institution meets state standards.

Providing the Least Restrictive Environment at School

Physical Integration

Largely as a result of P.L. 94-142, most education of handicapped children takes place in a neighborhood school and is carried out by the professionals I describe. There should be small rooms for various staff members to work with kids on a one-to-one basis, as well as large classrooms (resource rooms), containing specially designed materials and equipment, where special-needs children can spend part of the day. As I discussed earlier, the law requires that resource-room students spend more than half their day in regular school activities.

Most facilities have been adapted from spaces formerly used to house regular school programs, and their quality and the manner in which they are used usually reflect both the creativity of the system and its commitment to special education. Because of the emphasis on the least restrictive environment, most handicapped children should participate in some normal activities and share many of the school's regular facilities. More and more school systems are developing programs that integrate handicapped kids with nonhandicapped youngsters, achieving not only a physical but also a social integration. This requires imagination, scheduling initiative, and, sometimes, fortitude on the part of the school (fortitude because sometimes parents of nonhandicapped children resist such efforts).

Integration's success, or lack thereof, can often be felt simply by walking through the school building. It can be implemented at several levels, all the way from a token compliance with the law to a deeply rooted commitment to the philosophy behind the law so that it permeates all of school life. The latter approach works on the assumption that what benefits handicapped students will eventually benefit all students, and that special education is not just a holding action but a dynamic program committed to children who are going somewhere.

During the early years after the passage of P.L. 94-142, many schools sought compliance merely by grouping a number of similarly handicapped students together and assigning them a classroom off the beaten track but with easy access to exterior doors and bathrooms. This was merely a limited physical integration by which handicapped children were moved from an institutional or home setting into the local public school building. The change of setting was sometimes all the change there was.

Imaginative administrators, on the other hand, moved the special students out of the shadows and into central locations where regular student traffic was heavy and such facilities as cafeteria, student lounge, and auditorium were nearby. Such creative engineering meant that classroom location in itself offered real opportunities to merge the worlds of the handicapped and nonhandicapped students. They shared such common facilities as lockers, snack bar, library, and school store, offering a realistic but sheltered laboratory for handicapped children to learn such life skills as making change, choosing from a cafeteria menu, using appropriate table manners, being on time for class, using coin-operated vending machines, and operating locks under realistic, integrated conditions. Today, more and more schools are following this pattern. It beats the show-and-tell classroom approach every time, and handicapped children prepare for the adult world you hope they will eventually enter. This is the kind of school most parents are looking for.

Real Integration

The final stage that committed special program management can encourage is the real social integration that takes place when handicapped and nonhandicapped people get to know and understand one another and build personal relationships. Centrally located classrooms and the shared use of common facilities help this kind of ultimate integration, but they're still not enough. The school administration must see to it that in every way possible handicapped students are brought into the mainstream of school life, by urging them to attend outings, class days, school affairs, dances, games, and assemblies. The North Eugene High School, in Oregon, initiated a peer tutor program in which nonhandicapped students worked as teachers' helpers in the classroom with their handicapped "peers," offering small-group instruction and support. In the process, both groups got to know one another, with the result that handicapped youngsters enjoyed the wonderful new experience of being able to call other students by name and to socialize with them in the halls and in the cafeteria. Real integration, not just physical tokenism to comply with the law, can make the school a better place for everyone. (In 1986 the U.S. Office of Special Education and Rehabilitative Services launched a "regular classroom initiative" that supported even more complete mainstreaming of special students. It's sometimes called "unified education"; ask your special education people if your state is participating—and if not, why not.)

What Makes a Good School for Your Child?

Few parents have a choice of school systems, although in extreme cases parents have pulled up stakes and moved so their child could participate in a special program. We did, but this kind of disruption should no longer be necessary. As the result of P.L. 94-142, parents have many opportunities to work positively toward improving their public schools if they believe change is desirable, and most systems welcome their participation. However, we live in a mobile population; statistics indicate that people, on average, move and select a new home every five years. More often than you might suspect, the selection of the new home location is influenced by a parent's evaluation of the school system serving the area. How can you tell if an LEA places a high priority on special education and is doing an imaginative and committed job? Here are some indicators and suggestions. (The nature of your child's disability will determine which are applicable to you. You may think the time required for investigation is excessive, but the knowledge acquired and acquaintances made will be helpful later if you decide to locate in that LEA.)

1. Contact a local parents' support group. If you currently belong to one and it has national affiliation, there may be a local group in your area of interest. The Association for Retarded Citizens, for example, has many local affiliates. The social worker at the nearest hospital or representatives of governmental agencies may have the names, addresses, and phone numbers of contact people for local groups. If you are being transferred or are moving to a new job and are looking for feedback, ask your company's personnel manager for the names of employees who have children in local school systems.

2. Contact the school system you are considering and arrange a conference with someone knowledgeable about its special education program. Explain your youngster's disability to the secretary and ask him to put you in touch with a qualified person. Try to evaluate how school officials respond to parental participation. Do they welcome you enthusiastically as equals or do they treat you as a necessary but irritating part of their professional responsibilities? Visit during school hours, and try to avoid doing your school planning in the summer (the people who can give you the best information may not be there). It may also be helpful to chat with the school nurse, to find out how medical treatment and such problems as catheters and colostomies are handled. Faculty attitudes in and out of the special education program can affect your child. Some classroom teachers have reservations about handling duties they consider not in their job description. I can sympathize with the staff in this regard. Had I been a stranger to Owie it would have been difficult to deal with his involuntary and chronic soiling problems. While we sent all our kids off to school with a smile and a lunch box, we sent Owie off with a smile, a lunch box, and a second set of underwear. For the most part the staff have been understanding, but sometimes irascibility shows through, and I can't blame them much. Feedback from other parents can be a valuable source of information on faculty attitudes.

3. Try to get a sense of the school's ambiance, particularly how the school community seems to respond to minority groups and handicapped students. Have they held assembly programs geared to understanding disabled people? (This is a common occurrence in many schools I've visited.) Is there an active student community-service program? This in itself can offer an indication of how much the school population is concerned about others who may not be so fortunate as

they. Are nonhandicapped students encouraged to help out at Special Olympics or to participate in holiday dances or fairs for residents at nearby institutions for the mentally retarded? Such activity is currently so common that I would wonder about a school in which there was none. Drop in to the cafeteria. Where do the handicapped students sit? By themselves? Or are they, at least to some extent, accepted and part of the regular crowd?

4. In a conference with the local school people, or by mail if a visit is impossible, find out what particular services are available for students like your child. Even if your youngster has already been declared eligible for special education services, you probably will have to go through the process again in your new school, although you will already have collected most of the necessary information. In general, eligibility is nontransferrable. If your child has mobility problems, you will want to find out how handicapped children are transported and whether the facilities at the school he will be attending are accessible. Ask to see any printed material the school has available on the special education curriculum—a parents' bulletin, for instance—and inquire about the programs that are offered preschool children and at what age such services begin. Even if your child is older, it is often interesting to see what schools are doing on a preschool level, particularly in a state where such services are not required by law.

Ask what provisions are made in the school's curriculum to facilitate the transition from school to community and in what ways the administrators reach out for help beyond the school walls. This attention to concerns that go beyond the traditional academic routines, no matter what age group is involved, is the sign of a well-run school that cares for all its children.

Does the school have a work-study program for mentally retarded students? Is its guidance department involved with special education students? Do staff members help parents plan for postschool employment or education? (Such help can be an indication of the system's commitment to special education in general and to integration in particular.) Have school staff gone further than they had to? How they have responded in the past may give some idea of how they might behave in the future. Another indication of alertness in a system is whether they have received or have applied for any special grants for special education purposes. Are their resource rooms and special education facilities well maintained, attractive, and in the mainstream of student life, or are they tucked away somewhere? How many due process appeals have been filed in that LEA and what kinds of problems were involved? Does the staff treat older handicapped students as the adults they are, or as perennial children?

5. Find out about the LEA's other out-of-school programs. Do they have home-based outreach activities? Will they tutor your child at the hospital or at home? If he is chronically ill and is subject to frequent absences, find out what kind of tutorial services state law requires. If your child needs special individual services, it is important to know if they are available at his school or if he will have to be transported to the specialist. In addition, if students are "tuitioned out" to special programs offered by other systems, consortiums, or state or private schools, how is transportation arranged, what kind of equipment is provided, how much time will be spent on the bus, and what mainstreaming opportunities will your child miss at school while he's away?

6. Budgetary commitment can be misleading, since many factors can influence finances—some beyond the system's control. However, the quality of the equipment and rooms and the willingness of a school to go beyond the minimal staffing required by state law can be an indicator of excellence. And a well-financed system with an enlightened parent body may be more disposed to make the necessary commitment to special education than one with constant budgetary problems.

7. Ask for information about the training and experience of the special education staff and, if noncertified teachers are involved, find out how they are supervised. Teaching ability is not necessarily a function of advanced degrees; paraprofessionals, student teachers, and graduate students can be very effective. However, they should be well supervised by experienced professionals in a balanced and constantly evaluated program. An extensive in-service plan for the special education staff is another sign of a first-rate program supported by the administration and the board of control.

8. If possible, visit the program you believe your child might enter, paying particular attention to the following questions: Do the students appear to be getting enough individual attention? Is the room well lit and large enough for the number of students? Is its atmosphere upbeat, with creative displays? What is the teacher's attitude toward his students? Is there indication of plentiful, appropriate instructional materials and adequate equipment?

9. Are other skills besides the academic emphasized (recreational and daily living skills, for example)? Do the handicapped youngsters have a social life? What specifically is the school doing to coordinate school services with the social service organizations that, you hope, will take over when your child leaves special education coverage? Is career and vocational education an important part of the curriculum? Has sufficient equipment for shop, home arts, and the whole range of prevocational studies been adapted or acquired for use by the handicapped students? Speak with the guidance department. Do they have a pro-

gram to offer guidance that takes in the full range of career and post-secondary opportunities?

In the final analysis, if you are able to look carefully at the LEA you're considering, you will probably end up not so much with a large body of facts as with an overall feel for the program. Trust your instincts. As a special parent you probably have developed sensitive antennae to identify schools in which your child will thrive and feel at home.

20

Postsecondary Education for Disabled Students

Today many disabled students are continuing their education after high school. Although further education after high school is out of the question for students like Owen, for an increasing number—even those with severe orthopedic impairment or mild mental retardation—it can be a realistic option. The term *postsecondary education*, as used in the discussions that follow, means all education that follows high school and includes education in universities and colleges, vocational-technical schools, junior and community colleges, and adult education courses. The course of study can involve a full-time commitment working toward a degree or a single night course taken to acquire or strengthen a particular work or leisure-time skill. Postsecondary educational options for severely mentally handicapped students are *extremely limited* and, when available, usually are offered only through local programs at community colleges or adult education courses. They often concentrate on basic independent-living skills and, occasionally, modest vocational training, with some emphasis on leisure-time interest and skill development. However, educational horizons have expanded for the majority of the disabled population, including physically handicapped kids, emotionally disturbed children, the learning disabled student, and some mildly or moderately retarded students. Parents should be aware of the many educational possibilities that only a few years ago were unheard of.

Attitudes of college administrators, too, have changed: many now realize that the ability of handicapped students to perform postsecondary work has been underestimated and that adapting the academic environment to meet their needs can be accomplished without lowering academic standards. (It can also be good business for the institution.) As a consequence of the educational effort initiated by such legislation as P.L. 94-142, there has also been a significant improvement in the educational capabilities of disabled students leaving high school as well as a heightening of their expectations for the future. Their need for additional education beyond the high-school level has increased along with the nonhandicapped population's need to meet the shifting demands of the workplace in a changing society. But probably more than any one single factor, federal law has again played the key role in changing what was once an abysmal picture, and an understanding of federal legislation should be central to your efforts to ensure that your child seizes every educational opportunity. Regulations of the Rehabilitation Act of 1973 (Section 504) provide extensive and specific protection so that handicapped students get a "fair shake." Know the law!

The intent of this law is that a disability shall not stand in the way of a qualified student's receiving a postsecondary education, and the key word is *qualified*. Your job is to help your child become qualified and to take advantage of whatever post-high-school option is best suited to his abilities and needs. This chapter discusses the academic transition from home to adult life and addresses the following questions:

- What are the higher educational possibilities?
- What postsecondary educational option best meets your child's needs?
- What preparation is necessary?
- How can you handle the admissions process?
- How can life on campus be made more enjoyable and rewarding?
- Is financial help available?

In this chapter I have drawn extensively from information published by the HEATH Resource Center (Higher Education and Adult Training for People with Handicaps; see Resources: Clearinghouses). This resource has proved invaluable to me and could be equally helpful to anyone seeking information in this area. Write for their current publication list.

Is Postsecondary Education Realistic?

In Chapter 18 I wrote of the need for both parent and child to be optimistic about what is achievable and to begin planning for graduation and the transition period early on. Planning for adulthood has been a mainstay of nonhandicapped education for years. It's normally called "career education" and has focused on what jobs (professions) are available and appropriate for the individual and on the education and aptitudes required to land and hold those jobs.

Such planning is equally important for handicapped students but it is considerably more complex. For them, a career may mean the whole business of living successfully. Some students will be able to participate unassisted in the regular high-school offerings, including counseling, career education sessions, college admission testing, cram courses, and so on, but the great majority will need special help. (Particularly in smaller schools, which often have limited support resources and little experience upon which to draw, additional effort will be required of students and parents.)

You may have to do much of the "digging" yourself, while at the same time educating school administrators, guidance staff, and college counselors (at least the special families following after you will have an easier time!). Try to think of this process more as an opportunity than a frustration, but always remember that a special education student has as much right to the benefits of postsecondary counseling as his non-handicapped peers.

The IEP process should provide the framework for much of the planning and preparation, so make sure that the IEP committee addresses this problem in a timely fashion. One of the first steps is to decide whether postsecondary education is, in fact, a realistic possibility. Again I urge you to be optimistic. Your child's ability to cope with the intellectual demands or to profit from the experience may be in doubt, but if there is a possibility, keep the options open! A vocational rehabilitation counselor drawn into the IEP process early may be able to provide insights, since one of his main concerns is helping disabled people become productive members of society.

If there is a question in your mind, ask the interdisciplinary team to consider, at your child's next evaluation, the appropriateness of postsecondary education. The regular evaluation process required by law should be invaluable both in reaching the decision and later in supplying necessary information to the postsecondary institution. Whether any kind of traditional postsecondary education is a possibility is a factor of individual circumstances, which play a critical role. For example, certain physical disabilities can be so severe and the supportive services needed so extensive that they preclude participation on campus, despite the fact that the student's mental abilities are unimpaired. (Correspondence or televised courses might be an option.)

Even if postsecondary education is included in the IEP's long-range goal, the plan may call for an educational track that doesn't live up to what you see as your child's potential. For example, the committee may recommend a vocational program that precludes admission to a four-year college. This conflict should be rare, but remember, a parent enjoys specific appeal rights and a difference of opinion about appropriate career paths for your child may be significant enough for an appeal. Once it is decided that some kind of postsecondary education is realistic, plan an appropriate curriculum that includes all the prerequisites for admission to that particular postsecondary program.

The Many Options

Colleges and Universities

Universities have professional or graduate schools associated with them and are usually larger, offering a wider selection of courses and often a more diverse student body, while colleges are apt to be smaller, with a more intimate climate, but generalization is difficult. There are many exceptions, and it is best to see for yourself. Both kinds of institutions can be either public or private, with the tuition at the public school generally being lower. Some colleges specialize in particular fields, for example, Gallaudet University in Washington, D.C., has a curriculum that is geared to students with a hearing impairment.

It is common for both colleges and universities to require preadmission testing as well as a high-school diploma. However, a successfully completed high-school equivalency exam can meet the diploma requirement and ordinarily can be adapted to meet the needs of eligible handicapped students.

In the early 1960s the University of California at Berkeley opened a residence program for severely disabled students. In the years since, the university, supported by a fast-growing permanent resident handicapped population and the nearby Center for Independent Living, has provided leadership in efforts to remove barriers to postsecondary education for intellectually capable handicapped students.

The University of Illinois at Urbana-Champaign, through its rehabilitation education program and rehabilitation education center, offers a comprehensive program that extends into every corner of campus life. It provides a model of what can be done where there is the will. Every year approximately two hundred handicapped students, more than half of whom permanently use wheelchairs, are enrolled in the program. "As of August 1984, there have been 1019 graduates including many with advanced degrees. Over half of the graduates are confined to wheelchairs. There has been nearly 100% placement in positions with salaries averaging in excess of $20,000. . . . In the thirty-seven-year history of the rehabilitation program, the [academic] results of disabled students' efforts have been somewhat above average when compared with all other students. Many have succeeded, some have failed, and some have been honor students."[1]

Regular university residence halls at the Urbana-Champaign campus offer specially designed or modified furniture, toilets, and showers. A driver training course is offered by the physical therapy

1. Pamphlet from the Division of Rehabilitation Education Services, p. 1, Rehabilitation Education Center, General Statement, University of Illinois.

staff, and the rehabilitation center's Braille and tape library contains Braille editions of encyclopedias, English and foreign-language dictionaries, mathematics tables, etc. A prosthetic shop that works with the prescriptions of professionals to iron out difficulties in equipment, and a chapter of Delta Sigma Omicron, a coeducational service fraternity of disabled students, are affiliated with the university.

The program at the University of Illinois provides an example of what is being accomplished by forward-looking universities, and so can act as a frame of reference in college selection. Keep in mind that both the University of California at Berkeley and the University of Illinois at Urbana-Champaign are large institutions and are able to provide services that are unrealistic for small colleges. On the other hand, in many small schools the handicapped student is more thoroughly immersed in the mainstream of "normal" school life.

Most four-year academic institutions emphasize the maintenance of academic standards, and as a result the adaptation of programs to compensate for the student's handicap is carefully monitored so as not to "water down" the course content or represent a double academic standard. These schools are for students who have the intellectual potential to perform the work expected of all students.

Junior and Community Colleges

Many handicapped students choose two-year, usually public, institutions (a survey of American college freshmen by the American Council on Education indicates that more than 50 percent of handicapped students enroll in these educational options). Although both junior and community colleges involve two years of study, they differ significantly. The junior college is usually a privately funded liberal arts school that offers either a certificate or an associate of arts degree (AA). One of its primary goals is preparing students who are not yet ready for a four-year college.

Community colleges, on the other hand, are publicly funded. Although many provide liberal arts courses, they often offer special vocational and occupational programs for preparing such specialists as X-ray technicians, dental assistants, auto mechanics, and secretaries. Since many are new and of relatively recent construction, they tend to be more barrier-free and provide campuses specially designed to accommodate the handicapped student.

Community colleges offer some advantages. Tuition can be less, there are many institutions to choose from, and they are common enough that a handicapped student should be able to locate one near home. The admission requirement is often limited to a high-school diploma or its equivalent, with admissions testing rarely required. Several states have what is called an "open-door policy" for community colleges that allows a high-school graduate or equivalent or anyone who is eighteen years old to be automatically granted admission.

> Persons with learning disabilities who wish to take the high school equivalency exam can obtain special accommodations and editions of the exam through the GED (General Educational Development) Testing Service. The Chief Examiner must be provided with professional verification of the disability. Special editions include braille, large print and audio cassettes. Special accommodations include additional time, quiet surroundings, low-glare lighting, etc. The fact that the test was taken under special conditions generally will not be included on the student's record. For more complete information, contact the State Department of Education in your state.[2]

Because of public control and the large number of handicapped students enrolled in recent years, community college administrations have become sensitive to the needs of handicapped students and are experienced at meeting these needs. Kingsborough Community College of the City University of New York is an example. Kingsborough students who have certified physical, emotional, or learning disabilities and need supportive services to pursue their academic career are eligible for special services, including counseling, tutoring (students receive 1–4 hours weekly), special adaptive testing, depending upon disability, and a streamlined registration process that takes into consideration room accessibility and between-class mobility, the student's level of physical and intellectual endurance, and special degree requirements. Efforts are also made to establish close faculty–student understandings and to resolve issues of concern to professors working with disabled students.

Vocational-Technical Schools, Technical Institutes, and Trade Schools

These schools specialize in preparing students for specific jobs or in upgrading the basic skills already acquired. Their curricula involve from a few weeks to more than a year of study, and usually they offer a certificate upon completion, although state certification or licensing may require further study or passing a written exam. There is usually no admission requirement other than, in some instances, a high-school diploma or its equivalent. Vocational-technical schools, usually publicly supported and therefore relatively inexpensive, cater to a wide va-

---

2. HEATH Resource Bulletin, "Learning Disabled Adults in Postsecondary Education," 1987 edition, p. 6.

riety of occupations, with particular emphasis being given to local job opportunities. Technical institutes offer educational preparation for such specialists as medical assistants, industrial technicians, computer technicians, and dental technicians. Trade schools usually offer courses in one trade or a group of crafts within one occupational cluster. Here are some things to check out early in the game from the HEATH Fact Sheet "Education Beyond High School: The Choice Is Yours!"

What are the admissions requirements? Do you need to have a certain reading or math level, or pass an entrance exam?

What are your interests? Will jobs be available in your area after you've received training? If not, are you willing to move to where the jobs are? Will the school help you find employment?

Is the school licensed by your state's post-secondary school licensing bureau? Most states require a license, but a few do not. You can find this information in the school's catalogue.

Is the school accredited? This is important. It means that the school has passed a thorough examination by an accrediting agency recognized by the U.S. Department of Education. The school is evaluated in such areas as educational quality and teaching ability.

Does the school make use of laboratories or shops so that most of the training takes place in a setting that resembles the real work environment?

Is there anyone in the program who can help make accommodations for your specific needs?

Home Study or Correspondence Courses

A student can study a wide variety of subjects and even earn a bachelor's degree through this educational alternative, which is particularly attractive to homebound students. (Televised classes have become more common and offer expanded options for the homebound student.) The material to be mastered is prepared in sequential units, including written assignments that can be returned through the mail for correction and comment. The corrected assignment is then sent back with the next assignment, and the cycle is repeated until the course is completed. Take particular care to evaluate the quality of the school and to make sure it meets your child's needs. A directory of schools accredited by the National Home Study Council can be obtained from the HEATH Resource Center.

Adult Education

Adult education programs provide educational opportunity up to college-level courses to any student, often sixteen or older, who is no longer included in P.L. 94-142 coverage. They cater to the part-time student population and, therefore, ordinarily meet in the evenings or over weekends so as not to conflict with regular job responsibilities. Tuition is normally low, and programs may include several general categories, such as preparation for the high-school equivalency (GED) test, basic courses in English composition, reading and math skills, and English as a second language (ESL) courses. Your LEA or the state director of adult education should be able to furnish more information.

Another academic alternative is continuing education. The courses, which are usually not graded and receive no academic credit, cover an extremely wide range of interests and include occupational, academic, and leisure-time subjects. Your LEA, community college, or department of recreation may offer these programs. They are advertised through direct mail, on local radio and TV spot announcements, and on publicly posted bulletins and schedules.

Choose the Postsecondary Program that Serves Your Child's Needs

Many institutions of higher learning now go to remarkable lengths to make postsecondary education a realistic possibility for the disabled student. It's important, however, that the handicapped student and his parents make a thoughtful decision about which type of institution best meets his needs and that they determine which particular school seems most likely to be right for him.

This decision should take into account four factors: the student's ability to perform academically, his career goals, his special needs, and finally the institution's ability to meet his needs. The IEP evaluation (involving the interdisciplinary team, the vocational rehabilitation counselor—whom you may have asked to be involved in certain IEP meetings—and the regular school college-career counselor) should have helped you determine your decision by the time your child completes high school. For example, the conclusion might be that a four-year college isn't a realistic possibility but that a local community college makes sense. I recommend the HEATH Resource Center bulletin *Education for Employment* (prepared by Nancy L. Stout and Maxine T. Krulwich in November 1982) for additional information and resources.

Helping your child select the most appropriate school will probably take time and patience. The high-school guidance office ordinarily is the place to start. (It begins the route followed by all college-bound nonhandicapped students.) You should invite the college counselor to attend an IEP meeting to discuss the situation, particularly your child's ability, needs, and career goals. It's important, if a four-year college is in the cards, that a general preliminary meeting be held no later than the end of the tenth grade, so that academic provision can be made to meet minimal college admission course requirements. Your college counselor may advise that you select several schools to apply to if you are interested in four-year schools in which admission is competitive.

No matter where your child's postsecondary educational interests lie, you should consider certain criteria:

1. *What is the institution's admission policy?* Are admissions tests required? The most commonly used tests are the Scholastic Aptitude Test (SAT) designed by the Educational Testing Service of Princeton, New Jersey. Both testing services provide special accommodations and/ or editions for students with learning disabilities. Cassettes, readers, extended time, large type, and marking assistance are typical of adaptations offered. (For details, see Resources: Testing.) The SAT makes note of any test taken under nonstandard conditions, while ACT makes special notation only if "extended time" is allowed. Parents will want to think over whether their child's disability warrants his taking the special test. Although an additional expense is involved, students occasionally take tests in both the regular and the special versions.

2. *Do the school's physical characteristics meet your needs?* The school's size, location, and campus characteristics are of importance to all students, but they have special implications for the handicapped student. If he has close ties with home, attending a nearby college can make the transition easier. A large urban school may have more handicapped students and special facilities, whereas a small rural school can seem more relaxed and personal. Visit if you can. Many colleges require or strongly recommend admission interviews.

3. *Is the campus, particularly the dorm, accessible?* Before you visit, set up dates to meet with the dean of students, special services director, or the person charged with handicapped students' concerns (he's sometimes called the "disabled students services officer"). Ask if a handicapped undergraduate can take you around the campus. Get a feel for the place. Can a wheelchair fit through the doors? If the buildings have elevators, can you use them? Will your child need to have rails installed in the shower? Do such obstacles as turnstiles in libraries, bookstores, or cafeterias present problems?

4. *What about the physical terrain?* Is it hilly? Will there be snow and ice? Some schools have orientation sessions to acquaint incoming

disabled students with the lay of the land. If the campus is large, find out if the school has accessible vans. Is public transportation accessible? Can your child get into the stadium to watch athletic contests? What about the swimming pool and the theater? Some institutions offer special campus maps that identify accessibility characteristics and areas of particular interest to the handicapped, i.e., the location of curb cuts, accessible entrances, reserved parking. Some even have three-dimensional "tactile maps" written in Braille or large print. Take a trial run. Make up a schedule. Is just getting around a problem?

5. *How does the institution feel about disabled students?* What resources are available? To a degree, the provisions an institution makes to accommodate disabled students reflect its interest in them. It might help in your thinking to draw up a checklist of the special things important to your child and then compare that list with the resources a particular school has to offer.

Ways Your Child Can Help Himself

The HEATH Fact Sheet "Make the Most of Your Opportunities" by Susan J. Sorrells, Lois Hertz, and Maxine Krulwich offers thoughtful suggestions to make your child's college life more productive, some of which I have drawn upon in this section. Your youngster can do much before he leaves home. It may be helpful and reassuring for him to discuss his postsecondary plans with persons with whom he has established close relationships—teachers at school, a counselor at an agency, a physical therapist, a doctor. You should also contact local sources of financial support to see if they can continue their assistance.

Your child should list the equipment and aids he has found helpful (Braillers, talking calculators, tape recorders, TTY equipment) and find out if they will be available at his new school or whether he should bring them with him. (If so, what arrangements must be made?) Since registration routines may prove difficult for your youngster, most schools have preregistration periods. Ask how this option is arranged. Your child may wish to participate as much as possible in the mainstream of campus life. If this is the case, be sensitive; let go, and allow him to exercise his independence.

Since considerable lead time may be required, contact the new academic institution early and arrange for such things as taped texts, required reading lists for courses, readers, attendants, and any adaptive equipment necessary. Make an appointment, if possible, before the semester begins and *before* everyone gets frantically busy, to make arrangements. Locating readers or arranging for attendant care may be difficult. Advertising on a school bulletin board or in the local newspaper is often productive, and some schools keep lists of applicants. Perhaps work-study students are available; the financial aid officer should know. Local service organizations (the Rotary, Kiwanis, or Lions clubs, an area affiliate of Easter Seals, or the state Commission for the Blind) sometimes offer organizational or financial assistance. If the school is on the ball, it should make many of these arrangements for you, but you must make your child's need known and give the school time. (If your youngster qualifies for services, the vocational rehabilitation program may be a source of help.)

Other organizations besides the school can be helpful. For example, a local independent-living center (discussed in Chapter 22) is an excellent resource for locating accessible housing, prescreened personal care attendants and counseling and advisory services. The Independent Living Research Utilization Project (see Resources: Independent Living) has sponsored a computerized listing of independent-living programs and their services, on a national basis. Another resource available on an increasing number of campuses (particularly large urban ones) is a disabled-student support group. Like many peer-support organizations, it can offer advantages difficult to obtain through any other resource. If none exists, ask the dean of students for the name of disabled upper-classmen whom you can contact for advice and counsel.

Although the special student may have to wait till he's on campus, I suggest he contact his instructors to introduce himself and acquaint them with his special needs. He is asking for no advantages—only an even break. For example, if he has a communication problem, it may be helpful to sit toward the front of class where there is good light, or to get advance lecture notes. Accessibility, nondiscriminatory testing, and course requirement modification, discussed earlier, also apply on the postsecondary level. Postsecondary degree programs are designed as one-, two-, or four-year programs, but special students may require additional time to complete requirements. Arrangements should be made as soon as it becomes evident that an extension is necessary.

Students with learning disabilities may encounter special problems, and schools—particularly large institutions—often offer comprehensive programs that include diagnostic testing, special learning centers, tutorial help, individualized education plans, and instruction by specialists in the field. If your child is diagnosed as learning disabled, consult with his current secondary-school teachers; decide what specialized support he needs and make it an important consideration in your college selection. At the University of Illinois the emphasis has been upon the physically handicapped rather than the learning-disabled (LD) student, but research in postsecondary instructional methods for LD students and their accommodation on campus is receiving national attention and prospects continue to improve. LD students can bring particular academic problems to a college and require specialized resources; parents should make sure that the institutions they consider have expertise in this area and a willingness to provide the additional help sometimes required. However, before special help and curricular adaptation are provided, most institutions require medical confirmation of the disability. A whole variety of popular books geared to the college-bound community is available at most bookstores and should be no farther away than a high-school college counselor's office. *Lovejoy's College Guide for the Learning Disabled*, by Charles T. Straughn II and Marvelle S. Colby (see Resources: Education), is one example, and I have drawn from it for certain general information contained in this chapter.

Paying the Bills

Postsecondary education is often extremely expensive, and getting help can be a complex process that changes annually. Ask your child's high-school college counselor for up-to-date information. Occasionally, college admissions directors or financial aid officers visit high schools to speak to parents' groups about financial assistance. See if visits can be arranged at your school; then, during the coffee hour, pump the speaker about special provisions for handicapped students. Postsecondary financial aid is currently available in three general categories:

- **Grants:** scholarships and gifts that do not have to be repaid; for example, on the national level, federally supported Pell Grants and Supplemental Educational Opportunity Grants, and on the state level, programs that vary from state to state.
- **Loans:** money borrowed to cover direct school costs. Loans carry interest charges (usually low) and must be repaid over a specified schedule; for example, Guaranteed Student Loans and National Direct Student Loans.
- **Student jobs,** usually school-oriented, that enable the student to earn money to help cover his educational costs (for example, a college work-study program).

The federal government assists needy students in a variety of ways, but budgetary cutbacks make this a rapidly changing area. Write to the HEATH Resource Center and ask for its latest financial aid update on federal/state student assistance. Two other valuable sources of information are the National Library Service for the Blind and Physically Handicapped's Reference Circular "From School to Working Life: Resources and Services" (October 1985) from which I have drawn in this chapter, and "The Student Guide: Five Federal Financial Aid Programs," which may be obtained from the U.S. Department of Education, Office of Student Financial Assistance (7th and D Streets, S.W., Washington, D.C. 20202). A recording describing student financial aid for the visually impaired can be obtained from the same department, free of charge.

Most academic institutions centralize their financial aid program in one office that coordinates overall student assistance, often by combining all resources available into one package. To determine how much any one family should contribute to their child's total educational costs, involves a complex formula. The family must supply the information needed to make this projection on a standardized, confidential form; most schools use either the Financial Aid Form (FAF), published by College Scholarship Service (Princeton, NJ 08541), or the Family Financial Statement (FFS), published by American College Testing, Student Need Analysis Service, of Iowa City, Iowa 52243. Information and blank forms are available at a high-school college guidance office or at the college's financial aid office.

The magic formula that determines financial need is simple, at least in principle. Expenses (tuition, fees, books, board, transportation, etc.), less the family contribution (the amount that the FAF or FFS forms indicate the family should be able to pay), equals the financial need that should, if possible, be met by the institution's financial aid package. Whether the need will be met depends upon several factors— for example, the financial resources available to the institution, campus jobs available, and the latest status of the government student-aid programs.

The formula can include certain handicap-related costs, such as transportation, special equipment, interpreter, note-taker, reader expenses, and noncovered disability-related medical costs, which, if accepted, will correspondingly increase the financial aid package. Ask the financial aid office what documentation is required. As I have mentioned, at some institutions special services are already available. Check with the network of disabled students, the student services office, or the 504 coordinator for information. Irrespective of what services exist, notify the financial aid office of the details of your child's disability so that they can be a factor in the financial aid package.

Vocational rehabilitation, Supplemental Security Income (SSI), and Social Security disability income are significant sources of financial aid for many qualifying handicapped students. In addition, state funds and private scholarships may be available in your location. Some service organizations (Kiwanis International, Lions Club, Federation of

Women's Clubs, Elks Clubs, Rotary Foundation, and the American Legion) have in the past offered scholarship assistance. Check with your local high school's college counselor. The financial aid office at the postsecondary school you are considering, however, is your most up-to-date resource for financial aid information. Advising students on resources is part of their job.

Dos and Don'ts
for the Formal Education Years

1. *Become familiar with key material.* Get copies of: P.L. 94-142, Section 504 of the Rehabilitation Act, the Buckley Amendment to the Family Education Rights and Privacy Act, your state and LEA special education regulations, as well as their policies on management of confidentiality of records. For quick reference, your parents' group, your state's advocate office, or state or local education agency may publish parents' manuals that outline and simplify the law. Be sure you understand your rights and responsibilities under the law, the individualized education program (IEP), and the concepts of least restrictive environment, due process, and evaluation.

2. *When in doubt, find out.* If your child (from birth to age 21) is not receiving special services and you think he may be eligible, contact your LEA and ask what their procedures are to determine who qualifies.

3. *Get involved.* Develop a positive relationship with your LEA. Get involved with your school. Visit and see the program in action. Establish informal and relaxed contacts with your child's teachers. Don't just complain. Compliment the teachers when a job is well done, and don't lose contact as the years pass.

4. *Know your own child.* Be sure that your child's evaluation tests all aspects of his abilities in a nondiscriminatory way; that a complete physical is included; and that his IEP is written so that you understand it and in such a fashion that its success can be objectively evaluated. Never sell your child short. Existing strengths should be the foundation upon which future progress is based.

5. *Be a part of the IEP team.* Take an active part in the development of your child's education. The law makes you a member of the IEP team. Take advantage of this. Attend all meetings, but take a supportive, knowledgeable companion with you. When in doubt, ask to be included when critical decisions are made. Always keep in mind that the goal of your child's education is a fruitful adult life. Don't fall into the trap of thinking of your son or daughter as a perpetual infant.

6. *There is power in numbers.* Consider joining a parents' organization.

7. *Keep your notebook up to date, with all important information.* This is a period when having dated, complete records is most critical.

8. *Set goals for your youngster.* Work toward developing in your own mind ongoing goals and objectives for your child and a concept of what constitutes an "ideal" program within an "ideal" school. This concept can be a starting point for developing specific educational programs for your child. Sometimes you must live for today only, but don't postpone thoughtful, appropriate plans for the future.

9. *Work for your child.* Become an informed advocate for *all* handicapped children, but avoid "shooting from the hip" in your relations with caregivers. Avoid creating adversarial relationships; as much as possible, work with, rather than against, others involved with your child and assume that the school people, the professionals, and the bureaucrats are also acting in your child's best interests. Listen thoughtfully to what they have to say but make your own decisions. Be an advocate for such things as complete birth-to-21 coverage and an effective, comprehensive transitional program between school and the adult world if your school doesn't currently offer such coverage.

10. *Learn how to appeal.* Use due process or litigation as a last resort and then only after you have exhausted other means to reach a satisfactory conclusion to your differences, including mediation. Sometimes compromise brings about the best result for your child, but don't hesitate to exercise the basic due process right when the interests of your child are at stake.

11. *You can do only so much.* Participate actively in all aspects of school life, particularly in the IEP process, and reinforce your child's program as much as possible at home, but let the school know the limits of your capabilities.

12. *Keep working.* Don't lose interest in the IEP as time passes, you grow older, and the novelty wears off. The last few years—the transition stage—can be the most critical of all.

13. *Education doesn't necessarily end with high school.* Postsecondary education is a realistic goal for millions of disabled students. A wide range of academic possibilities exist. Think seriously and early about whether postsecondary education is a possibility and plan early to meet any prerequisites.

NOTE: Extensive checklists to help you with preparation for and involvement in the IEP process are included throughout Part Four. Refer to them whenever necessary.

PART FIVE

May you live all the days of your life.

JONATHAN SWIFT

Life in the Adult World

Prologue

Parents' Weekend in May is the high point of the year at Stewart Home, Owen's school near Lexington, Kentucky. Residents and staff spend weeks in preparation, and families gather from all over the country for the three-day event. It's held right after the Kentucky Derby, and the bluegrass country our son sees from his dormitory window is bursting with life as mares and their foals dot the rolling hillsides.

The program hasn't changed much since we began going ten years ago, yet it's never boring and we look forward to the trip more each year. It's given us a great deal: a circle of friends with whom we have much in common, and a widening pool of memories. Since Mary and I expect our other children will look after Owen when we're gone, we invite one or two of them to join us, to get acclimated to Owie's world and to meet his friends.

The program always begins with a reception at the large Southern mansion that serves as the administration building. It's often hot and always crowded; the food trays are loaded with mountains of cookies and there's punch. The kids (they're called residents) love cookies. Every year I'm convinced that someone has finally ordered too much, but when I work my way through the jostling crowd to the refreshment tables, I find everything with icing or chocolate has disappeared and only crumbs remain. I help myself to a vegetable dip. (Vegetable dip doesn't go fast.)

The reception is traditionally followed by a parent–child softball game, which is characterized by heated arguments over ground rules and alleged ringers. Sometimes caps get thrown on the ground and bases get kicked. Overconfident parents who begin the afternoon by cautioning one another to "let the kids have a chance to hit the ball," end up sprawled on the ground. They get dusted off by the school's pitcher, who happens to have Down syndrome—he's called "Vapor Ball" by his buddies.

After the game comes a parade, led by a police cruiser with its siren and blue flasher on. There's usually a fire truck, a National Guard tank-recovery vehicle, and a local beauty queen (who smiles and waves from the back of a convertible). The mayor of Frankfort is always there as

323

well as a representative of the governor, who later reports that the governor "wanted very much to be here but is unavoidably called away on state business." The disabled onlookers respond to the pageantry in highly individualized fashion as the spectacle rolls by, but they really get excited when the huge flatbed truck, festooned with ribbons, comes rolling around the bend carrying Stewart Home's newly elected Parents' Day King and Queen surrounded by their court. The flatbed rolls and pitches on the uneven ground and the court has trouble keeping their balance. Parents of special kids can fill in this picture without further details.

And then there's a fair—a fair with balloons that the kids break and booths run by student volunteers from the local high school. The residents get their faces painted with flowers and half moons, or throw a ring on a hoop and win a prize. But the handicapped children's favorite is the dunking game. This perennial feature of fairs and firemen's musters involves an ingenious arrangement of hinges and pulleys so constructed that an accurately thrown ball plummets a victim, seated high above a water tank, down into the water below.

At Stewart Home the "victim" is always one of the popular teachers, and if the young thrower isn't successful at first, he edges up nearer and nearer to the target till he is. Last year I watched, interested, as Owie sprayed softballs in the general direction of the tank. The teacher, who was making an effort to appear to be having the time of his life, was dripping wet and had skinned his right elbow. Occasionally he looked over his shoulder at the line of kids behind Owen waiting a chance to throw. It was growing longer and it was still early in the afternoon.

Last year a National Guard helicopter flew over from Lexington for the events. Getting the landing site cleared caused general excitement, and each time the teachers got their charges temporarily under control and off the field—and the pilot was waved in—an awkward figure would dart out of the crowd waving his arms and jumping up and down in excitement. Landing took quite a while.

Later, everyone trooped up a ramp and through the helicopter's cockpit for a closer look. Two airmen kept a sharp lookout near the control panels. They kept repeating something to the crowd as it pushed by, and occasionally would glance up at the large rotors moving slowly overhead. No one paid any attention to what they were saying, and it wasn't until we stepped into the cockpit and walked by the banks of instrument controls and blinking lights that we could understand their words—"Don't touch the switches everybody. Please don't touch the switches."

I don't know which of the annual events is the high point for me, the talent show or the dance Friday night. The show is the kind of event that once experienced is never forgotten. Picture a typical high-school gymnasium decorated with colored crepe paper and Special Olympics banners. Three hundred parents, friends, and guardians wave and call out from the audience. Despite the heat (it's always breathlessly hot), they jump up to take a flash picture, point in recognition at friends across the room, wave at their kids, and, in general, make delightful fools of themselves. Their children, attired in costumes that defy description, wave back, call out, and jump up and down on the stage. The one-man orchestra consists of "Butch," a blind pianist who can play anything you can whistle and play it well! Butch may have serious physical handicaps, but he has given others more pleasure in his evenings of music than I, in my normalness, will ever give in a lifetime.

The Friday night dance is also an experience not to take lightly. With the exception of the physical characteristics of the resident dancers, and the fact that the fifty-year-olds are often more abandoned than the teenagers, the dance is very like the ones that Mary and I remember as kids. There's the disc jockey, who apparently speaks in tongues, darkened lights, girls whispering, boys watching, and mysterious comings and goings. Originally, I was disconcerted when my dancing partners—Owie's girl friends—tired of my conservative dancing technique and drifted off into the shadows, leaving me alone in the middle of the swirling dance floor. Family pride was salvaged two years ago, however, when Mary and Owen won the mother-son dance contest.

In many ways, Parents' Weekend represents a wonderful and joyous acceptance of life as it is for disabled people, without loss of hope for the future. In the eyes of the families I have grown to know, I see acceptance of a handicap no matter how severe, without loss of one's sense of humor or loss of love. I see a willingness to meet the world without embarrassment or posturing. It's a wonderful weekend, a wonderful school, and a place and time when you mustn't take yourself too seriously, and whatever you do, "Please don't touch the switches."

21

The Transition from School to the Adult World

What happens when your child grows too old to be eligible for the benefits of P.L. 94-142? The formal school years were no picnic, but school is not an end in itself, and the time comes, often when your child reaches age 21, when a new life begins. This section deals with this life and preparation for it. It discusses living arrangements (from the traditional residential/custodial institution to almost completely independent living), leisure activities, sexuality, religion, advocacy, and, finally, preparation for that day when you must pass the responsibility for your child to someone else. Educational issues continue to be a significant factor in this chapter, since for many youngsters like Owie, the educational component of transition continues well into their post–P.L. 94-142 adult years.

The transfer from school to adult life, called the "transition period," is critical, since relationships with new support systems must be established that could continue for most of your child's life. The need to reorganize and to adapt to new personalities, regulations, and conditions comes at a developmental period when profound changes are taking place as a natural consequence of the youngster's physical growth. Often the transition period begins with the child living at home as a teenage student almost completely dependent upon parents and school, and ends four or five years later when he has moved away and established a new life for himself both emotionally and physically. Even for the nonhandicapped young adult, the process of establishing a new identity is a big order.

For parents of physically handicapped children, it's particularly important during the transition years to keep in touch with their child's health-care team and to keep abreast of new technological developments in orthotic and adaptive equipment. There is an unfortunate tendency for parents to relax as years pass and to assume that the arrangements they made years ago for their child are still the best available. This probably is not the case. Everyone concerned with special students must remember that more careers are possible than you might suppose. Did you know that Stephen Hawking, one of the most brilliant physicists ever, has made major contributions to science and humanity in spite of severe handicaps?

For years, the special education establishment emphasized the elementary years, and paid insufficient attention to the period when, as handicapped youngsters grow up and require progressively more skill proficiency, they need specially trained teachers and preparation for the transition to the adult world. A generation of handicapped students paid the penalty for this oversight. Fortunately, in recent years federal and state governments have increasingly acknowledged what most parents already knew—that both the educational and support services needed during this period were inadequate. At long last efforts are being made to improve the situation.

The shift of attention to the secondary educational years and coordination of education with adult service providers was given momentum by important legislation. Public Law 98-199 expands P.L. 94-142 to provide planning for the transition from school to work. P.L. 98-527 (the Developmental Disabilities Act of 1984) emphasizes community integration and nurturing the independence of people with qualifying disabilities, and amendments to the Vocational Education Act of 1976 encourage state-level coordination of vocational education, special education, and vocational rehabilitation. In addition, the federal Office of Special Education called for a nationwide "initiative," part of which involved awarding grants to develop transition models.

Several states have already moved to coordinate the postschool period. For example, on the state level Massachusetts' Chapter 688 provides "for continuity of services to developmentally disabled persons whose age no longer entitles them to service under special education programs." On the national level in the late 1970s, such cooperation was encouraged by a joint memorandum from the Commissioner of Education and the Commissioner of Rehabilitation Services, which ruled that students may be eligible for services from more than one federal agency simultaneously, and an agreement was made in 1978 to encourage cooperative planning and programming in vocational education for handicapped students.

The legislative details change from year to year and often are implemented differently, but it is important that you understand the basic ingredients of applicable federal and state legislation and keep current on their significant amendments. The momentum has grown and more and more resources will be available to you.

Transitional Goals

Throughout this book, I emphasize long-range planning and timely skill development to avoid a last-minute flurry of pregraduation activity. The goals for which all the earlier years have been preparing and upon which transition programs must build are:

- **Independence** and the freedom for a young adult to live his own life and make his own decisions.
- **Involvement** in the everyday affairs of his community to the extent he finds congenial.
- **Fulfillment** in such nonwork areas as social intercourse, recreation and leisure activities, religion, and sexual satisfaction.
- **Productivity** achieved through many avenues.

It's wonderful if gainful employment is a possibility. Getting and holding a job is a natural goal for most people. For a disabled person it has a variety of benefits that go beyond money earned: it provides a natural setting to learn acceptable social behavior. It offers the opportunity to perform satisfactorily some task that is valued by society. (Never underestimate the importance of having a place to go after breakfast where you are expected—where your participation is valued.) Finally, a paying job can offer some financial independence and the self-esteem that is of prime importance in a work-centered culture. These goals are a large order, but aren't they ones we all seek? How can we exclude any of them from our children's future if means are at hand to secure them?

Letting Go: Prerequisite to a Successful Transition

As children strike out on their own, they become less dependent upon their parents. This process can be painful, and for many parents decisions about when and under what conditions to let go their hold can be delayed, often to the detriment of the child. Some parents never let go. (If your child is mentally competent, you'll have little alternative, since when he reaches legal majority, he enjoys the basic right to make his own decisions.) Some professionals suggest parents are often overly protective and underestimate their children's potential. I have heard statements like: "They [parents] worry so much about what bad things might possibly happen to their kid in the outside world they guarantee that nothing good can happen to him in either world," and "Parents seem to think they'll live forever."

On the other hand, mothers and fathers sometimes see professionals as "insensitive to our concerns," "expecting too much too fast," and "never around to help pick up the pieces when too much freedom backfires." It's natural for parents to think in terms of "what if," and safety should always be a concern as a youngster is given more freedom. One of our constant worries is that Owen will get lost, and one night he did, but a mobilized neighborhood eventually found him safe and sound. (Everybody was worried except Owen.)

Participation in society involves some risk for all, but risk-avoidance shouldn't be a lifetime preoccupation lest it control our lives. Thoughtful parental planning can usually reduce risk to acceptable levels. Your LEA or social service agency should be responsible for safety within certain limitations, but you should know what the limitations are. If you're concerned, discuss the issue at the IEP meeting or with your social service agency representative—not in a negative way that might discourage program initiatives, but constructively. It's a tightrope we all walk, but, at least with older children, I'm convinced more harm is done by apathetic parents who abrogate their responsibilities than by those who are overly protective. On the other hand, if we had been preoccupied with a fear that Owen's airplane might get snowbound in Cincinnati, he and we would have led less interesting lives and missed much. My advice: be a prudent risk-taker.

As you approach the transition years, bear in mind that the fundamental changes that occur in your child's life will place emotional stresses on everyone in the family. This is particularly true if he acts out in response to new pressures. Although Owen apparently enjoyed the experience when he first entered an outside work program, he began to lose weight and, until his new schedule became routine, for the first time he had a behavior problem. As a family we found talking things over helped us understand what was happening to him, and helped us acknowledge openly that Owen's success in his new environment depended upon our wholehearted support. To have overreacted as his weight loss steadily increased and said, "See, I knew it wouldn't work; he belongs back at school" would have been a singular mistake. When a handicapped child begins to venture into the world, whether it be from home or from school, he gradually loses routines and structures with which he is familiar and upon which he still depends. Letting go does not mean letting go of love or support. It must be a measured and continuing process for the good of all concerned.

Independence requires that certain basic skills be acquired. Throughout this book I have stressed the importance of developing skills in personal management, decision making, hygiene, and grooming, without which even minimal independence is impossible. Along the way you have had an opportunity to nurture these skills by involving your child in home chores of increasing complexity, by taking him with you into the community, by giving him decisions to make, and by exposing him to the reality and demands of society's basic competency requirements. You have also prepared him for independence if at IEP meetings you insisted that his skill mastery be addressed early, both in his total curriculum and in a broad spectrum of school activities, curricular and extracurricular. His abilities—mechanical and attitudinal—will have a maximal opportunity for success if they are based on local expectations ("community referenced") and if they are developed on a continuing basis, progressing from the most simple to the more and more complex ("longitudinal skills"). If our experience with Owen and his friends is typical, as many severely handicapped people fail to integrate into society because of unacceptable social behavior and lack of motivation as are rejected because they lack the basic motor skills or intellectual ability to operate a machine or complete a task.

The problem is not limited to physically handicapped or mentally retarded persons. Even learning-disabled people may find social integration difficult. Frustration caused by a lack of academic success may spill over and negatively influence relationships with others, or his disability may cause the LD student to react in ways his companions find inappropriate, since his disability makes it difficult for him to read the social sign language that is so much a part of life. (A smile may appear to be a sneer to someone with a learning disability.) It is your job and that of the school system to face and, as much as possible, correct these problems while your child is still in school and before the last push is begun to move from the controlled and protected environment of the school and home to the freer and more challenging adult world.

The final integration of skills considered part of prevocational education may be taught at various academic levels in special education, depending upon the nature and severity of the child's handicap. (Some special students spend the rest of their lives in the process—Owen is in his late twenties and is still attempting to learn these skills.) For the mildly retarded or physically handicapped child, such instruction often is done during the junior-high years. However, for those with more severe handicaps, the experiences may not occur until the later stages of transition, as preparation for a sheltered workshop or other limited work activities.

The IEP and a Transition Curriculum

The IEP remains the foundation for special education through the last years of P.L. 94-142 coverage. Your active participation in the meetings that construct, adapt, and evaluate your child's curriculum is his best hope for a successful transition. Although the composition and scope of the IEP meeting remain fundamentally the same as during the elementary years, significant differences exist.

First, your concerns become more pressing as time runs out and the program must be brought to a conclusion. In addition to the transition goals already mentioned, your child must meet graduation requirements (discussed later in this chapter).

Next, because successful transition must draw upon a number of agencies, the IEP has more resources available and therefore more work to do. A coordinated program must be drawn up—some states call it an individualized transition plan (ITP)—and many agencies can be involved, including your state's vocational education program or the state organization receiving federal vocational rehabilitation funding (sometimes called rehabilitative services) or the state agency concerned with mental health and mental retardation. Depending upon your state's regulations, either they *can* or they *must* be involved in developing your child's ITP. Find out which agencies are involved in your state. Remember that, whatever agency or combination of agencies is involved, all the provisions of the IEP must be in compliance with P.L. 94-142. When there is a multiplicity of agency responsibility, make sure that one and only one person is responsible for overall coordination.

To ensure that you are taking advantage of every opportunity, ask your director of special education or IEP chairperson three key questions, perhaps phrased in your own words:

- What rights does my child have under federal, state, or local laws, programs, or regulations to help him prepare for transition?
- Are any other organizations (besides the LEA) mandated to provide assistance or interagency coordination during this period?
- What organizations are required to provide assistance once the LEA no longer offers coverage, and how early can their representatives be brought into the picture? (An increasing number of states now require that all IEPs contain transitional plans to help with employment and independent-living arrangements.)

Part Four considered ways you can best represent your child's interests in the IEP meetings. Here are additional areas you should explore during the transition period:

1. Is the staff aware of the many resources available to promote transition education? Have they thought about applying for a grant to support a demonstration project? The Texas Developmental Disabilities Council, for example, funded a grant to "develop a public school curriculum on employment and independent living skills beginning with early intervention (ages birth through three) through age twenty-two."[1] Do they know of work being done in other places—university-

---

1. "Transition After Education? Yes! The Role of Developmental Disability Councils," by Joellen Simmons, *Exceptional Parent*, December 1986, p. 27.

affiliated programs, for example—to stimulate faculty training in this area, particularly in prevocational and vocational education?

2. Are IEP members familiar with recent developments in special vocational curriculum and teaching methods applicable to this period? Many traditional approaches have proven ineffective. Share the information you have gathered. For example, one new instructional approach, called "task analysis," takes a particular activity, say supermarket shopping, and breaks it down into many small component parts—appropriate dress, comparison shopping, public transportation, budgeting, handling money, etc.—which are taught separately. Then the skills are linked together and reassembled to form the total task. Although some handicapped people may make these linkages slowly, many can eventually achieve remarkable proficiency.

3. Examine your child's program. Have specific skills been identified that he must master in the transition stage and have strategies been developed for how they will be taught? Are the skills based upon a knowledge of local community experience? It doesn't really matter whether the teaching technique employs terms like *task analysis, sequential skill development,* or *chain of generic responses* as long as they have been successful in the past. The track record of transition programs geared to helping severely handicapped persons move into the mainstream of society, particularly the world of work, has not been good. Find out what skill-development techniques will be used (make sure they're described in terms you understand) and ask what kind of success rate your LEA has experienced with them in the past.

4. Again, I emphasize that you must insist upon qualified instructors. Although it can be a touchy subject, your child has the right to be instructed by teachers competent in the field they teach, particularly in secondary special education, which in the past was neglected. Inquire about the background of those who will teach such areas as vocational education. Have they had recent training in the field? Is a specific state certificate required (broken down into elementary and secondary special education), and if so, in what area is your child's teacher certified? Find out what kind of in-service training programs your school has offered in recent years. Be particularly sensitive to the availability and credentials of the school's career and/or college guidance counselor. Perhaps your parents' group can organize a fund raiser to support special teacher travel to observe model programs or to bring in experts to speak on recent curricular developments. No matter how small it is, a school system can remain alive and receptive to change.

5. Request that key people participate in IEP meetings as your child approaches his last years in school. One member of the committee who is knowledgeable about the needs and resources of the local com-

munity and familiar with state and federal agencies should act as the "linkage person" and facilitator to smooth the transfer of responsibility to adult services. He should be helpful in identifying the skills necessary for integration, play a key role in setting up and coordinating community-based instruction programs, and, finally, be invaluable in hooking you up with the service providers responsible for your child's posttransitional life. Your school may already have designated such a staff person. If not, a competent member of the counseling or guidance staff or a resource room teacher could fill the bill.

A second critical resource person is the local representative of your state's vocational rehabilitation program. Since one of the goals of this state-administered program is to help the disabled student enter the world of work, the representative may be able to arrange for a vocational aptitude test and supply you with information and counseling service. He certainly can supply details about how the services his department has to offer might help your child. The Rehabilitation Act of 1973 authorizes grants to state vocational rehabilitation agencies to provide services for a limited period to handicapped persons to help them develop the skills that would make them employable if there is a reasonable expectation that such employment is possible. The services available are varied and include: evaluation and diagnosis of rehabilitation potential, books and materials, counseling and guidance, and vocational services.

Discuss with your IEP chairperson how these two resource people can most effectively be used in planning and implementing your child's entry into outside community life. (Our experience with vocational rehabilitation, which came before interprogram coordination was emphasized, was not fruitful. Although a trial placement was arranged for Owen with Goodwill Industries, our local school system, and the state school for the deaf, Mary and I felt communication with the agencies was frustratingly slow and loaded with bureaucratic red tape.)

6. When a prevocational program is offered off school grounds, visit the site, meet the supervisor, and find out how program—home communications are handled, what kind of clothing is appropriate, how lunch (including beverage) is handled, and if snacks should be brought. Make sure the staff know about your child's special background, his nickname, medication needs, self-help ability, and other personal details. (The profile describing your child developed in Appendix A should be helpful.)

7. Examine programs carefully before giving your approval, and satisfy yourself that the placement suggested—school or community-based—meets your child's needs. Ask the professionals what specifically is to be gained through the program, and what success other stu-

dents have encountered. Is there a parent with whom you can speak whose child has participated? Have other programs been considered as alternatives? Is the program designed with local work conditions in mind? What safety precautions are in place? How will the program's effectiveness be judged? Could your child function in society without such placement?

8. Last, and most important of all, don't allow your child to leave P.L. 94-142 coverage without specific plans having been made for his next step in life.

Preparation for the Work World

Despite the fact that efforts to help severely handicapped people find and keep productive employment have been disappointing, too much is at stake for parents to slacken their efforts. Even part-time work or volunteering, combined with leisure activities, can be a satisfactory alternative. Before examining some educational programs commonly available, let's consider ways *you* can help your child prepare for possible employment.

- Through your actions and words, be positive about the world of work. When out in the community with your child, point out workers, describe what they do, and spell out how they benefit your community.
- Help your child attain good health and grooming habits and develop as high a level of physical fitness and stamina as possible.
- Encourage good work habits, particularly thoroughness and punctuality, by expecting him to help you in responsibilities requiring these characteristics in home chores.
- Be optimistic about your child's future. Identify and reinforce the positive characteristics of the world he will be entering.

Educational Pathways to Work

Many educational programs attempt to prepare students for the work world. There are too many to mention here, and they vary from state to state, but a few are common to most parts of the country.

Vocational Education

Every state offers some form of vocational education in its regular secondary education curriculum. The term can refer to any education geared toward occupational preparation and/or to the specific state organization responsible for such preparation. In the past, students involved were predominantly nonhandicapped, but, today, if vocational education is offered to the nonhandicapped student, it must also be provided for the handicapped student. Utilizing the pre-existing local or area educational network offers "special" vocational education all the advantage of a ready-made pool of teaching staff and facilities. In some instances it's helpful if representatives of both the state's vocational education network and the federally funded vocational rehabilitation program participate in the IEP meeting that plans work-oriented programs. Since many states have cooperative agreements, cooperation should be enthusiastic. Find out what facilities your LEA offers in vocational education and what access disabled students have to these facilities.

Work-Study Programs

This approach, which covers many variations, encourages the student to develop general job concepts and skills in the classroom and then to put them into practice in real, although often part-time, job settings. Ideally, work-study evolves from a series of vocational experiences that lead the student through progressively more demanding levels of work training toward a final point where he can function as an independent, paid worker. (His on-the-job experience can be paid or unpaid, depending on circumstances. Owen's pay was nominal and only enough to cover direct expenses.) Work-study can involve working at jobs in the school building, such as assisting elementary teachers, custodians, librarians, or office staff. On the other hand, it can mean traveling to a community site to learn about a job by actually working at that job or by observing a veteran employee in action (called job shadowing).

Another alternative is to become familiar with one or more occupations through presentations organized by a potential employer (called job observation, job exploration, or job orientation). Work-study programs do not normally offer indefinite *ongoing* support at the work site by staff assigned to supervise the student; therefore, participating students must be able to function "under their own steam" at a satisfactory level of independence.

Supported Employment

This is an important, fairly recent, grouping of programs directed toward less functional students who currently need, and may always need, considerable ongoing assistance if they are to perform satisfactorily in regular, competitive employment. Support usually involves a "coach," who originally trains and later assists the handicapped worker on the job in whatever areas the handicapping condition requires help. Special equipment may also be necessary to adapt work conditions. (Feedback I have received suggests that the program is more successful when the coach is an experienced co-worker who will be a continuing supportive presence than when an outside staff member is utilized.) Although continuing funding is required, the costs involved in transforming a severely handicapped individual, who otherwise might be on public assistance, into a productive member of the work force can represent a significant *net savings* to society. The human savings and benefits to everyone concerned are immeasurably larger. (Funding for this program can range from 100 percent paid by the employer to a maximum of 50 percent coming from such government subsidy as the Job Training Partnership Act.)

Another approach to occupational preparation is to identify occupations that currently exist in a community and then to train handicapped students from that community to fill the positions. This approach can be organized by the school's linkage or community resource person as the consequence of an individual IEP, or it can be institutionalized on an ongoing basis. In the latter instance school staff identify and contact cooperating area employers and develop a job bank containing descriptions of so-called entry-level jobs available, including a task analysis (skills needed for these beginning, lowest-paying jobs). Training may then be carried out at the same school or area vocational center, matching job specifications to the characteristics of student applicants.

When a student has developed competency in the skills required by the task analysis and is judged to have mastered work-related attitudes and habits, he may actually be placed on the job for a limited period of time, perhaps with temporary support. Although such experience doesn't guarantee continuing employment, it makes it a real possibility (social worker friends of mine say parents can help out by assisting their children in mastering the transportation skills required for getting to and from the job assignment—apparently a common problem area).

The goals of this approach, and of all work-oriented programs, are to develop both the manual skills necessary and the work ethic and attitudes required to land and hold down a job. With parental support, programs should work toward developing the discipline and stamina required if the student is to be punctual and regular in attendance and a contributing team member in the employer's organization.

The degree of effectiveness of any program will depend not only on the student but also on the commitment of staff, on its ability to match students with available jobs, and its willingness to get out in the community to locate appropriate job opportunities. (Parents of young children should be interested to know that some research suggests that there is a direct relationship between job success and whether students have participated at home in household chores and assumed family responsibilities.)

One personal observation, gained from our experience with Owen, is that many children with admittedly limited employment potential are stalled too long on the bottom rung of the work ladder, where everything is simulation and nothing is reality. Sometimes well-meaning staff will caution that your child is not ready to take the big step—to move on past simulation, that he is not ready to test the skills he has been learning for years, supposedly for only one purpose—to put them to use. Sometimes staff are right in their concern; however, there is a critical moment when the youngster must be given a chance to stand on his own, to see if he can move on, or whether he is forever to be stranded at the bottom of the work ladder. It is possible that by being too conservative, one can take the highest risk of all. (Parents must be willing to be thoughtful risk-takers.)

The End of P.L. 94-142 Coverage

When and under what conditions a disabled student "exits the system" varies from state to state, and even among individual school districts. Remember that P.L. 94-142 services remain in effect until your child graduates, or he leaves the school system early (when minimal state regulations permit) at parents' request or his own, or he has reached his majority, or he reaches the age when benefits for handicapped students in that state expire.

No disabled child may be forced to leave school at an age earlier than that required by state law for compulsory attendance for all students, although under certain very special conditions a handicapped child may be suspended or expelled for disciplinary reasons. When a handicapped child legally becomes an adult and no guardian has been appointed by the courts, he is entitled to make certain decisions for himself, including those concerned with school attendance. Check with your LEA to learn local regulations, or if you are concerned that your rights have been infringed upon, get in touch with your state's advocacy office.

Graduation

Usually the courses students must successfully complete to receive a diploma are determined by the local LEA, although often state regulations set a minimum standard. (Since P.L. 94-142 services extend to age 21, some special students may not "graduate" till late in their transition period.) Neither federal law nor the Fourteenth Amendment gives a handicapped student the right to a diploma. The intent of equal rights legislation is to eliminate barriers to fulfilling graduation requirements caused by a student's disabilities, not to lower standards for one special group. To comply with reality, some schools grant various types of diplomas reflecting a variety of levels of academic performance.

The importance of his receiving a diploma depends upon the nature and severity of your youngster's disability and the prognosis for his future. For example, Owen's problems were so extreme that an academic diploma was of no significance, and a certificate of attendance better reflected reality without negatively affecting his future. However, for many handicapped students a diploma represents an important psychological victory and is of real significance in their postsecondary life in either college or the job market. (On the other hand, parents have suggested that it's a mistake to push for graduation and resulting termination of educational benefits before transition plans are made. It may be, they argue, a case of being all dressed up with no place to go.)

Ask about local requirements at an IEP meeting before your child's secondary school years begin and be sure the requirements are a factor in committee planning. Early planning is essential, since graduation requirements are often based on course credits acquired over the four conventional high-school years. The IEP meeting should play a central role in clarifying requirements and in determining whether curriculum, time limits, or teaching methods and materials need to be modified.

The IEP can make specific provision to reduce the impact of a disability and may also be empowered to adjust certain graduation requirements that present particular difficulties to a handicapped child if this can be done without changing the basic intent of the requirement. For example, if a course in music appreciation is required, an art course might be substituted for a hearing-impaired student. "Whenever a student's handicap makes participation in a course inappropriate, unduly difficult or meaningless, another course should be substituted which satisfies the intent of the requirement."[2]

Once set, however, standards must be met. If specific IEP goals in a special program are accepted by the school as satisfying graduation requirements, these goals must be satisfied before the student can graduate. Therefore, it's critical that your child's progress be checked regularly. Additional effort or a change of methods or goals may be necessary before it's too late to meet graduation deadlines. Also, normally, if a handicapped student is enrolled in a regular course without a

2. "Relationship of the IEP to Grading and Graduation Requirements" (Fact Sheet 146), prepared by Josephine Barresi and Jean Harris Mack (produced by ERIC Clearinghouse on Handicapped and Gifted Children, Reston, Va., 1980, p. 1

special education provision, he will be expected to meet the requirements of that course as they exist, and grading standards will be the same for him as for any other class member. A student may still receive certain obvious support, such as Braille books or additional time on exams to compensate for his handicapping problem, but in no way can he be relieved of meeting minimal academic requirements. Grading standards must be the same for all students in a regular academic class.

22

Living Arrangements: Independent and Not So Independent

Because of circumstances beyond our control, Mary and I often moved Owen from one residential arrangement to another. Each time we were forced to face the same problems you face when it's time for your child to leave home for what you hope will be a more independent life. We've become experts in the field. For most parents the transition involves an acceleration of the search begun earlier for a least restrictive environment. This chapter concentrates on residential placement (where your child will live) and day activities (what he will be doing during the normal 9-to-5 workday). (For simplicity's sake, in this chapter the decision maker is assumed to be the parent or guardian, singly or in concert with some agency.) Some families must also consider the ultimate question: Is institutionalization the best solution?

Early on, Mary and I learned several things about leaving home and independence. We learned that successful independent living doesn't depend on facilities alone, but is the result of a combination of many ingredients. We learned that a parent cannot expect to ensure his child's happiness simply by arranging a program and signing a form. We learned that independent living is a relative thing and that meaningful independence can be achieved even in custodial institutions in which appropriate decision making and opportunities to participate in the community's activities are incorporated into a child's day. Finally, we learned that the job of providing for a child's future is more than any parent can handle by himself, that it requires help from outside the family, and that the process is easier, and therefore more effective, if you're able to put independence into perspective.

Few people can or should lead completely independent lives. Possibly the early homesteaders, who built their own houses, grew their own food, chopped wood, educated their own children, and buried their own dead, came closest to pure independence, but even they looked to one another for help. Today, most of us depend upon others. Friends and family offer emotional support; the church can be a source of spiritual strength. Often the government or private agencies provide us with more concrete assistance. To resist help, to be embarrassed, or to feel guilty can be counterproductive and may work against the interests of your child.

Getting General Information and Assistance

Let's examine national sources of help and information. An "independent living program" is a term you often hear in this context and should understand. It refers, in general, to any program that helps handicapped persons live more independent, self-governed lives and is, in part, an outgrowth of P.L. 95-602, the Rehabilitation Act Amendments of 1978. P.L. 95-602 provided funds to promote independent living and established an authority for this purpose whose direction and management came primarily from disabled people. (The independent-living movement also reflects the national concern for transition coordination, discussed in Chapter 21.) The National Institute on Disability and Rehabilitation Research supports research that "helps assure the integration of disabled persons into independent and semi-independent community life." Write them for information (see Resources: Federal Agencies).

What began as spontaneous, local, self-help efforts by disabled people to break away from institutional and parental control suddenly flourished. Despite the good start, however, governmental support to date has been insufficient to fund necessary programs, and continuing citizen lobbying is required if activities are to expand or even to continue at present levels. But parents should remember that this movement seeks independence from *all* unnecessary outside control, *including* parents. Note that the independent-living movement limits its organized activities to the concerns of individuals whose handicap is *not* so severe as to require complete custodial care or hospitalization.

Title VII of the Rehabilitation Act reinforces three principles central to the concept of independent living. First, an independent-living program should be a community effort utilizing the resources of the community it serves. Next, it should be consumer-oriented, depending upon the people who receive services (the handicapped consumers) for leadership. Finally, it should provide not rhetoric and promises but services needed to help its constituency attain maximal independence: transportation, education, job promotion, attendant care, housing, peer counseling. Unfortunately, Title VII is currently only partly funded, although many independent-living organizations are aggressively tapping local and state funding sources and even generating their own income through consulting work for the private and public sectors.

Independent-living organizations answer many needs and can be structured in a wide variety of ways, and they may have many names and fill many functions. They can provide or coordinate such necessary services as transportation, housing, and attendant care and may be called independent-living residential programs. They can be called transition programs and offer halfway housing for severely handicapped people moving from some restrictive environment to more independent living (this is also called an independent-living transition program).

The name isn't important. It's performance that counts. A first-rate independent-living center, such as Alpha One in Maine, can offer wheelchair sales and service and on-site accessibility surveys for public and privately owned buildings. It can recommend equipment and modifications to the home and workplace needed to enable an individual to operate more effectively. It can act as an advocate to see that public buildings and transportation authorities observe required standards. It can operate driver education and assessment programs with specialists (an occupational therapist, for example) who not only teach driving skills but also recommend adaptive equipment to make driving safer and easier for the individual (see Resources: Suppliers). It can be an educational center where business management, consumer and legal knowledge, safety, healthy sexuality, and personal-care management skills are taught.

Such programs, run by disabled people for disabled people, are the wave of the future and represent a primary and expanding resource. Parents, however, should be sensitive to the ground rules of the organization—and to its justification—and participate, when appropriate, with discretion.

Throughout the area of independent living, activity is expanding and interagency coordination is improving. Some states have established independent-living programs for the blind and a number of mental health and mental retardation agencies have initiated local community programs to support independent living for mentally retarded as well as mentally ill citizens. Resources are increasingly combining forces to meet needs when one resource, alone, would have been insufficient. (Housing and Urban Development (HUD) loan/subsidy programs in combination with state funds and federal SSI funds are an example.)

In my efforts to locate information I found Independent Living Research Utilization (ILRU) of Houston (see Resources: Independent Living) particularly helpful. ILRU describes itself as a "national center for information, training, and technical assistance in independent living." If you are interested in this area, contact ILRU and ask for a listing of resources available. It responded to my request promptly with an avalanche of excellent material, including a listing of independent-living programs in my state. The Center for Independent Living, in Berkeley, California, is another fine resource.

Plotting an Overall Program

Who will be responsible for your child's program and how can you help make it the best available? In planning your child's adult living arrangements, certain broad responsibilities must be provided for. Someone must:

- Find out what agency is responsible.
- Arrange for an appropriate plan and see that it is implemented. If satisfactory facilities are not available, participation in the creation of facilities that meet the need might be considered.
- Monitor and evaluate progress.
- Provide for continuing family support.
- Make financial arrangements.

Finding out whom to contact is the first step. Years ago, when it became obvious that Owen could no longer live at home, we approached state agencies for help. Frustrated by delays and not knowing what agency, if any, was responsible, I became convinced that no satisfactory state placement was available. In desperation, we decided to move Owen to an out-of-state school at our own expense. Today, such a drastic, expensive, and often unsatisfactory step should not be necessary if parents take advantage of resources available.

You may already have established a relationship with a social service organization and/or your state may already have legislation mandating support. If not, or even if you need only general information, the following resources should give you a helping hand and information about whom to contact. (Chapter 21 also dealt with establishing contact with adult service organizations.) Contact:

- The LEA's special education director or a member of your child's medical team.
- Your state's advocacy or developmental disabilities office.
- The area department of human services, the agency concerned with mental retardation, or a local hotline.
- Your parents' support group, nearest independent-living center, or national organizations, such as ARC.

These same resources provide information peculiar to your state in a wide variety of areas affecting posttransition living arrangements; for instance, there may be a consent decree imposing special conditions on a program, or there may be low-income, accessible housing in an area appropriate for your child. Armed with such information you should be ready to contact the agency you hope will replace the LEA as your institutional partner.

Making the Approach

Now, as you enter an area in which a productive partnership with professionals is critical, I'm going to reiterate some adjectives I used earlier in describing exemplary parental behavior. I suggest you be courteous, considerate, reasonable, positive, and cooperative. Don't overdo: don't be pushy, overly assertive, or a chronic complainer. In all your efforts, remember that your primary job is to serve your child and to be responsible for his interests, and public servants have a similar responsibility. Neither the parent, guardian, nor public servant should forget the complementary nature of these responsibilities.

Initial Contact

Whether you phone or write depends upon which approach is most congenial to you. I found it usually quicker to phone on the first contact, although it may prove more frustrating, since you may encounter prolonged waits while the appropriate person is found and brought to the phone. By following up the call with a letter, you can enjoy the best of all possible worlds, since you create a record confirming details for your notebook and are almost ensured a response (most agencies require that all correspondence be answered within a certain time). Some advocacy groups suggest that sending copies to your correspondent's superior will stimulate attention. I would refrain from such potentially abrasive action until I had exhausted all normal channels; more than attention may be stimulated. Another advantage of direct phone contact is that, psychologically, you feel you're on top of things, whereas it could be weeks before you receive a written response, and meanwhile you stew.

Before you telephone, refer to my earlier suggestions (see "Telephoning" in the index). Think through what you'll say to the switchboard operator. For example, "Please connect me with someone who can supply information on residential placements and day programs for an adult mentally retarded man." Once you have been referred to the correct department, describe your child's situation briefly. For example, "My son has Down syndrome. He's 21 years old and lives at home. This arrangement is no longer possible, and I would like an appointment to discuss ways in which your agency can assist me in providing housing and a program for him."

Be prepared to supply your child's Social Security number, age, address, and your phone number as well as any public services he may be receiving, particularly if he or you participate in any program under Social Security. Ask that you be sent written material describing the services the agency renders, if available, including a description of procedures required to obtain services. Record the name and title of the person with whom you speak, the date of your appointment if one is arranged, whether your child is expected to attend the preliminary meeting, and the material you should bring to the meeting or send in advance.

If you are told that this is not the agency designated to serve you, ask for the name and phone number of the one that is, and the name of the individual with whom to talk. In the unlikely event an agency will neither meet with you nor refer you to another agency, ask for a letter setting forth the reasons for the rejection (in case you appeal its action). Read carefully the material sent you as well as other material mentioned later in this chapter. It will help you make the most of the first meeting and suggest questions to ask.

The Individualized Program Plan

Most state and some private agencies follow procedural patterns similar to those used under P.L. 94-142, and many of the general suggestions made earlier pertaining to educational services are applicable here as well. Occasionally, at transition time, IEP team and individualized program plan meetings can be held together, or representatives of one committee can attend the other meeting—by invitation, of course. Your child must be found to qualify for services—usually on the basis of medical evidence and financial need. Eligibility may be established at the first meeting, although you may have to sign a form so your doctor will release medical records. (Obtaining medical records may take longer than you expect. Don't hesitate to remind your doctor if records are slow in coming; it's often a case of no records, no services.) If your child qualifies for services, a group of individuals, in some states called an interdisciplinary team (IDT), makes specific program and placement recommendations, and you and your child, if he is capable of understanding what is involved, should be key members of this team and play an important part in decision making. Sometimes the handicapped child is present at meetings but is *ignored* and talked *around*. If your child has the ability to participate, see that the staff acknowledges him and treats him like other committee members.

The total package of services is sometimes called an individualized program plan (IPP), and your youngster is usually euphemistically referred to as the "client." (The IPP is similar to but more comprehensive than the vocational rehabilitation individualized written rehabilitation program (IWRP).) More than most federally supported programs, vocational rehabilitation programs vary from state to state, so you *must* find out what services are available locally.

Similar to the procedural protection guaranteed under P.L. 94-142, the appeal process follows the general requirements of due process as to which areas can be appealed and the fashion in which the appeal is to be made. Often even eligibility decisions may be challenged, but the IEP analogy is not completely valid, since there is currently no federal legislation similar to P.L. 94-142 covering all adult human services operations. Of course, the rights of every citizen are guaranteed by the Constitution, and if any state program receives federal funds, the protections of Section 504 also apply.

Since social service regulations vary from state to state, to understand what rights you and your child enjoy in your relationship with state agencies, familiarity with your state law is necessary. Every agency with which you deal should (upon request) furnish and explain the regulations under which it operates. Ask for a copy. You should know what happens to your child's plan during the time an appeal is in process, what agency actions require your approval, and what right you have for legal representation.

Agency regulations should provide for regular revision of the plan as well as explanation of conditions under which IPP meetings can or must be convened. As in the IEP, your child's strengths as well as weaknesses should play an important part in IPP construction and determine his needs, which in turn will set the goals and objectives required to meet these needs. An initial assessment will arrive at recommended placement services and a program, and regular re-evaluations will monitor progress and adapt the program to changing circumstances.

Examination of past medical and educational records, professional consultation, and input by staff will help establish the foundation for the program. The final written IPP, like the IEP, should describe in detail all the special services required, by whom they will be provided, and the nature of the participation by the client, parent, and representatives of any facility or agency involved. It should consider the total client and address all his basic physical and emotional needs. The importance of appropriate skill development, often a vital ingredient of the IPP, has been emphasized throughout the book and will not be repeated here except to reiterate that skills taught need be realistic and practical.

Evaluating the Program

Almost every agency has a formal evaluation requirement, often in the form of an annual IPP review. You, as a parent or guardian, should be part of that process; if not, ask that you be included. Some critical points to consider are:

- Have objectives been met? If not, why not?
- How does your child feel about himself, the program, and his progress so far?
- Does it appear that real movement toward more self-sufficiency has been achieved?
- Have all the services contained in the IPP been provided?
- Have community resources been utilized to the maximum?
- Has the program kept you informed?

Routine Services

In general, the IPP should be individualized for your child. Whether he is placed in a residential facility that provides its own daytime activities or remains living at home or in a group home and participates in a separately organized day program, in many states certain standard services will be provided to him and *all* other handicapped participants. These services act as a foundation upon which the IPP is built.

In Maine the basic services are called "routine services" and include, if your child is in a residential program: an annual physical, dental care, continuing medical treatment, sex education, access to religious activities, and instruction in personal and home management, grooming, travel, safety, and nutrition. If your youngster's in a day program, routine services include supervision of health and safety, sex education, diet/nutrition, and participation in the individualized program plan. Helping your youngster find a home (a better term than *residential facility*) where he has the best chance of being happy is a pivotal point. You should know what's available, both nationally and within a visiting radius of your own home.

Housing

On one end of the housing spectrum are the custodial institution and intermediate-care facilities, which represent the most structured and restrictive environment. Fortunately they are rarely required. Many possibilities, however, exist for those whose capabilities make more independent living possible. Although a great deal of overlap exists among categories, and names and organizational details vary from state to state, most living arrangements are similar nationwide. Here are a few:

- **Home care, foster care, and family care:** A child may remain in his own home or in the home of a friend where adaptive construction can make living quarters pleasant and convenient and daytime activities and transportation can be arranged through local agencies. In addition, the client is not required to leave familiar settings and established relationships. Foster families or families who board one or more clients on a less structured basis commonly receive remuneration from the state and assume a more or less parental role, although overall supervision is usually provided by some agency.

- **Halfway houses (sometimes called "hostels"):** These are temporary residences for those waiting for or preparing for a more permanent independent-living option, although the stay can, under certain circumstances, be extended to more than a year. Therapy, instruction in independence skills, and counseling are often provided.

- **Group homes:** This common arrangement consists of a group of between 4 and 10 residents who, under the supervision of a live-in counselor or house manager, share homemaking responsibilities and function much like a family. Sites are often residential houses. Many group homes and hostels offer 24-hour supervision; some provide highly structured living and close supervision (even one-on-one) for the severely handicapped individual whose needs do not require a medical facility. Homes are often located so clients can walk to nearby resources or take advantage of local transportation. Community access is vital!

- **Supervised and/or sheltered apartment programs:** This is another traditional arrangement in which the resident, living alone or with a partner or partners in an apartment, receives varying degrees of supervision, assistance, and counseling, depending upon the nature of his handicap. In some instances, a regular program of skill development is offered in such areas as money management, meal planning and preparation, general housekeeping, and personal hygiene. Supervised apartment living can be a transitional step to more complete independence, although such placement can also become permanent. Sheltered apartment living with a resident manager is similar to the supervised approach except that counseling is often less frequent and the expectation is that the arrangement may be an end in itself. The difference between the two can be in the eye of the beholder.

- **Lodge programs:** Sometimes hospital staff members or other professionals organize a number of handicapped persons as a group to operate a business together and share both living and financial arrangements. As is discussed later, many thriving enterprises have begun in this way.
- **Independent living with a personal care attendant (PCA):** This option is particularly appropriate for physically handicapped individuals with little or no mental impairment. It offers maximal independence; since the client hires and directs his own attendant, the residence is really the client's home turf, and to that extent he is master of his fate.
- **Unsupervised living accommodations with no structured supervision or assistance:** This possibility is usually realistic only for the mildly retarded and those with moderate orthopedic impairment. I urge caution, since even the most independent youngster can fall prey to people who take advantage of individuals who are in any way vulnerable.

Independent Living with Attendant Care

This option is wonderful for those who have the potential. For many it can be the ideal solution. Some physically disabled persons—and under certain circumstances those with mild mental disabilities—can live more independent, unsupervised lives in an adapted physical environment if occasional help with certain tasks can be obtained. For a book that describes thespecifics involved, I recommend *Design for Independent Living: The Environment and Physically Disabled People* (see Resources: Independent Living).

For many physically handicapped persons, the help of a personal care attendant (PCA) can tip the scale and make independent living a reality. The PCA is hired by the disabled person and works directly under the disabled person's supervision to help him in the activities of daily living. Many handicapped persons find this relationship refreshing, because the PCA allows them, perhaps for the first time in their lives, to become the masters of their lives, free of the overriding authority of parents and professional caregivers.

In general, PCAs can be utilized in two ways. Either the PCA can be retained personally to work when needed in the disabled individual's own quarters, or a group of handicapped people can join together—perhaps in the same apartment or in clustered residences—and organize a pool of attendants. The handicapped community in Berkeley has pioneered the use of PCAs and has flourished there possibly because of them. Whether PCAs must be licensed varies from location to location.

In many states listings are available, although sometimes difficult to obtain. Your state's department of human services, bureau of rehabilitation, or, particularly, the nearest independent-living center should have information in this area. If circumstances make the use of PCAs impossible, or if organizational work presents a problem, commercial organizations such as Upjohn Health Care Services can provide somewhat similar services.

Finances

Unfortunately, the costs of the PCA must often be borne by the individual. Occasionally health insurance will pay benefits, and in some states Medicaid benefits can be applied, although rarely will they cover the entire cost. (If your child qualifies for Medicaid, ask the nearest Medicaid office about their "waiver" program, which can provide significant financial support. The local independent-living center should also be up to date in this area.) State benefits vary, so check for yourself. In Texas, for example, the Department of Human Resources pays for a portion of attendant-care costs for qualifying individuals.

Handicapped persons seeking independent housing can approach the problem of rental payments in a variety of ways. Many facilities are so organized that the rental charges required can be covered by the SSI benefits of qualifying clients. In other homes, sliding scales fix the rental on the basis of the ability to pay. Low-income and handicapped individuals may be eligible for housing assistance payments from the U.S. Department of Housing and Urban Development. Payment is made by HUD directly to the rental property owner and amounts to a monthly payment that will:

> make up the difference between the HUD-approved rental amount and the amount the tenant is required to pay. Tenants pay an average of 30% of their adjusted income (gross income less certain deductions). Rental assistance payments under this arrangement are not considered additional income to the tenant who is also eligible for Supplemental Security Income payments from the Social Security Administration. For further information on rent assistance or other housing programs benefitting disabled persons write to Special Advisor for Disabilities, U.S. Department of Housing and Urban Development, Room 10184, Washington, DC 20410.[1]

1. *Pocket Guide to Federal Help for Individuals with Disabilities*, Publication No. E-87-22002 (Clearinghouse on the Handicapped, U.S. Department of Education, Washington, D.C. 20202), p. 22.

Another invaluable resource in the area of housing is the HUD User, an information clearinghouse under contract with the Office of Housing and Urban Renewal. HUD User helps citizens like you find the most recent information available from HUD (it has an 800 number— see Resources: Clearinghouses). Become familiar with HUD User's services before making long-range housing plans for your child's future. Some of its manuals, as well as other material, are listed in the Resources section under "Adaptive Housing and Equipment."

Starting a Facility on Your Own

Today a large number of citizens, many of them parents frustrated by the lack of adequate housing, are creating residential facilities either on their own initiative or as part of a group. An example is the Langton Green Development in Anne Arundel County, Maryland, where twenty apartments were built as part of a supervised living program conceived by a group of families in cooperation with ARC. In some instances I know parents who have given housing to their children and made arrangements with an organization to provide supervision. This is a good idea, but in your planning take into consideration the income limitations that might make your child then ineligible for federal programs. (See Chapter 27.)

Although circumstances vary, and each carries with it particular challenges, five generalizations may be helpful if you are considering such an undertaking.

1. Gather a sample group of interested people and examine the possibility together. Try to include an attorney, an accountant, and at least one handicapped person in this group, as well as a successful businessperson. The handicapped group member is a *must*; it would be great if he eventually served as chairperson. Some organizations receiving federal money require that handicapped citizens constitute a stipulated minimal percentage of the board of directors. At the beginning keep the study-group small, so that if the idea makes sense, more members can be added without making the group unwieldy.

2. Collect information, paying particular attention to the state licensing agency's regulations as well as the requirements of the agency that may refer clients to your facility (department of human services, bureau of rehabilitation, etc.). Your state's independent-living center (it can go under various names) should be a source of this information. Since funding will be critical, become familiar with possible sources of building or renovation loans. In addition to the HUD User services, two manuals will come in handy: the *Summary of Existing Legislation*

Relating to the Handicapped, and *Pocket Guide to Federal Help for Individuals with Disabilities* (see Resources: Guides).

3. Ask the accountant or businessperson on your board or committee to draw up a rough budget of anticipated expenses and income on the basis of your estimate of the average number of clients to be served annually. If this estimate looks promising, you're ready to move forward.

4. Consider forming a tax-exempt nonprofit organization.

5. Once you have established a formal organization with a board and officers, you are ready to make specific plans. Consult with the applicable state agency and/or a nearby independent-living program. ILRU, in Houston, Texas, may be able to offer advice.

Mary and I considered starting such an organization but were discouraged by the financial picture and the considerable amount of bookkeeping involved. Don't undertake such a move unless you are totally dedicated and ready to put a great deal of yourself (including some of your own money) into the project on a long-term basis. Some key points:

- Know staff requirements and certification.
- Understand the safety and health-code requirements.
- Remember to provide for ongoing supervision. Sometimes arrangements can be worked out with a human services provider, which could have financial benefits for both client and agency.
- Find out if you can accept private nonagency clients.
- Determine how much control state agencies will have over your operation.
- Check to see how frequently you will be reimbursed by the agency providing most of the clients.
- Know what obligations you have, morally and legally, to supply a day program.

If you find all the variables satisfactory, and you and your group determine to move ahead, Godspeed! There is a tremendous need for this resource.

Final Decisions

When the IPP reaches the decision-making point, here are some housing questions you should have answered:

- Do the clients participate in community activities and services?
- Are transportation arrangements satisfactory? (Try them out yourself.)

- What provisions have been made to promote fire safety? What kind of attention is paid by staff to problems of street safety—drugs, alcohol, forced prostitution, and sexual molestation (both on the street and in the facility)?
- What are the admission policies? Must applicants be city, county, or state residents or a client of a particular agency? If there is a waiting list, where does your child stand and does any other class of applicants receive priority? (Some agencies reserve a certain number of spaces for their clients, which can work against the interests of a parent who must arrange his own child's placement. It did for us when a placement we desperately wanted was not available because a state agency had "reservations" that effectively closed that placement to private clients.)
- How are ongoing and emergency medical problems handled? Will someone check to see that medication is being taken?
- How are residents involved in household chores and planning? Do activities encourage independence or dependence? (Unfortunately, it's often easier for staff members to do a task themselves than to teach it to a client.)
- If counseling and various therapies are offered, on what basis are they provided?
- How are leisure-time activities and unoccupied hours of the day handled? See for yourself what goes on by dropping in at odd times, including the weekend.
- Are there published visiting hours and rules, particularly pertaining to sexual conduct on the part of residents? If so, look them over to see if they're reasonable (see also Chapter 25). Ask if there is a policy on restraining residents with behavior problems and whether staff has received training in this area.
- What is your impression of staff members? Are they enthusiastic? What is their training? Has there been much turnover?
- How are finances arranged? Is it a private or publicly funded program or facility? How will you be expected to pay, and what are considered extras?

Probably the most important advice I can offer is never to agree to a placement you have not personally visited. We were always surprised at the number of parents who never bothered. So much can be learned by seeing how current residents react to one another and to staff members. To get information about residential possibilities available in your state, contact your local bureau of mental health/retardation, the nearest independent-living center, the area chapter of ARC, a local parents' support group, or national organizations, such as Easter Seals or Independent Living Research Utilization (ILRU).

The Work Day: Posteducation Work Activities and the Real Thing

Earlier I stressed the importance of seeing that your child's 9-to-5 day is filled in a way that is meaningful to him, and suggested that daytime activities could be the pivotal ingredient of a successful life away from home, even more important than residential placement. Several options are available, but don't impose your own value judgments on your youngster. Getting and keeping a paying job in the competitive marketplace offers the least restrictive environment, the closest approach to the normal world, and, for that reason, is the most desirable alternative. However, for many, like Owen, this option is not a realistic possibility, although many programs as well as federal initiatives and dollars have been directed toward such placement. On the other hand, being responsible for housekeeping duties in a group home or working on even the simplest task in a sheltered workshop—for a lifetime, if that's all that is possible—can be as meaningful to a child with a severe mental disability as working on a computer at a big company downtown is for a hearing-impaired youngster who suffers no mental limitation.

Finding the right program or employment can be more difficult than locating acceptable housing. Don't be easily discouraged or reluctant to make changes if you're dissatisfied with your child's situation. It may require a great deal of effort, but it could be worth your while. In the pages that follow I mention many resources, some that may help you promote your child's interests, others that will be helpful *only* if you are interested in taking a larger advocacy role. Be selective. You can't be knowledgeable about every resource and law. I mention them only so they will be there if you need them.

Earlier I urged you to become generally familiar with federal legislation bearing on vocational education if work is a possibility for your child. Some of the same laws also have the effect of ensuring that handicapped citizens are encouraged rather than discriminated against in the job market. The Rehabilitation Act of 1973 speaks to this point, particularly in Section 504, which as I have pointed out forbids any program or activity receiving federal money to discriminate against persons who are "otherwise qualified."

This means not only that handicapped workers enjoy equal job-related benefits and activities but also that reasonable accommodations will be provided to help them overcome their disability in the performance of their job. Accommodation can mean anything from giving a blind worker oral rather than written instructions to adding a $150 speech synthesizer or a comparable peripheral device to a computer.

One small nonprofit company specializes in working with industry to adapt jobs to handicapped employees.[2]

Section 501 of the same act requires federal agencies to make an effort to hire qualified handicapped employees, to see that they receive fair advancement opportunities, and to have an affirmative action plan, spelling out these rights and setting forth exactly how they will be guaranteed. Section 503 requires affirmative action in the hiring of qualified employees for any company involved with federal contracts in excess of $2,500. Words like *reasonable, qualified,* and *affirmative action* sound fine in general but are vulnerable to different interpretations in the particular. Consequently, several federal agencies are responsible for enforcement. If you have problems, contact your state advocate (see Chapter 24).

In addition to prohibiting discrimination, the government encourages employers to hire qualified disabled workers by offering tax incentives, Targeted Jobs Tax Credit (TJTC), by earmarking on-the-job training funds through the Job Training Partnership Act (JTPA), and by encouraging businesses to make their premises accessible through Tax Credit to Business for Barrier Removal. The government has even entered into partnership with private business by sponsoring joint hire-the-handicapped projects and, as we have seen, one of the primary responsibilities of the federally sponsored vocational rehabilitation program is, in cooperation with industry, to place disabled citizens in appropriate jobs. Outside the government, organizations like the Association for Retarded Citizens, the United Cerebral Palsy Association, and the Epilepsy Foundation of America (write them for information on TAPS, their Training and Placement Service) are active in providing job-training services and disseminating information.

A recent encouraging development is the willingness of local parents' groups and area associations to take matters into their own hands and to create actual jobs for their own children in their own towns. The Shoreline Association for Retarded and Handicapped Citizens (SARAH), in Connecticut, began its operations, which now include a wide variety of services to handicapped people, by starting businesses for its clients to operate: the Apple Doll House Tea Room, a gift store, a landscaping operation, a restaurant, a maintenance company, a concrete products operation, etc. SARAH even leases the town golf course and maintains and runs it (see Resources: Support Groups). The February 1987 issue of *Exceptional Parent* featured work opportunities initi-

---

2. Some information taken from "Jobs for Disabled People," by Frank Bowe, in *Public Affairs Pamphlet No. 631* Public Affairs Committee, Inc., March 1985.

ated by parents' groups: the Stepping Stones program in California, which, as part of its training program, operates a small business on a profit-making basis, and Independent Opportunities Unlimited (I.O.U.), of Oregon, whose mobile crew of handicapped workers runs a groundskeeping and maintenance company.

For physically handicapped individuals, the transition to employment may be made easier by the use of adapted and special equipment and reading materials. The National Library Service for the Blind and Physically Handicapped Reference Circular "From School to Working Life: Resources and Services," compiled by Merrillyn Gibson, is a marvelous resource. By all means get a copy. It's free! Here's an example of its content: "Many devices and tools, particularly in the computer field, are currently on the market to aid in matching skills of the disabled persons with the requirements of a specific job." (Many can be helpful in postsecondary education and in the home as well.) The circular proceeds to list and describe this equipment and concludes with a bibliography of books and periodicals dealing in more detail with the subject. Devices include Braille translation software programs that "instruct computers to transcribe material from print to Braille," and talking terminals with a "speech synthesizer [which] converts digital information to recognizable speech." Did you know there are such magazines as *Bulletins on Science and Technology for the Handicapped* or *Aids and Appliances Review*?

Educate yourself so that you can be a resource person not only for your own child but also for other handicapped youngsters in their efforts to enter the workforce. Use the Reference Circular "From School to Working Life: Resources and Services" just mentioned and the resources it lists as a springboard for learning about vocational rehabilitation, job-search techniques, the Multiple Sclerosis Job Bank Program, the Job Accommodation Network (JAN) of the President's Committee on Employment of People with Disabilities, and all the federal programs related to training and employment of disabled persons. Many federal acts and programs deal with the area of work: the Randolph-Sheppard Act, the Wagner-O'Day Act, the Equal Employment Opportunity Commission (EEOC), the Office of Personnel Management Selective Placement Programs, and even NASA's Handicapped Recruitment Program, Office of Equal Opportunity programs. Not every parent will, can, or should become even superficially familiar with all this legislation, but for those who wish to be helpful in the area of employment opportunities, knowledge of the assistance the federal government can offer is important. Much digging is required, but the reward could be great if you help a handicapped child or children make something of their lives. (The nearest office of your federal congressional delegation should be able to provide information on any of the programs I have mentioned.)

Your child might be interested in developing a home-based business. If he uses a wheelchair but has good fine-motor control, he could learn the skills of metal engraving, calligraphy, or trout fly-tying. I know from experience that there's a shortage of competent professionals in these fields, at least in my state. The Small Business Administration in Washington offers tips on how to get started. Write them. There should be a field office in your state. If your child would rather work for someone else but operate from his own home, ask your nearest state Vocational Rehabilitation office to help you locate responsible companies who "farm" work out to home-based workers (in many states the Vocational Rehabilitation Department will help shepherd your child through the entire job-placement process). But before your child gets involved with unknown people in any business relationship, check them out through the local chamber of commerce or your city's Better Business Bureau. There are creative ways to generate jobs, but it will require more than thumbing through the help-wanted ads to locate them.

Compiling an effective résumé and preparing for the job interview are important steps for which help is available. Ask your reference librarian for written material on the subject, or contact the President's Committee on Employment of People with Disabilities or your local independent-living center for suggestions. In preparing for the interview, I suggest you follow the same sensible guidelines anyone would use. Your child's potential employer is interested in hiring someone who is organized, enthusiastic, appropriately groomed, pleasant, reliable, and independent. He will want to know how a handicapped employee will handle the problems that appear to be associated with the disability, for example, transportation to and from work, communications, and health (a statement from your doctor could be helpful but certainly is not necessary). You know, and I guarantee the employer knows, the mandates of the law, so don't remind him of them. Be upbeat and straightforward about your problems. He shouldn't be as interested in your problems as in your solutions. For heaven's sake, don't be confrontational. One thing he doesn't need is a new employee whom he sees right off the bat to be a potential problem.

If Competitive Employment Is Not an Option

An often overlooked alternative to full-time paid employment is volunteerism, which, on a regular basis, offers many of the advantages of the competitive marketplace and can be a stepping stone to a regular job. Through it your youngster can make contacts with the outside world, learn work skills, and gain satisfaction from a job well done— all in a less stressful environment. Don't underestimate the importance of his having a place to go where people are glad he is coming and thank him for having been there. Many urban areas now have coordinators whose job it is to hook up willing volunteers with appropriate openings. Your local chamber of commerce will probably know if such a person exists and, if so, how he can be located.

Most custodial arrangements and intermediate-care facilities include a round-the-clock structure for their residents. The majority of group homes and even some sheltered apartment facilities provide in-house or affiliated day programs that may consist of activities with such names as work or day activity centers, sheltered workshops, supported employment, transitional living, or volunteering programs. (In some private programs, regular classroom instruction continues to provide academic training long after residents are past the normal school years.)

Whatever their name, often the focus of these programs is not so much on eventual placement in competitive employment as it is on providing living skills to improve the quality of the residents' lives by making them more self-sufficient, and on broadening their participation in such leisure-time activities as arts and crafts. Sometimes arrangements are made with area agencies to provide programs, and contact is made with local organizations (churches, the YMCA and YWCA, community adult education and recreational programs) to integrate residents into community life. With Owen, we were much more concerned about whether he seemed to enjoy the activity than with the quality of his work—the weaving, the painting, or the lettering that he produced. But no matter how successful residential and day programs are, some ingredients vital to successful independent living can be provided by you and your family better than anyone else.

Paradoxically, in his attempts to live more independently, your child needs the continuing support of his family more than ever. It's possibly one of the few stabilizing influences in his life, which is full of change. Do you visit and write him regularly? Have other family members been involved in his attempts to gain independence? Aside from the pleasure that their presence furnishes your child, it's important that close relatives be familiar with the details of his program and the personalities involved so they can carry on if you become unavailable. Even though you may have no legal responsibility after your child has reached his majority (the law varies from state to state), you still have a moral obligation. If he is living out of town, weekly letters, birthday presents, and holiday cards are important. Visits home and to the homes of adult siblings should be arranged often.

23

The Institution

The Trauma of Choosing Institutionalization

Few words have as many negative connotations as *institutionalization*. It strikes at the core of how we view ourselves and our responsibility to the handicapped child. When Owen was a baby, few options existed for parents with severely disabled children. There were large state centers, a very few small private institutions, and the possibility of keeping your youngster at home during your lifetime. Institutionalization and home segregation were the norm. Before the drive toward the least restrictive environment and normalization, a parent who tried to work his child into the "mainstream" was often criticized by neighbors for "pushing the kid into a competitive environment where he'd only suffer." Today the opposite is true, and even the suggestion of custodial placement is frequently viewed as a sentence to a hopeless life in a forgotten backwater.

Fortunately, although some state institutions have been closed or reduced in size, the spectrum of alternatives has dramatically grown since those early days and their quality has improved. Families with disabled children are able, without guilt, to take advantage of many of the options available to normal families (day-care programs, summer camp, vacations away from the children), and the percentage of children who actually require the services that only residential placement offers has declined. However, for a significant number of people, institutional life still is the best alternative, and this alternative should be explored as dispassionately as any other option.

The trauma created by the ordeal of sending a child away is still not easy to bear. Often father and mother view the decision from conflicting perspectives, and differences can be so wide as to threaten their marriage. Fortunately, Mary and I were in agreement—this option was so obviously the right one for Owen. Our decision was based primarily upon what we thought was best for our son, but we were also convinced that the move was the right one for the entire family, because the time came when we felt our son was threatening the entire family structure. He took up our whole day, and when left alone for a minute he would sit and stare, sometimes in the dark, until we came back. We got to the end of our collective rope. It wasn't so much that we couldn't cope, although perhaps we couldn't. Our dilemma was that there seemed to be no advantage to Owen in our coping. He seemed happiest when he was with others who operated in the same world as he. Although Mary and I reassured one another this was true, in our heart of hearts we feared such thinking might be self-serving rationalization.

One of the most debilitating characteristics of residential placement is that it often isn't a final solution but one that must be faced again and again through the years as the child is forced to move from one location to another. There is rarely an emotional closure. Even today few facilities offer lifetime services. Another wrenching characteristic that "goes with the territory" is that rarely can a parent look back with pleasure and say with unwavering confidence, "This was the right thing to do." Even in our family, with all its support systems, we have memories of those early days that never grow dim: the joy of having Owen home on vacation, followed by the despair of vacation ending. Despite the bleak moments, institutionalization proved to be a success, and today, although Owen comes home with a broad smile, he is always anxious to get back to his buddies. His school provides an environment where there is much for him to do, much that he can do, and where he feels at home.

Making the Decision

Although every family faces a different situation, on the basis of our experience I note a few general observations applicable to most situations: Take enough time to make a thoughtful, informed decision, but don't allow thoughtful delay to lapse into procrastination. Gather as much professional advice and information as possible and look objectively at the pros and cons as a mother and father seeking the best option for their child and for the entire family.

Often the decision will come as the result of an IEP meeting and interaction with professionals. The least restrictive environment principle and financial concerns can be persuasive influences arguing against such a move, and school officials rarely recommend or agree to residential placement unless appropriate educational services obviously cannot be provided to the student by the LEA in the home environment. However, if after carefully examining local programs you are convinced that an institution is the only answer, stick to your guns. Remember, you must agree to the IEP before it can go into effect. In the event of an apparently irreconcilable disagreement, I suggest you consider initiating the appeal process. The character of your child's handicap, the adequacy of transportation to local services, the availability of specialists in the field, long-term goals, behavioral problems, and the home situation all should be evaluated. If you are one of those fortunate people who can afford the high costs involved in private placement, LEA agreement is not necessary, but your decision will still be difficult.

Selection and Evaluation

Literally hundreds of institutions across the country offer residential placement. Unfortunately, private facilities can be expensive and public placement can be complicated or even impossible, particularly if your child doesn't meet specific state admission criteria. Porter Sargent's *Directory for Exceptional Children* (see Resources: Directories) lists institutions by disability served and separates them by state into private and public categories. It includes considerable information on individual institutions as well as speech and hearing, psychiatric, and guidance clinics, along with the names and addresses of federal and state agencies and U.S. and Canadian associations, societies, and foundations listed by disability. This sourcebook is helpful if you're interested in a general survey of residential placements.

Other useful resources are *The Directory of Members of the National Association of Private Residential Resources* and the U.S. Department of Education's *Directory of National Information Sources on Handicapping Conditions and Related Services* (see Resources: Directories). The latter is an outstanding source of information but may be eliminated by federal budgetary cutbacks. If so, petition your congressional delegation to reinstate it or to see to it that it is replaced by *one* federal agency responsible for compiling a similarly comprehensive, national directory of resources for handicapped citizens.

If these directories are unavailable in your local library, the reference librarian may be able to identify the nearest library where they can be found. Even then you must usually travel to inspect the directory, since reference material rarely is available through interlibrary loan; occasionally, if you know exactly what you want, selected material can be reproduced and sent to you.

Contrary to popular opinion, some institutions, often church affiliated, specialize in preparing clients for integration into society and act in a transitional capacity. Regulation, certification, and state/federal approval vary from state to state, but in general all institutions are subject to local governmental regulations pertaining to health and safety. In addition, most, public or private, fall under some kind of supervision by the State Department of Education and/or Human Services or by some federal agency, particularly if public money is in any way involved. This supervision can be either a blessing or a disadvantage depending upon the competence and dedication of the controlling bureaucracy.

Owen's school is privately owned, and Mary and I have been extremely pleased with its flexibility and freedom from often-inhibiting educational regulation, which allows it to operate in the way the staff see as best for their clients. The expense of private institutions, however, excludes them from consideration by many parents, and in their relative freedom from governmental red tape can be vulnerable to the problems that such regulation attempts to avoid.

To encourage high standards, many private institutions participate in voluntary accrediting organizations, sometimes along with public institutions. For example, the Accreditation Council for Services for Mentally Retarded and Other Developmentally Disabled Persons (see Resources: Facilities, Schools, Institutions, and Clinics) is sponsored by such national organizations as the Epilepsy Foundation of America, the United Cerebral Palsy Associations, Inc., the Association for Retarded Citizens, and the American Association on Mental Retardation.

The National Accreditation Council for Agencies Serving the Blind and Visually Handicapped (NAC) in New York City and the Commission on Accreditation of Rehabilitation Facilities (CARF), in Tucson, Arizona, are two other accrediting organizations (see Resources: Facilities, Schools, Institutions, and Clinics). Listings of accredited schools may be available from these organizations to help in your search for suitable residential placement. Such accreditation, however, is voluntary, and an institution's absence from the list does not necessarily have negative implications.

Although both residential facilities and the goals parents have vary greatly, some generalization about how one can prepare for the decision-making process is possible.

1. Be sure your goals are clearly defined. Do you prefer an institution that is large or small, single-sex or coed, rural or urban—and what's the basis of this preference? Do you have strong feelings about educational philosophy, sex education and human sexuality for the handicapped, institutional structure, physical restraint, religious practices, specialized staff required, and policy on visiting and correspondence? Too large a staff can pose a problem if management feels they must be constantly utilized, particularly if additional charges are made for their services. Organize your thinking and establish priorities.

2. Get feedback. Although parents are apt to give the truest picture, institutions are not apt to refer you to dissatisfied clients. Sometimes it's possible to get grass-roots feedback from an area parents' support group, such as ARC, especially if day students are enrolled. One

reliable way of gauging resident sentiments is to be on hand when the youngsters return after a vacation or weekend home. When Owen is happy, he leaps from the car and rushes into the building without a backward glance. If a large percentage of children return long-faced and silent, I would want to know more about the institution. Accreditation by an established organization is certainly a good sign. If a facility isn't evaluated by some accrediting body, ask why it isn't; if it is, ask to see the summary of its most recent accreditation report.

3. Attempt to judge the quality and continuity of leadership and staff turnover. One problem Mary and I faced in our relationship with institutions was the frequent turnover of staff, and one of the great strengths of his current "home" is its stability. If a transitory environment is upsetting for parents, think how it must affect the child. Inquire about in-service training for staff. Sometimes the school representative you meet during the initial interview will not be involved with your child, so don't be too influenced by the impression he makes—if the institution is smart, he will be one of their brightest lights. Judging the abilities of top administrators is important, but meeting the staff who work daily with the clients is key and should be insisted upon. In particular, ask to speak with the houseparent who will be responsible for your youngster's physical well-being.

4. Find out how communications between parent and child and parent and institution are handled. Will a staff person—sometimes called a "correspondent"—be assigned to keep you posted on a regular basis? How will medical emergencies be handled, and how often and in what form will clinical progress reports be available? Good communications are of particular importance if the school is far away from your home.

5. Determine how long your child can stay. If your goal is not limited to short-term institutionalization, a facility that offers the possibility of care through the adult years has much to recommend it.

6. If the institution represents itself as a bridge to eventual integration into society, try to determine how successful it has been. An attitude that focuses on the least restrictive environment and on teaching transition skills is vital. How extensively is the program integrated into the local community? Such integration is beneficial for the handicapped client, and it's an excellent way to spread public awareness and understanding.

7. Examine the details of your financial responsibilities. What charges are not covered by the base fee? What has been the history of tuition increases? Is there a plan through which lifetime services can be guaranteed? Such an arrangement is not available at Owen's current

home and usually is not available because of the unpredictable nature of inflationary forces.

8. Finally, visit the place! You can learn more about an institution by seeing it in action than by reading its brochure. (If possible, visit sometime other than regular visiting days.) Mary and I always felt one key ingredient of an institution was the degree to which it was able to make its clients feel at home, comfortable, and good about themselves. Owen's physical and mental well-being flourish in environments where staff and other clients care about him and show it. Walk the grounds of the institution. The body language of even the most severely disabled individual will tell you a story if you will only "listen." (Unfortunately, it is sometimes a story the accreditation committee never sees.) After you have addressed these questions, you should have a realistic feel for the institution you're considering and whether you want to entrust your child to its care.

Public or Private?

Because of financial considerations, deciding between public and private care is rarely a factor, although LEAs and state agencies occasionally utilize privately operated facilities. On the other hand, many church-affiliated institutions require only a modest tuition or one that is adjusted on the basis of a family's ability to pay (a sliding scale). Our family selected a private institution for many reasons, the most important of which was that it appeared to meet Owen's needs far better than any other organization we knew of, and fortunately we could afford it. Experience has confirmed our judgment. Of secondary long-range importance, but key to us at the time, was that we would have had an indeterminate wait for admission to the only acceptable state-sponsored alternative, a group home more than 100 miles away which had not particularly impressed us on our visit and which left the management of daytime activities to the parent to arrange.

Parental Responsibilities

Whether your child's institution is public or private, you can help make institutional life happier if you:

- Visit as often as possible, preferably on a regular basis so your youngster can look forward to seeing you. If the institution has special parent affairs that other parents attend, make an extra effort to go.
- Write regularly. This means a lot to a child, even if he can't read. To be the only one not receiving mail is awful. I buy dozens of out-

landish, out-of-date greeting cards (it doesn't matter what their subject—bar mitzvahs or golden wedding anniversaries do just fine) and Mary makes some cards out of recycled Christmas cards. I add my own stick drawings. Owen apparently loves them.

- Join the parents' organization, if there is one and if the distance to be traveled makes participation realistic. Such groups, a potential agent for helpful support and change, are usually underutilized. We started one, but it requires work, an upbeat view of human nature, and a thick skin.
- Give the staff feedback, but make it positive and constructive. It is difficult for them, particularly in an institutional setting, where parents are often far away, to correct unsatisfactory situations if they don't know that they exist and that parents are interested.
- Don't assume an institutional placement will always be best for your youngster. Both he and circumstances may change. Keep an open, inquiring mind. Don't assume that the services he needs won't someday be available in a less restrictive environment.
- Finally, admit you will not live forever. Make plans to cover the responsibilities that must be shouldered by someone else after you're gone—financial, emotional, and decision making (see Chapter 27). This is a problem for which there is sometimes no foolproof solution, but avoiding it won't provide any solution. Arranging for siblings to pick up the reins is an obvious approach for some families. Friends or other relatives may also provide help.

24

The Advocate

There are times in our lives when we need a helping hand, and an advocate is a person who tries to provide this help. He may defend you, provide you with information, or work for your best interests in any number of ways. When referring to the handicapped population, *advocacy* means acting for the individual to see that he receives a fair deal. Because of the unusual problems handicapped citizens face, however, special efforts must be made to see that their rights are protected. As we have seen, several laws and court decisions detail these rights and set forth specific procedures to ensure they are not violated.

A lawyer is an individual advocate who defends his client in court, but an advocate may also be a whole group of people. The Pennsylvania Association for Retarded Children—now Retarded Citizens—acted as an advocate in May 1978 when it brought a class-action suit against the State of Pennsylvania arguing for the right of all handicapped youth to an equal education. (A class action is a legal suit representing an entire group, or class.) Your local parents' group could act as an advocate for the handicapped population in general and for your child in particular were it to seek a zoning change to allow a group home to be established in your town. (This is an informal class action.)

Advocates can help your child in different ways at different times, and this chapter discusses when and in what way advocates can be useful, and how to obtain their services. Remember, however, that well-informed parents remain the most effective advocates for their own children.

When a Parent Needs Help

Sometime as your child's live-in advocate you'll need help. For example, you may feel unqualified or you may lack free time because of the pressures of your job, especially if you're a single parent. The problem may be legal, medical, or educational and it may require expert advice. Your natural impulse will be to contact the professional with whom you are already associated, and ordinarily this is the sensible thing to do.

Sometimes, however, particularly if you have a complaint, the people you would ordinarily turn to for help are part of what you see to be the problem. In this case an independent consultant is almost a necessity. Typical of this kind of advocacy is the psychologist who provides a second evaluation for an IEP, the lawyer who advises you of possible grounds for a malpractice suit, or the doctor who testifies that your child's handicap qualifies for agency services. At one time our family retained a psychologist to represent us in our attempts to arrange respite care through state agencies. Such private advocacy can be out of the reach of many people for financial reasons, although sometimes professional advice is available either free or on a sliding-scale basis. Public advocacy, on the other hand, is always free. Although laws change and are constantly amended, I am convinced there will always be at least one federally designated agency responsible for providing advocacy protection. Your challenge is to locate it and use it wisely. I am also convinced that funding provided under the law will always be withheld from states not guaranteeing equal rights protection, although, sometimes, states may be allowed to spend federal funds in different ways.

Advocacy Services

Certain Advocacy Services Are Required by Law

Federal legislation (including P.L. 94-142, P.L. 94-103, and the Rehabilitation Act of 1973 as amended by P.L. 98-221) makes explicit provisions so that disabled citizens are not denied access to federal programs, and state laws usually reflect or implement such action. P.L. 98-221 (Sec. 112a) authorizes grants "to establish and carry out client assistance programs to provide assistance in informing and advising all clients and client applicants of all available benefits under this Act, and, upon request of such clients or client applicants, to assist such clients or applicants in their relationships with projects, programs, and facilities providing services to them under this Act, including assistance in pursuing legal, administrative, or other appropriate remedies to ensure the protection of the rights of such individuals under this Act."

P.L. 94-103, the Developmental Disabilities Assistance and Bill of Rights Act, establishes the same type of safeguards for the "client" (your child or you as his representative; we are now also called "consumers") and mandates that the advocacy system established by the state "must be independent of any agency which provides treatment, services or rehabilitation to persons with developmental disabilities."

This independence from influence is vital; you wouldn't ask the fox to guard the chickens.

The details of how this advocacy is provided are left to the individual state, and the agency responsible goes under different names in different states (for example, Advocacy Services in Arkansas, Protection and Advocacy in California). There are several ways you can locate help if you believe you're not getting a fair deal and have been unable to work things out with the agency involved. Your state's Developmental Disabilities Office is one of the best sources of up-to-date information, and the community services listings in the phone book may offer leads under such headings as "Advocates," or "Disabled." In some states all public advocacy is located in one department (see "protection and advocacy agency" in your NICHCY State Resource Sheet), and many states publish lists of their toll-free hotlines and have computerized listings of all services available, publicized by TV and radio public-service announcements. (NICHCY also publishes a directory of national toll-free numbers.) These advocacy organizations may be called ombudsmen or protective services and cover such diverse areas as mental health advocacy, accessible housing, child or adult abuse, civil rights violation, and so on. When you inquire, be sure you make clear in what area you desire assistance.

Advocacy's General Characteristics

Although the details differ across our country, there are certain services your child can expect from most agencies. They should:

- Tell you if he qualifies for their services. (If your request for help is rejected, they should inform you how you can appeal *their* decision.)
- Explain the services they offer.
- Listen to your problem (even that may help) and explain your child's rights under the law.
- Provide expert opinions or advice, if requested.
- Investigate your case, get the facts, and try to work out a solution agreeable to you.
- Help you, or even represent you, in a formal hearing or appeal, if your child's problem can't be solved in any other way.

Protecting your child's very basic, but general, right to fair treatment on a day-to-day basis involves some specific rights that are generally agreed to by everyone in theory but violated occasionally in practice. (If it weren't for the violations, advocates would be out of business.) Among them are the rights to free appropriate education, equal housing opportunities, equal employment opportunities, a life in the least restrictive environment, nondiscriminatory treatment in transportation, freedom from intrusive treatment and neglect, effective utilization of the judicial system, privacy, dignity, appropriate medical treatment, recreation services, and physical safety—in short, the right to be free to live as normal a life as possible.

Other rights often mentioned by professional advocates are still controversial when applied to those with severe mental disabilities and can be causes of bewilderment to parents. For example, the right to parenting services, sexual expression, and marriage; the right to vote; and the right to acquire and control property. The problems that these rights generate are too complex and too personal for treatment in this book, although I do discuss the question of sexual rights in Chapter 25.

The Advantages of a Public Advocate

Public advocates (sometimes called "case-manager advocates") should be qualified on the basis of statewide criteria and up to date on all the benefits to which handicapped citizens are entitled. Their services are free (if you qualify) and confidential, and they should work solely for your interests. Public advocates are often supported by a large department with financial and staff resources that individuals lack. Their services are client-directed, which means that the client does not relinquish control of his own affairs but, in consultation with the advocate, decides the basic approach to use in negotiations and the goals sought. Remember that the client is the handicapped person—your child—and not you, and the client makes the final decisions unless he is a minor or a legal guardian has been appointed by a court.

Although this book assumes that the parent speaks for the child, in practice you must determine whether you have that legal authority. The age when "children" reach legal majority is a state matter; usually it's 18 if they are mentally competent. In most instances the client can terminate the advocacy arrangement at any time and resume representing himself directly. If you have retained an attorney in the matter, check with him before going to a state advocate for help, to avoid confusion about who represents the client.

Public advocacy organizations are vulnerable to the pitfalls to which all bureaucracies are subject. They may have more demand for the services you require than available resources. You may have to wait your turn, although they will probably have a priority system. (When you make your initial contact, check on this.) You may find that the advocate assigned your case is often out of the office and unavailable. My experience is that staff turnover can be high, and you have no guarantee that one advocate will be with your case throughout a long, drawn-out affair or that you will see eye to eye with him. Another possible disadvantage is that he may focus on settling disputes, and probably can't guarantee that your complaint will be taken to court.

It's important that you have confidence in your child's advocate and that he clearly understands your objectives. Although we opted for private consultants, I often came in contact with public advocates as I made my rounds on Owen's business. Many were, in my opinion, first rate and effective. A few, however, seemed to confuse their own agenda with that of their client, particularly in the area of sexual rights. Be sure your advocate fights *your* battle and represents your child in a fashion you feel appropriate. One advantage of retaining a private consultant is that you have absolute control over selection and can change advocates at your option. (Another advocacy option that may be worth considering is the American Civil Liberties Union (ACLU), but I suggest you contact them *only* after exhausting the other advocacy resources mentioned in this chapter who are specialists in problems faced by citizens with handicaps.) On the whole, if your state advocacy agency is well run, the advantages of utilizing their services outweigh possible disadvantages, and you can't beat the price.

Here are a few suggestions to help you when applying for assistance from your state advocacy agency:

- Locate your nearest advocacy office and find out if it has a toll-free number.
- Contact the advocacy office. Ask the staff to send you information describing their services (including the appeal process) and any other material dealing with your problem or interest.
- After looking over the material, you may wish to apply for services. Call the office, but be prepared to provide information it is almost sure to require: name, address, telephone number, information about your child's disability, and the problem you want help in resolving. Be sure to record the date, time, and the name of the person with whom you spoke in your notebook, along with the 800 number, for future reference. If you feel comfortable writing, by all means write a dated note and keep a copy. If your situation is an emergency, contact the agency right away and make sure the person with whom you talk knows the nature of the emergency. Ask when you can expect to receive an answer.
- If you don't hear within a few days of the date given you over the phone, call again to ask when you can expect to be contacted.
- If your request for services is rejected, you may utilize the appeal process that most state agencies have available.

If you are unable to get satisfactory answers, contact an office of your congressional delegation; the staff should be familiar with federally mandated advocacy programs. In unusual circumstances in which a child is at risk, a state government board or council can step in to establish a guardianship or a trusteeship, a kind of protective services advocate to safeguard and represent the child. (A number of professionals may initiate this chain of events: a hospital social worker, a juvenile service officer, or an official from the educational system.) In other instances in which it is felt the public sector should step in to protect the interests of a disabled individual, an ombudsman may be appointed to act for that person.

The Citizen Advocacy Movement

Professional advocates aren't the only option. Increasing numbers of organizations are training volunteers to serve this function. Some parents' groups have initiated "teaching chains": a professional advocate trains one parent in advocacy skills, who then trains another parent, and so forth. Parents can make good advocates. Their sympathies lie with other parents, they speak the same language and share similar experiences, and they may not be associated in any way with the bureaucracy. However, volunteers may find it difficult to be available at the times when the client most needs help.

Another approach to citizen advocacy is the child advocacy project. Sponsored primarily by the Association for Retarded Citizens, the program uses core training materials to help people start state and local programs and it provides a standardized package on citizen advocacy to train citizen advocates. Their activities have now spread into many states, and your local ARC chapter should have detailed information. Although volunteer advocacy is a relatively new movement nationally, I suggest you establish contact with a local group that offers such services to see if their program suits your needs. My experience with such an organization, although not extensive, has been positive.

Parents as Advocates

A continuing refrain throughout this book is the key role that parents play as supporters and defenders not only of their own children but also, as best they can, of all handicapped children. Not all parents will be able—or want—to extend their activities beyond their own families. What might be possible for the well-to-do parent whose child has grown and lives in a residential facility is worlds apart from what is possible for the single working parent who has all she can do to hold things together. Your primary responsibility is to be an effective advocate for your own child; it is far more important to continue this role through the years than to support a variety of outside causes.

Do be an advocate for *all* handicapped people if and when you can. It shouldn't be difficult to locate a cause to help; in all probability your life has been peppered by "there ought to be a law" thoughts. Any group of citizens who band together to right what they see as a wrong is involved in what could be called "class advocacy," although they might call it lobbying, political action, or a parent coalition. Many of the reforms that we benefit from today were brought about by such groups, and I have found that generally the groups are made up not of wild-eyed radicals but of people just like you and me.

Never assume that your voice doesn't count or that things can't be changed. Not only will you feel good to know you are helping others but you may advance your own practical interests beyond the particular issue you are fighting for at the moment. Here are three potential benefits:

- It is often easier to become acquainted with the resources available and the procedures necessary to utilize them (on both the local and national level) if you are personally involved in evaluating and attempting to improve these resources and procedures for others.
- The group of advocates with whom you become involved, not all of whom will necessarily be parents, can act as a natural support group for you when you seek solutions to your own problems.
- In working with a cross-section of the community, you can develop a better understanding of other people's points of view and problems, which often can make you more effective when dealing with these other people later when promoting your own child's welfare. However, these practical advantages will be advantages only if you have acquitted yourself in a professional, thoughtful, and adult manner. If you are extreme and unreasonable, the chickens you release in anger are apt to fly home to roost in unexpected ways.

Maximizing Your Personal Advocacy Potential

Your effectiveness ultimately will be determined in two ways: by the actions you take and by the way you take them. Your strategies will be controlled by local conditions. You can become involved in the political scene by running for the school board, PTA, town council, or planning board. If you lose the election or don't feel public positions suit you, you can attend hearings on issues affecting the handicapped, help start a needed parents' group, or apply positive pressure on decision makers about specific issues by writing letters or sending telegrams.

is the transportation situation in your community? Are day-care centers available for special kids? Are there respite-care facilities, a Ronald McDonald House?

You can expand community understanding of handicapped persons by starting or joining a group that stages puppet shows and other presentations for schools and civic groups. The presentations show in dramatic visual terms a nonstereotyped picture of the disabled person. You can demonstrate that disabled people are warm, flesh-and-blood human beings who have grown beyond their handicap. Just working in your community to change destructive stereotypes could be a lifetime occupation.

How do you find what needs attention in your community? Listen, read the papers, and look around. Several excellent booklets deal with the subject of community advocacy, and parent and advocacy groups will develop and make others available. Whether or not you are the advocacy type, get some of the current material and add it to your own reference library. The *Advocacy Handbook: A Beginner's Guide to Affecting Change*, a publication of the Parent Information Center in Concord, New Hampshire (see Resources: Support Groups), has been helpful to me and is a handy resource in this area.

How You Do Things Influences Your Effectiveness

Your attitude and abilities will determine the effectiveness of your efforts. The skills involved in running a meeting, speaking in public, starting an organization, and negotiating a settlement are not within the scope of this book, but there are ways to improve your abilities in these areas and books are available if you are interested. Whether you wish to be an advocate for all handicapped kids or only for your child, the attitude you have when you put the technical skills to work is vital.

Throughout this book, optimism, perseverance, cooperation, and intellectual curiosity are emphasized as characteristics you'll need. Assertiveness is another. When kept under control, it is almost a necessary ingredient of successful advocacy. The manual *How to Get Services by Being Assertive,* by Charlotte Des Jardins, provides excellent and comprehensive coverage of this subject, offering both general approaches and specific techniques in the pursuit of personal effectiveness (see Resources: Advocacy). The areas covered are indicated by such chapter headings as: "Let Your Body Language Say Positive Things about You," "How to Get Off the Guilt Trip," "How to Get Around the Runaround," "How to Negotiate with Bureaucracies," and "How the Press Can Help You Get Services." I recommend that you get a copy.

25

Sexuality and Sex Education

Originally I approached the subject of sexuality with discomfort and almost didn't include it in this book because of four concerns.

First, I was bothered because the topic intrudes into a highly personal and controversial area about which parents and even professional caregivers often feel uneasy and unqualified. A generation gap exists between some younger professional advocates and parents whose values were established before the sexual revolution. In some cases, religious beliefs run counter to the positions promoted by those who advocate complete sexual equality and freedom of expression—including homosexuality—for the handicapped person.

When Owen was young, my view of sexual fulfillment for the disabled person was unfortunate in that I grouped it and the sexual act together, associating both only with procreation and sensual gratification. In those rare moments when I thought about it at all, I believed that handicapped individuals should be prohibited from all overt sexual activity and that they were uninterested in or incapable of participating in any meaningful human relationship that involved sexual intimacy.

Second, when I was forced to make decisions concerning Owen in a sexual context, I found there was little helpful literature on the subject, and for the small amount of research available, results were often contradictory. As a consequence, limited factual information was available upon which to base opinions.

Third, even if a parent was concerned enough to seek help, counseling and support resources were generally unavailable—and what good is a chapter on resources if there aren't any resources to report?

My fourth concern was that, never having come to grips with my own son's sexuality, I feared I would be a poor advisor for others. Unfortunately, my experience is typical of that of many friends whose primary concern is to protect their children from the negative by-products of human sexuality rather than to help them struggle to gain its positive benefits. For years I scrupulously avoided thinking of Owen as a sexual being. Having no communication at all with him except the most elementary body language complicated an already complex and, for me, distasteful subject. It's characteristic of the environment in which I moved that at no time in all my conversations with educators, institutional administrators, or parents over a more than twenty-year span did the subject of sexuality arise except in the context of possible abuse, pregnancy, venereal disease, or similar concerns.

I eventually changed my mind, partly because, as I read through current literature, I saw that progress is being made, that resources are gradually becoming available, and that whatever the difficulties, sexuality has been too long swept under the carpet and ignored. I also concluded that I, as a battle-scarred participant, might bring something of value to the subject. Times have changed and so have I. What is the situation now and what about the areas that originally concerned me? (*Sex Education for Disabled Persons* [see Resources: Sexuality] was extremely helpful to me in the preparation of this chapter.)

Let me begin with the caveat that the potential for meaningful sexuality, like so many other areas involving people with handicapping conditions, is dramatically affected by the nature and severity of the disability and that what may be possible or appropriate for one person could be out of the question for another. Only the individual parent will be able to determine if any of this chapter is helpful. The generation gap and a reluctance to confront their children's sexuality are common among many parents, but time and the sexual revolution have mellowed sensitivities.

Many, like myself, now understand that sex for people with disabilities is not necessarily limited to achieving sensual satisfaction but can be a first step toward reaching an intimate emotional and physical relationship with another human being that is helpful in many ways. A handicapped couple can make an effective team and give each other better support than their professional caregivers can. An opportunity to form a close relationship of any kind can be rare for many handicapped people. Owen has had few during his life. "Sexuality and self-esteem are intimately connected. For those whose learning skills will never carry them into law, medicine, music, or science; for those whose uncooperative bodies will never accept discipline, or grace, success and satisfaction in personal relationships are particularly vital in giving a great sense of self-esteem and self-worth. There is little left for one who has cause to feel permanently outside the circle of things that matter."[1]

What resources can we provide that offer our children as much happiness as this kind of relationship, and on what basis can we deny them such an opportunity? Many parents' response to the problem is to

1. Dr. Sol Gordon, "Disabled Children Are Vulnerable," in Irving Dickman with Dr. Sol Gordon, *One Miracle at a Time* (New York: Simon and Schuster, 1988), p. 300.

try to shield their children from all sexual exposure, but is this isolation possible, even if it were desirable, when every TV set proclaims its own kind of lurid sex education? And can you imagine a group home or institutional lounge without a TV set? Having always assumed mentally disabled people were incapable of satisfactory sexual responses, I was surprised to learn that for a significant number of those with mild retardation, a meaningful sexual relationship and sometimes even marriage are possible and that even some individuals with moderate intellectual impairment can, in varying degrees and in supervised situations, receive pleasure and benefit from sexual activity. With marriage or whenever sexual intercourse is involved, particularly where participants have chromosomal disorders, the possibility of passing on the condition to offspring must be considered, and I strongly recommend counseling, sexual and/or genetic. The degree to which the parent participates depends upon the age and condition of the special child (who obviously is biologically no longer a child).

With more severe degrees of mental retardation, sexual control decreases and the possibility of sexual activity acceptable to society decreases proportionately. In short, in my opinion, expanded sexual experience is not desirable for all, and some severely handicapped people can be upset by new personal contacts and find disturbing any factor that threatens to change the order and regularity of their lives.

Examining my own experience, I find the most persuasive argument for a parent to take active interest in his child's sexuality expressed in one question: Can I bar him from participation as a sexual being, irrespective of his potential, knowing that this may be one of the few experiences in his life that will link him to the mainstream of life and proclaim his humanness?

Examining my second reservation (lack of reliable information), I find that, although research is still limited, more and more helpful literature is becoming available every year (see Resources: Sexuality).

I still find little reason to be overly optimistic about the third reservation, lack of sex counselors and resources. Sex-education courses for disabled persons remain largely inadequate, and professional counseling resources are either scarce or nonexistent in many areas and probably will continue to be so for the foreseeable future, particularly in rural regions. But despite the lack of resources and continuing public apprehension, the situation improves steadily and the environment is better now than in 1962, when Owen was born. I have learned a great deal, and, if I were to lead my life with Owen over again, I would do things differently:

I would not automatically assume my son incapable of any meaningful sexual experience. Such may turn out to be the case, but too much is involved to act on the basis of simplistic judgments. Society has fluctuated between two contradictory and unfounded myths—one suggesting that handicapped people are perpetual sexless Peter Pans, the other that their elementary drives are overpowering and beyond their control.

I suggest that a parent does not have the right to dismiss sexuality as a taboo topic or to foster either myth. If one assumes that the child develops many sexual attitudes by the age of five, there is very little time to make the informed judgments concerning his sexual potential that a parent must make if he is to be positive and supportive. In many instances the youngster should be able to look forward to a life in which, with parental support, sexuality can play an important and constructive role. Don't make any hasty assumptions. A child is not deprived of sexual drives because he can't walk or talk or see normally, or even do simple math problems. "Urinary incontinence does not mean genital incompetence. Absence of sensation does not mean absence of feeling. The presence of deformities does not mean the absence of desire. Inability to move does not mean inability to please. Loss of genitals does not mean loss of sexuality."[2]

If your child is severely handicapped and you have questions, as we did, seek advice. Time is important; some vital matters should certainly be faced before puberty. Embarrassment may be unavoidable but, embarrassed or not, go ahead. A frank conversation with your child's doctor is a natural first step in obtaining information. Your question might be, "Doctor, in view of my youngster's condition, how do you evaluate his future life as a sexual being? How can I best support him? The last thing I want to be is destructively inhibiting."

Your desire for this information is as normal as are questions concerning other developmental issues. Impress upon the doctor the seriousness you attribute to the problem and that you want to find out if a sexual life is possible and if not, why not. If the doctor feels unqualified to answer, and he well might, ask him to refer you to someone who is qualified. Your source of information doesn't have to be a professional sex counselor who specializes in matters concerning the handicapped. A respected professional in some other field can be helpful. A lawyer, a nurse, a clergyman, or a social worker who is a close friend or one with whom you have established a close relationship and with whom you can speak freely can act as a sounding board or refer you to appropriate resources. There may be no definitive answer for you, but you are ac-

2. Ted and Sandra Cole, as suggested to Dr. Sol Gordon in *One Miracle at a Time*, p. 301.

customed to living with unanswered questions, and at least you've done all you could.

Try not to be rigid or judgmental. The sexual revolution and the movement for deinstitutionalization have precipitated many changes for the disabled population, not all of which have necessarily been good. Parents must make difficult decisions. I don't suggest they can arbitrarily change attitudes held for a lifetime nor do I assume that administrators or professionals have all the answers. I do suggest parents be open to examining these concepts when they affect their children's future and evaluate them thoughtfully, particularly since in some fundamental areas even the experts disagree.

Professionals tend to be of two minds about sexuality. Some (often institutional administrators) believe that severely handicapped people should be protected and consciously steered away from sexual involvement, since "they are happier without it, and only frustration and vulnerability can result. So often the kids get hurt needlessly." Some professionals suggest that to encourage sexual expression, or even to allow it, is purposely creating an unnecessary complication—that it's looking for trouble. On the other hand, some suggest that many areas of sexual experience constitute a basic human right and that mentally retarded citizens, for example, should enjoy the same freedoms as other people living in our society. One writer[3] has presented a list of eight basic sexual/social freedoms for mentally retarded people:

1. The right to receive training in social-sexual behavior that will open more doors for social contact with people in the community.
2. The right to all the knowledge about sexuality they can comprehend.
3. The right to enjoy love and to be loved by the opposite sex, including sexual fulfillment.
4. The right for the opportunity to express sexual impulses in the same forms that are socially acceptable for others.
5. The right to birth control services which are specialized to meet their needs.
6. The right to marry.
7. The right to have a voice in whether or not they should have children.
8. The right for supportive services which involve those rights as they are needed and feasible.

3. W. Kempton, "The Mentally Retarded Person," in H. Gochrus and J. Gochrus eds., *The Sexually Oppressed* (New York: Associated Press, 1977), as quoted in *Sex Education and Counseling for Mentally Retarded People*, Ann and Michael Craft, eds. (Baltimore: University Park Press, 1983), p. 2.

Some professionals express attitudes widely at variance with those of many mainstream parents, occasionally in language unnerving to parents: "With these concepts, the client should realize that guilt is an inappropriate feeling, not because the individual is less able, but because no standards for anyone, disability or not, are legitimately imposed. One needn't worry about being different sexually because anything goes that is functional and mutually acceptable. Oral-genital stimulation, manual stimulation, anything that the couple or the individual can find satisfaction in doing is okay, and we as professionals and agencies have to make our permission and sanction (because we have the power to grant such) very clear."[4]

Being nonjudgmental and open-minded is difficult. At many professional meetings of those concerned with providing services to handicapped persons, I have heard the complaint that, in matters concerning sexuality, parents often block the way to more independent living by being overly conservative and protective. As we saw earlier, letting go is difficult, particularly in areas that challenge some of our fundamental beliefs.

As a first step, you should attempt to become well informed. To make intelligent decisions and to function effectively as your child's advocate, you need a broad knowledge of sexual matters that may affect him. This knowledge will help you to know both when it's important to get expert advice and where it can be obtained. Parents can't become knowledgeable in every area, nor should they try to, but some information can be critical. For example, the information gained from genetic counseling can be important when providing sex education and counseling for your child if he or she is thinking about marriage.

If your child's handicap is physical, you can be of help by being familiar with the many orthopedic devices now available to make the sexual act, or sexual gratification, possible. (The Resources section lists suppliers of this type of equipment and national organizations that might furnish helpful information.) Physical and occupational therapists also are potential resources. Seeking information about this sensitive field may be embarrassing for you, but it may be impossible for your child. Raising the subject and exploring it with him may be too difficult for you. One alternative is to have someone else, a member of the medical team or a friend—preferably a contemporary—or a sibling of the same sex, engage your youngster in a candid conversation and even act as his ombudsman.

4. Milton Diamond, *Sexuality and Disability*, from an address, "Sexuality and the Handicapped," presented at the National Rehabilitation Association meeting in Honolulu, Hawaii, in 1973 and now published by the National Easter Seal Society, 1981, p. 4.

When legal questions arise concerning such matters as marriage of two retarded people, homosexuality, and sexual abuse, self-education can be tricky. I feel it's prudent to seek professional advice, and if I were the parent of a child who had the physical potential of becoming sexually active, particularly if he were institutionalized or capable of limited independent living, I'd seize the opportunity to ask our attorney about the kinds of exposures a parent should be alert to. The issue of involuntary sterilization of a young woman with a severe handicap is particularly complex. In many states there is, for all practical purposes, no way in which this can be legally done unless proof is offered that her life or health is in severe danger during pregnancy. My only advice, if sterilization might be a consideration, is for parents to address the issue early so as to allow time for appropriate professional consultation.

Similarly, parents often can obtain little assistance in the areas of sexual counseling or in dealing with unwanted pregnancies. The courts offer little or no assistance at all, but some guidance may be available from social workers with whom you have established personal relationships.

Many years ago the state arbitrarily withdrew funding from an institution Owen was attending. Although to my knowledge formal charges were never made, it was suggested that the state took action because of child-abuse allegations (possibly of a sexual nature) lodged by former employees. Mary and I had to decide whether Owen would remain there or move with the other dislocated children to an undisclosed institution somewhere "upstate." It was a difficult decision, but, after consultation between ourselves and with a lawyer, Mary and I decided to have Owen stay put, primarily because we felt the school was being falsely accused and our son had been and would remain safe there. I eventually retained a lawyer and took legal action against the state in the name of the school's owner on the grounds that the government had closed the school without observing due process. We won the suit, but the state appealed, and the owner refused to pursue the action. I was disappointed. Legal fees had been expended; the owner's reputation had been sullied; many children's lives had been affected; and the state was never legally required to explain its actions.

One of the reasons human sexuality has long remained a taboo subject is that it means different things to different people, and sometimes major misunderstandings occur. The effects of sexual activity fit easily into two categories: First, those having public ramifications, such as marriage, procreation, birth control, sex education, genetic counseling, and legal involvement (e.g., indecent exposure, sexual abuse, and prostitution); second, those activities that are personal and private. The second category includes all sexual behavior that should go on behind closed doors and has to do with sexual gratification, and the effect a successful sex life has on an individual's happiness and self-esteem. One problem for parents is to determine what their role should be in these significantly different areas.

I would attempt to act upon my knowledge in a timely fashion. Parents can be supportive in more areas than one might expect. Parents can help their children in a minor way by being straightforward and by using correct labels to describe intimate body parts and functions. Males have penises; people urinate; females have vaginas and breasts. Euphemisms and cute codes aren't helpful to a youngster who already feels different from his peers and "out of it." He can be embarrassed at school if he doesn't even understand the adult sexual vocabulary.

It's even more important that you teach your child proper behavior and don't allow activity to be inadvertently taught that encourages the negative image sometimes associated with mental handicaps. This is more difficult than it may appear. For instance, behavior that you innocently encourage when your youngster is five—hugging, kissing, patting—will be inappropriate when he becomes a young adult. You can indicate in a kind way that grown-ups don't hug and kiss strangers; they shake hands and look one another in the eye. Owen lost his job at a sheltered workshop partially because we hadn't corrected his practice of patting people's behinds. While acceptable at one stage in life, this mannerism is suspect and misinterpreted later.

Both parents and society in general encourage unacceptable behavior when, for understandably practical reasons, we maintain double standards for our handicapped youngsters. It is not surprising that Owen has no idea that nakedness is inappropriate and that it's not O.K. for him to emerge from the bathroom naked or leave the toilet in a restaurant pulling up his pants and zipping his fly. For his entire life, both at home and in institutions, the niceties of sex-appropriate behavior have often been impractical; females have helped him in the shower and toilet, and an array of professionals—often complete strangers to him—have conducted endless examinations of the most personal nature without the benefit of explanation or introduction.

The remedy is obvious but difficult. Parents and caregivers should maintain the same environment in private that they expect the child to observe in public unless the child is able to understand the differences between the two situations. If he can understand, you should make a consistent effort to explain the difference and to see that it is observed. The entire question of what is acceptable in society's eyes in behavior and grooming can have sexual overtones and reinforce the unfortunate stereotype of the unkempt, sexually uncontrolled handicapped person. I find two articles helpful in this area: "Advice on Good Grooming," by Carol Tingey, Ph.D., in the April 1987 issue of *Exceptional Parent,* and "Learning Appropriate Social and Sexual Behavior: The Role of Society," by Dvenna Duncan and June Canty-Lemke, in the May 1986 issue of the same magazine. Duncan and Canty-Lemke suggested that the average citizen sees certain characteristics as typical of the retarded person: ill-fitting clothes, poor grooming, loud talking to oneself, over-friendliness, inappropriate touching, and masturbation in public. However, the authors suggested that "they are all behaviors which can be changed," just as nonhandicapped people learn acceptable behavior by getting negative responses from parents and friends when they transgress. Thus, when Owen misbehaves by patting a stranger's bottom and the family only smiles and excuses him on the grounds that "Owen's different," his bad action is positively reinforced, and Owen is given the message that it's not only not bad to pat bottoms but, in fact, rather cute.

In the long run it's cruel to excuse your child from society's norms. How much healthier it is to insist, in a kind but firm way, on his observing them. Help him make the most of his appearance and to look as attractive as possible. It's important for sexual reasons, among many others, that we help our youngster look as sharp as he can. In her article, Carol Tingey stressed the importance of grooming principles that apply to all, such as weight and dandruff control, and particular remedies for specific groups (e.g., for the Down syndrome child, lip balm or petroleum jelly can help eliminate permanent lip fissures). The author also emphasized developmental therapy to increase muscle tone and balance, exercises to increase muscle control of the mouth area, and, perhaps, most important of all, cleanliness of the body, braces, communication boards, and wheelchairs.

Sex Education Should Be a Priority

If your child has even a minimal ability to communicate and understand concepts, sex education is important, even though it may be controversial. (Owen's retardation is too severe for this to be a possibility.) Don't be deterred by those who argue that teaching the retarded about sex will only confuse and frustrate them, that what they don't know won't hurt them, and that since many can't look forward to marriage or child bearing, learning about responsible sexual behavior will stimulate them to participate in undesirable sexual activities.

Since the vast majority of retarded persons live in community settings, it's unrealistic to believe they won't be exposed to word-of-mouth sex education from their peers, which can be misleading and confusing and encourage unrealizable fantasies. One of the primary goals of P.L.

94-142 was to dispel the dangerous myth that "what they don't know won't hurt them." A controlled sex-education experience, specially designed for youngsters like your child, is vastly preferable to the uncontrolled ignorance of the "what they don't know" attitude.

The advantages of such a course seem to be too obvious to require justification, since the battle was fought and settled for the nonhandicapped years ago. Although most agree that the school, along with the home and church, has a special responsibility to teach sex education to the handicapped, this part of the IEP has received too little attention in the past. Your child has a right to such instruction, especially if sex education is a part of the curriculum for nonhandicapped students. And you have the right to expect that he will be taught by sympathetic, competent teachers, using special materials, who understand handicapped youngsters.

To help ensure that your child's sex education is effective, you should have a clear idea of the goals you seek and the curriculum that will reach these goals. A good sex-education course should:

- Help your child gain social acceptance and enjoy the company of both sexes by teaching him appropriate social-sexual behavior and conventions.
- Help him understand his responsibilities to himself and society in such areas as marriage, sexual relationships, and procreation.
- Help him protect himself against sexual exploitation. One of the few undesirable results of the normalization movement is that some disabled people can be easy targets for those who prey sexually on the weak. Such areas as sexually transmitted disease, prostitution, and sexual abuse should be addressed.
- Help him gain self-esteem and confidence by teaching him about his body, thereby providing him with another area of commonality with all other people.

Here are some units that could be included in the syllabus to reach these goals:

- Discussion of proper terms and vocabulary.
- Examination of myths and misinformation that often cause frustrations and fears (e.g., masturbation will cause your hair to fall out).
- A survey of society's expectations. Areas to be discussed should include what constitutes the difference between acceptable public and private behavior, why some behavior is acceptable at one age and not at another, and what kinds of actions should definitely be avoided.

- A discussion of basic rights and responsibilities, including the right to privacy and the responsibility to be a good, law-abiding citizen.
- Workshops on personal hygiene and grooming. In addition to teaching ways to make one's self as physically attractive and healthy as possible, this unit would include practical information about menstrual care, nocturnal emissions, obesity, and sexually transmitted disease (how it is contracted, what its symptoms are, how it is treated).
- Discussion of the physical and moral aspects of the sexual act and procreation.

Although I would take all steps necessary to safeguard my son against sexual abuse, I am willing to allow him to take calculated risks that are part of normal living. Of course, I recognize that parents' fears about their child's sexuality are not necessarily limited to physical exposure, and that many wish to protect their children from disappointments as well. But part of maturing sexually involves the risk of being rejected, of going to the dance and being a wallflower. I would argue that the right to fail is an inescapable part of the right to try, and is, therefore, a fundamental right that very few of us would relinquish.

I urge you not to forget the importance the sexuality issue has for many handicapped people and to consider using your support or parents' group as a vehicle for the dissemination of information. I also suggest that, no matter what your beliefs, you be supportive of a sex-education course that meets your requirements, and that you campaign to see that such a course is included in any curriculum with which you are associated.

We can't shirk our responsibility as our children grow up and difficult moments arise. Although most parents have a natural tendency to become less involved with their children in later years, handicapped youngsters in particular have a continuing need for support. In the normal order of things, as children grow older they demand independence, and usually by the time they reach adulthood they have little if any need for support. Eventually, as the parent grows older, the roles tend to be reversed, and it is the parent who begins to lose independence and depends upon the child for support. Unfortunately, the problems faced by special families can become more complex at the very time that parents are less able or willing to help their children face them. This is the period when questions about marriage, child bearing, birth control, and homosexual relations can arise.

Often it is difficult to know how to help your child—or if he wants or needs your assistance. There are few pat answers. Recognition of the rights of the handicapped population has tended to increase their independence, particularly as public financial support has become more common. In my opinion, however, complete independence doesn't always guarantee happiness. I suggest that parents work toward preparing their child to be a sexually responsible adult and that they remain available as providers of support when he reaches the period when independence may be possible. If independence is not possible, I suggest they make decisions for him on the basis of his happiness and welfare and not their prejudices. I also urge them to make provision for others to take up their parental responsibilities when they are no longer able or willing to function in this role and that they see that those who take over are prepared to assume a helpful and supportive role in the area of sexual conduct, which may be as difficult and awkward for them as it has been for you.

26

Recreation, Leisure Time, and Transportation

Leisure time well spent is important to everybody. How we spend our nonwork hours, in addition to offering obvious recreational opportunities, can help us in our physical and mental development and in our healthy integration into society. Effective use of free time is critically important for disabled individuals, who share the same basic needs as the nonhandicapped population but must face problems created by their disability. Furthermore, the majority of the severely handicapped population have too many, not too few, empty hours in their day. And, since they are almost totally excluded from normal society, they miss the benefits to be had from participating in its basic mainstream activities: working to earn a living, raising a family, joining a church or temple, and even serving in the armed forces.

Commitments that most of us take for granted make demands, impose structure, and require the assumption of responsibility that gives meaning and form to life. Interplay with society helps the nonhandicapped person find his niche in the community. It gives him assurance that his life has value, that it is worth living. For a bedridden person the effective use of empty hours is equally important for the same reasons, and can help him more than you realize.

Unfortunately, many parents do little to ensure that their child's days are filled in a meaningful way. Some hesitate to expose a child to possible failure or embarrassment. ("Suppose he soils his pants, or can't catch the ball, and the kids laugh at him?") Some underestimate their youngster's capabilities. Others are willing to let go and take a chance but don't know where to begin. Many, strange as it seems, are oblivious to the problem or refuse to admit the management of leisure time is important to someone who "has too much spare time on his hands already and just sits and watches television all day long." Mary and I used to fit into some of these categories and might still if it hadn't

Recreation in the Community: A Step-by-Step Guide for Parents of Children with Handicaps (1984) is a thoughtful resource that was helpful to me in writing this chapter. It was developed by the Parent Resource Project of the Center for Developmental Disabilities at the University of Vermont. The project director is Richard P. Schutz; the project staff are Gail Colton, Kathryn Y. Lenk, Lynn A. McGovern, and Leslie Pine.

been for an unexpected rainstorm one morning in Kentucky, and a sporting problem that bowlers call a "nine-one split."

For years, a Saturday morning bowling tournament has concluded Parents' Weekend at Stewart Home, and immediately afterward exhausted mothers and fathers hug their kids, wave goodbye, and return to their normal lives back home. (The kids, too, return to their regular routines, but already they're thinking about next year.) Not being bowlers, Mary and I never attended the game. The thought of Owen bowling sent shivers up and down my back, for in my mind's eye I saw black balls ricocheting from alley to alley and pin boys scurrying for cover. Besides, how could our son, who ties his shoes only with difficulty, benefit from a game that requires manual dexterity and some computation skills?

It wasn't until a few years ago, when a scheduled picnic was rained out, that we finally made it to the bowling alley. We sent Owen on ahead, and by the time we arrived, we had trouble picking him out of the crowd in the dimly lit building. And it was some crowd! Fifteen alleys were jammed with athletes with every imaginable physical and mental disability, employing every imaginable bowling technique.

Some leaned over, dropped the ball on the hardwood alley, sighted over the ball at the distant pins, and gave it a push. Some heaved, one even rolled the ball between his legs, but all did so with gusto and remarkably positive results. The noise drowned out normal conversation, and almost everyone seemed to be exhorting or congratulating someone else or shouting directions. (Just the body English involved while bowlers followed their balls' progress down the alley would have done justice to championship bowling on TV.)

Eventually I spotted Owen, and at the same moment he looked up and saw us. He was standing in his characteristic cross-legged stance, with the ball cradled awkwardly in both arms ready to bowl. (Later we learned he was about to attempt a maneuver bowlers refer to as a "nine-one split." I won't describe it, except to say that it's considered extremely difficult.) Owen waved, smiled his wide, buck-toothed grin, and pointed us out to his friends, who were too preoccupied to look around. Owen was obviously glad to have us there. He began swinging the ball in ever-increasing arcs and, while still looking back at us, sent it crashing down the alley. He didn't make the split, but he did knock down one pin with a pleasing crack, and he returned to his seat amid general applause.

For the next two hours, in the hurly-burly of that alley, I saw in practical application what recreation can mean in the lives of special people. Owen was performing physically, mentally, and socially in a way that pleased and surprised us. Admittedly, he still was withdrawn and clumsy, but that didn't hold back his friends, who thumped him on the back and pulled down his cap over his eyes when he succeeded. Owen was then twenty-three. His success that day caused us to regret the opportunities we had missed in the past and we resolved to do better in the future.

The Advantage of Recreation

Effective use of nonscheduled time can do many things for your youngster. It can help him to:

- Make new friends, handicapped and nonhandicapped, and bring him into contact with healthy role models. (To the extent that handicapped people participate in society, prejudices and myths can be eliminated and a more humane world gradually created.)
- Improve his physical fitness, learn lifetime skills, and even combine necessary physical therapy with pleasurable activity (ask your physical or occupational therapist how this can be done).
- Build confidence and self-esteem.
- Develop the social skills and understanding necessary to function appropriately in society in such areas as personal grooming, dress, and behavior. (The structure of a group activity, whether it be bowling, a game of chess, or a dance, provides a microcosm of the world in which on-the-job learning can take place.)
- Divert attention from the physical pain and boredom of his own situation by providing a time for activities to which he can look forward, have fun, and be immersed in another happier world.

How Parents Can Help

You can do a variety of things, many in your own home, to give your child some if not all of these benefits. One way is to schedule regular, inviolate, weekly family recreation times. To the extent your youngster's abilities permit, let him be "boss" and take charge of making decisions and arranging the details of the day's activity—perhaps using a newspaper or radio advertisement to locate the theater, ballpark, or restaurant to be attended; buying the tickets; finding the seats. If he's taken along as a nonparticipating passenger, he may enjoy himself but never develop the skills necessary to eventually assume responsibility for himself.

The "Let's Play to Grow" program, sponsored by the Joseph P. Kennedy, Jr., Foundation, specializes in helping families with special needs to enjoy recreation together (see Resources: Recreation and Travel). This is accomplished through a network of national and international clubs, and the group distributes a kit that includes a set of twelve play guides. "Each play guide contains suggested activities in a specific leisure area, e.g., sensory stimulation, rhythm, arts, nature, water skills, and a variety of ball activities." One of its goals is "to stimulate physical and social development, as well as the independent recreation skill of special persons."[1] Write Eunice Kennedy Shriver at the Kennedy Foundation if you wish to obtain more information. You may want to start a local club. Mary and I learned early the importance of regular family recreation that not just Owen but the entire family could look forward to.

Fill Your Child's Day

One basic value of shared productive leisure time is its contrast to and refreshment from the frustrations of a too-busy daily life. If too many hours are unfilled and life is not busy, leisure activities lose some of their impact, and apathy results. Our son falls into this category, and we try to ensure maximal leisure-time benefit when he's home by keeping his waking hours occupied. It's important to him that his day be filled with predictable events.

This is a challenge for us, and for many of our parent friends. It requires perseverance and imagination. Here are some suggestions that have worked for us: Routinely save for his vacation those projects and activities around the house that you know your child enjoys and can do (or be taught). Work with your child on the skills that further his independence and relieve you of constant supervision: management of his personal hygiene, making his bed, cleaning his room, washing dishes, bringing in the newspaper, taking out the garbage, helping you vacuum. To visualize graphically the shape of his day, draw up an hour-by-hour schedule. Don't forget the value of snack and nap times.

Ask a social worker, physical or occupational therapist, school guidance counselor, or psychologist to suggest positive ways to fill his hours. At school IEP meetings or at conferences at your child's institution, be sensitive to the empty-hour problem and urge staff to see that time under their supervision is filled. Don't reject activities out of hand. Any activity, even one that is less than perfect, is better than no activity at all.

After many attempts, even a sheltered workshop proved beyond Owen's grasp, and now a "work activity" fills his day. Despite my earlier misgivings, it's been worthwhile. Originally I saw it as a sham in

---

1. "Let's Play to Grow," a descriptive brochure published in February 1985. For information, write Eunice Kennedy Shriver at the Joseph P. Kennedy, Jr., Foundation, 1350 New York Ave. NW, Suite 500, Washington, DC 20005-4709.

which everyone played at setting up a program whose basic goal, eventual constructive work, was, for most of the participants, patently unrealistic. Although Owen's productivity is minimal, he follows a routine · similar to the outside world, which gives his morale a boost. He eats early, picks up his brown-bag lunch, collects his seventy-five cents for a coin-operated machine's soft drink, arrives at the bus pickup on time (constantly checking his wristwatch, even though he can't tell time), and spends the business day with a group of his peers engaged in activities that require his attention.

Never mind that his salary doesn't cover his expenses or that he soon loses interest in many of the assembly-line assignments, his day is full and he is able to enjoy the contrast and relaxation of leisure time after work. Who is to judge the relevance or meaningfulness of that day? Owen wouldn't miss it for the world.

Learn What Activities Are Available Locally

Become familiar with the local recreation resources for handicapped people and know which will meet your child's needs. Possible sources of information are: local newspapers of all varieties, particularly in their public notice sections (call or visit the editor in charge of local coverage and ask which activities encourage participation by handicapped individuals); your special education contact person; librarians; local clergy; leaders of 4-H clubs, the YMCA and YWCA, and Boy and Girl Scouts; respite-care providers; and the director at your community recreation center or continuing education program. Some communities offer special vacation facilities for disabled citizens: for instance, Ocean House of Virginia Beach, Virginia, maintains a Summer Holiday Program that is designed and operated specially for developmentally disabled citizens. The main purpose of Ocean House is to offer adults with special needs an alternative community-based recreation program (see Resources: Recreation and Travel).

The search can be interesting and fun. Make a list of possibilities, including contact people, with phone numbers and basic facts. Visit potential sites not only to see if they offer programs but also as an enrichment experience for your child. Some possibilities are riding stables, skating rinks, bowling alleys, summer camps, physical fitness centers, concert halls, museums, public beaches and swimming pools, nature and conservancy areas, and even sporting goods stores and stores offering coins and stamps for collectors. Some recreational facilities offer physical conditioning programs adapted for various handicapping conditions. Help can be found in unlikely areas. In our home town, an orthopedic surgeon heads a thriving ski school for handicapped citizens.

National Organizations

As you get to know local resources, you'll find some draw support from national organizations and offer services beyond the capacity of smaller local groups. The most comprehensive publications I know of dealing with countrywide resources are Reference Circular 83-3, *Sports, Games, and Outdoor Recreation for Handicapped Persons,* and 82-3, *Information for Handicapped Travelers* (see Resources: Suppliers and Catalogs; Recreation and Travel). They are excellent, and I have drawn from them extensively in this chapter. Here is a sample of what is available in the "Recreation" circular:

- Listings and brief descriptions of national organizations involved with sports and recreation, such as archery, baseball, hiking, fishing, swimming, and volleyball as well as table games. Included in this section are lists of suppliers of various table games that have been adapted to facilitate their use by handicapped persons. (Included are bingo, backgammon, checkers, chess, cribbage, Monopoly, Othello, Scrabble, and playing cards, many furnished by the American Foundation for the Blind.)
- Suppliers of specially designed equipment. For example, one company specializes in "sport and custom wheelchairs, skiing sleds, and bowling aids for handicapped athletes."
- Information centers and clearinghouses. The Recreation Information Management Office, Forest Service, U.S. Department of Agriculture, provides information about the location, accessibility, and use of recreation sites in national forests.
- Guides to camping facilities and wilderness training and expeditions. The Office of Communications, National Park Service, U.S. Department of Interior, publishes a free national map showing the park system and including information about accessibility features for handicapped travelers. This same organization offers a pass called "Golden Access/Golden Age/Golden Passport," which entitles "persons of all ages who are physically disabled or blind . . . to free entry to national parks, monuments, historical sites, and recreation areas and [to] receive fifty percent discounts on fees for recreational activities such as camping and boat launchings. . . . Disabled persons must apply in person at sites for a Passport and must demonstrate that they are receiving federal benefits for their disability."
- Periodicals dealing with recreation for handicapped persons: for example, magazines about chess (*En passant, Castle, Braille Chess Magazine*) and a variety of others, such as *Wheelchair Sports and Recreation* and *Sports 'n Spokes.*

Many of the organizations mentioned here offer a potpourri of services, including newsletters (*Boating World Unlimited*), local leagues and clubs (blind bowling and flying clubs for handicapped pilots). They provide technical assistance ("football rules and methods for handicapped persons"). They conduct workshops. For example, one organization "maintains a library of riding instruction materials, provides films on riding instruction and horse care and aids in establishing new riding instruction programs and facilities for horse care."

The emphasis is not necessarily competitive, and some organizations include instructional programs in such areas as physical conditioning, jogging, weight lifting, scuba diving, and gymnastics. Nor are they necessarily limited to one disability or to exclusively handicapped participants. One organization's "programs are open to anyone in the United States with any type of physical disability," and another "sponsors events to develop barrier-free interaction between disabled and able-bodied persons." There seems to be an organization to meet every need.

Nonphysical Recreation

Don't limit your thinking to activities that may be impossible for some even with adaptive equipment, for there are many table games, a number of which (chess and checkers) can be played by mail, and stamp and coin collectors from many countries offer both relaxation and interaction with the outside world. This is an activity in which a handicap may be no handicap at all.

Spectator sports viewed in person or followed through television or radio are obvious sources of relaxation, and video games can bring recreation to the bedside. For some, a telephone, amplified or attached to a speaker, offers recreational as well as employment opportunities. Reading and listening to music can provide pleasure even for the hearing and vision impaired. And bathing for therapeutic reasons can be enjoyable if facilities are well designed.

The potential of many of the more passive leisure activities, however, depends upon the availability of pleasant space. A place to sit in the sun and watch activities outside, a private nook for reading, and a bathroom specially designed for the handicapped person can add immeasurably to the pleasure of passive recreation. Never underestimate the importance of housing. It can maximize a person's strengths and minimize his disabilities (see Resources: Adaptive Housing).

Coordinate All Resources, Human and Adaptive

Don't allow yourself or professionals working for you to overlook resources that might open up recreational possibilities. Modern adaptive equipment makes participation in sports and skill-based games possible that were unthinkable twenty-five years ago. There are electric fishing reels, outdoor electric wheelchairs designed to look like an adult three-wheel bicycle, and a battery-powered sounding device that allows a blind athlete to follow a guide in such sports as hiking, jogging, boating, and cross-country skiing. Blind skiers were featured at the 1988 Olympics, and the 800-meter wheelchair race was a highlight at the 1984 summer games.

These activities not only show what is possible but also provide role models and present a healthy nontraditional image of the disabled person. Discuss with your educational or medical team the availability of equipment that might give your child a lift. It would be a mistake to suggest that his horizons are not limited, but it would be a more serious error to be unaware of how far they can be expanded.

Another resource of the human variety was touched on earlier in the discussion of respite care and personal care attendants. On a volunteer or paid basis, attendants can accompany and even instruct your youngster. Babysitters, respite workers, friends, relatives, buddies from school, the church youth group, and your local Scout troop or 4-H club are possible sources of volunteer help. Students from a nearby teacher-training college may be interested, qualified, and available. Sometimes help can come from unexpected places, with far-reaching results.

The friend of mine in Greensboro, N.C., mentioned earlier when I discussed religion, had such an experience. When searching for some way to expand the activities of her son, John (who, you remember, has Down syndrome), she heard of a young high-school boy who gave swimming lessons in his backyard pool. John's mother explains: "This opened up the activity which John has most enjoyed. The young instructor became interested in the challenge of teaching John to swim. At the end of the summer season he asked if I would join the Y and let him continue to work with John throughout the fall and winter. Many cold nights that winter this young man came to pick up my John at 6:00 and take him to the Y to swim. Great was the feeling of joy and accomplishment on the evening when I was invited to see John swim in the deep side of the pool. Another joy was the feeling of accomplishment observed in the young instructor, who, a victim of cancer, died in the spring a bit short of his high school graduation. . . . To see the friendship between those two young people was such a beautiful thing." In the summer of 1983 John won two gold medals at the Special Olympics in Baton Rouge, Louisiana.

As is the case with all those who work with your child, paid or volunteer, you should satisfy yourself that each is dependable, competent, and aware of your child's needs and interests (see the profile in

Appendix A). Employ a briefing session (discussed later in this chapter) to pass on important information.

Offer Leadership

Imaginative parents can open new worlds for their children, but they must lead by example. As we have seen, most movement beyond the safety of the home entails some risk, real and imagined, and little advancement is possible without a certain amount of exposure. Parents can help, not only by letting go of their child but also by being initiators and watchdogs. They can see that their child's IEP includes lifetime leisure-skill development and that he is integrated as much as possible into the community's mainstream of social activities—dances, clubs, and volunteer projects, all of which can be natural stepping stones to acceptance. Making the most of the natural interaction with the world of the nonhandicapped that leisure activities offer is an important building block in the process.

Parents of institutionalized children help when they're familiar with their children's total day, from waking hours till bedtime, not just the classroom experience paraded before them on parents' days. Ask specifically how leisure activities are handled and how your child spends his unscheduled hours. Better still, if possible, spend the day with him from breakfast on as I have. This may take some doing for both you and the institution, but I guarantee it will give you insights you didn't have before.

As a parent advocate, you can contribute by helping organize local leisure activities where none currently exist. A number of organizations listed in Reference Circular 83-3 encourage the creation of local affiliates. Learn ways both your LEA and community recreation departments can take advantage of such athletically oriented activities as Special Olympics and the broad grouping of organizations controlled by the Committee on Sports for the Disabled under the U.S. Olympic Committee.

The Special Olympics program is probably more extensive than you think. It doesn't limit its scope to the well-known winter and summer games (in which mentally retarded individuals eight years and older compete in a variety of sports at all ability levels), and it doesn't limit its efforts to the athletically able. Actually, kids who currently are involved in intramural or interscholastic competition are ineligible for the Special Olympics program. To prepare kids with low motor ability to meet the requirements of Special Olympics, a developmental sports skills guide has been prepared. The program is "administered by the regular physical education teacher, the adaptive physical education specialist, the special education teacher, the recreation leader or the therapeutic recreation specialist. . . . Each sports skills unit complies with the requirements of Public Law 94-142 and can be written into the athlete's individualized education program" (from page 3 of *Special Olympics Development Sports*; for more information, see Resources: Recreation and Travel).

You can also directly affect the local social climate. Others have. A number of groups plan regular monthly socials for the developmentally disabled population. Perhaps your parents' group could sponsor such a project. If the activities involved a predominantly handicapped population it would be worthwhile; if it also included nonhandicapped participants, it would be great! It's no Herculean task, but it does take organization and planning. Issues like sponsorship, transportation, bathroom facilities, finances, rules and regulations, location, entertainment, medical coverage, refreshments, and insurance all must be faced. My school in Maryland used to give an annual Christmas dance for residents of the state institute. As the kids said, "It was a blast." Everyone learned something and everyone enjoyed the affair. The organizational details involved in such a party are described by Kevin Conlee in "Social Events: Setting Them Up and Making Them Work," in the April 1985 issue of *Exceptional Parent*.

Select the Proper Leisure Activities

One way to choose an appropriate activity is to examine your youngster's needs, then to locate an activity that most closely meets these needs. In a way you would be drawing up a recreation profile, either informally in your head or on a scratch pad. Here are some considerations you might include: How mobile is he? Would group or individual activity be preferable? How will communication skills, mental ability, gross- and fine-motor coordination, behavior, or need for continuing individualized help influence selection? Does he thrive on competition? What kinds of activities does he enjoy? When he watches TV, what captures his interest?

Of course, if your child communicates, ask him what kinds of things he enjoys doing, but don't suggest unrealistic alternatives. For example, this might be a profile on our son: "Bowling is ideal for Owen, since he has good fine-motor control and enjoys company but finds it difficult to interact or initiate action. He is not a team player, loves the noise and stimulation of the bowling alley, and can sit for long periods and observe others without having to be a constant participant himself. In addition, this sport need not, when properly supervised, be unduly competitive but can be supportive to morale, and the knocking over of even one pin is a stimulating success and applauded as such."

Some factors that may influence your final activity selection include its location, the accessibility of its various programs, its cost, the amount and quality of support you can expect from staff members, and your perception of their attitude toward disabled children. The reactions you receive from parents and whether the facility is integrated with handicapped *and* nonhandicapped participants are important. You should be interested in learning whether the activity offers programs and staffing characteristics that particularly meet your child's needs, and whether it encourages a healthy rather than a potentially harmful competitive climate.

After you select an activity, make sure that those involved know as much as the situation warrants about your child. The detail necessary is determined by the nature of the activity and ranges from very little in the case of a chess club conducted through the mails to a thorough, in-depth, careful description in the case of a daytime activity. Here is the kind of information the staff may find helpful:

- A simple layperson's explanation of your child's disability, including his strengths and weaknesses, likes and dislikes (the profile in Appendix A could be helpful here).
- Emergency telephone numbers.
- Medical information, including medication, allergies, history of shots received (tetanus, etc.), and seizure description (particularly important if swimming is offered).
- Method of communication (with Owen, knowledge of a few basic "signs" is important).
- Any activities not appropriate for your youngster.
- Any possible behavioral problems and how they can best be handled.
- The kinds of help your child will require in various programs. If the staff are to encourage him to be as independent as possible (probably one of the program's goals), they must know how he feels about being helped and what he can't do for himself. Often regular activities are adapted through a change of rules or by using special equipment so a child can participate. It's good and often necessary to make use of such adaption to increase an individual's participation and his level of success, and as a temporary help until he can participate without any adaption at all.

The criteria for program selection should come as a natural result of thinking through your child's profile. Can the activity fill his needs, supply the stimulation he enjoys, and cope with the requirements his handicap creates? If you're considering an out-of-home activity, will your youngster need assistance in dressing and undressing, toileting, communicating, moving from activity to activity, getting to and from camp, or eating (Does he require a special diet?), and is he receiving medication? In programs designed for the general population, special arrangements will probably require planning on your part and consideration on the part of the staff and administration. Be realistic but optimistic. Leisure activity can be fun. It can teach skills, encourage a person to make friends, and present challenges. It's surprising what resources are available to individuals if they have the courage and tenacity to search for them.

Keep on Top of Things

Even the most perfectly designed project can run into trouble once it's in operation. Therefore, it's important that you monitor your child's activity to see if things are going as planned or if there is anything you can do to help. Some adjustments might be appropriate once you have an actual experience to draw upon. Temper the monitoring, however, with the realization that handicapped kids are just like other kids in that the last thing they want is a parent hovering around for their peers to make fun of. Once the program is in operation, parental participation beyond regular visits should be limited to what is absolutely required and then performed diplomatically and behind the scenes.

Travel

Travel can be recreation in itself, an access to recreation, or a requirement of everyday living, and there are ways to make it more trouble-free. Library of Congress Reference Circular 82-3, *Information for Handicapped Travelers,* is a comprehensive resource listing organizations that can help reduce travel costs, facilitate foreign and domestic travel plans, and supply information to the handicapped reader about appropriate travel-related equipment and accommodations. Occasionally the organizations listed offer discount fares to handicapped passengers, and, although travel agents are not specifically listed, a number of other organizations that do not make reservations themselves will suggest travel agents with experience in serving handicapped travelers. If you travel frequently, this circular is valuable.

As we have learned with Owen, most national public carriers have experience with disabled passengers, and when given reasonable notice, they will make special arrangements in a courteous and efficient manner. Many airlines offer brochures describing their services, but be sure when you make reservations to notify the airline of the nature of the disability and any special assistance needed (follow this same procedure with bus lines, trains, and ocean transportation). The Airport Operators Council International's *Access Travel, Airports: A Guide to*

Accessibility of Terminals lists accessibility characteristics of almost 500 air terminals in 46 countries (see Resources: Recreation and Travel).

I have always checked a day or so before Owen's departure to see that his information is recorded accurately on the airline's computers; we arrive at the check-in counter early enough before departure so I have time to speak to the ticket agent and confirm arrangements, and I make sure someone is at home near the phone when Owen makes en-route transfers. In large cities most companies have an agent assigned to assist special passengers on and off the aircraft before other passengers board, but I always get permission to accompany Owen so I can introduce him to the flight attendants and describe his situation.

Many major car rental companies will provide special equipment (for instance, automobile hand controls) with advance reservation. The President's Committee on Employment of People with Disabilities publishes a guide called *Highway Rest Areas for Handicapped Travelers,* and the American Automobile Association offers a booklet assisting disabled drivers to select "suitable equipment and services." Several independent-living centers provide driver education courses, including instruction in the use of adaptive equipment (see Chapter 22).

Major bus lines allow handicapped travelers to travel with an attendant on a single adult fare (a doctor's statement is usually required), and will provide help in boarding and handling baggage. Call the terminal ahead of departure to make arrangements, and check in early.

Amtrak offers several services, including a toll-free TTY number for the hearing impaired for information and reservations (obtain this number from the local Amtrak ticket agent). Local terminals can also provide toll-free numbers to make special arrangements, and discount fares are often available for handicapped travelers who have identification cards from a government agency or an organization for the disabled, or a letter from a medical doctor. Accessibility information for any train, including accessible bathrooms and bedrooms, can be obtained from reservation agents. Amtrak publishes, free of charge, a pamphlet entitled *Access Amtrak: A Guide to Amtrak Services for Elderly Travelers,* which is also helpful for disabled travelers (see Resources: Recreation and Travel).

Travel outside the United States should not necessarily be ruled out but may be inadvisable, depending upon the limitations imposed by your child's disability. Careful planning is necessary, particularly for the intellectually handicapped. If there is any chance, however, that your youngster is up to it, foreign travel is a glorious opportunity for him to broaden his horizons and try his wings. The Reference Circular *Information for Handicapped Travelers* lists organizations in many countries "that can provide special guidebooks and lists of accessible facilities." A national organization specializing in your child's handicap may have information on foreign travel or be able to refer you to another person with similar limitations who has made a similar trip. I suggest, however, that your first step be to consult your medical team to see if such an enterprise is advisable.

Mobility International (see Resources: Clearinghouses/Databanks/Information) functions as a clearinghouse for international travel for physically handicapped persons and has branches throughout Europe that encourage exchange visits. It and a number of other organizations listed in *Information for Handicapped Travelers* offer guides and access information and such special features as suggestions about how to take holidays abroad and an international phrasebook specially designed for the handicapped. The International Association for Medical Assistance to Travelers (IAMAT) is concerned with helping arrange medical attention in foreign countries from doctors who speak English, and the National Association of Patients on Hemodialysis and Transplantation publishes a guide to dialysis facilities and a glossary that includes technical dialysis-related terms in French, Italian, and German.

27
Planning for the Future

Why Plan?

Planning carefully to maintain the quality of your child's life after you're no longer available to offer support is a bit like buying life insurance; you hope its benefits will not be realized till you've lived a long life and done all the things that need to be done to protect those who depend on you—and meanwhile, you can enjoy a clear conscience and peace of mind. True, there will be unknowns when you plan early, and the plan must be updated regularly as circumstances change, but, in general, the earlier you begin to think about the future the better.

The alternative, doing nothing, can have unfortunate consequences. For example, adequate resources might not be available when they eventually are needed, or the individual charged with the conduct of your child's affairs—perhaps appointed by a probate court—may not be the kind of person you would have selected. Or possibly a family member or friend feels morally obligated to fill the vacuum you leave but is unprepared to do so. It's true that even carefully laid plans can't guarantee a trouble-free life for your child, but they can offer him the best chance in an unpredictable world.

Your plan should be influenced by several factors: the severity of your child's handicap; the characteristics of the family unit, including its financial circumstances; current federal and state assistance programs and tax law; and your feeling of responsibility to your child, to his siblings, and to society. Mary's and my planning strategy has been to seek maximal benefit for Owen consistent with maintaining the well-being and independence of other family members. (The disabled child is not the only family member to whom independence is important.) Your plan for one usually affects your plans for others, and it's easy to fall into a pattern of inadvertently sacrificing the interests of other individual members for the supposed best interests of the one who is handicapped.

Our planning has been based on the belief that the most valuable inheritance we can leave our children is not money but an unimpeded future, a future made possible by a plan that provides for their handicapped brother's needs so they will be relieved of the financial drain and possible moral dilemma that ultimate and complete responsibility for his care can entail. Relieved of the burden, they are free to chart their own lives and still have enough time and energy to monitor their brother's care and provide him, by ongoing visits and correspondence, reassuring evidence that he remains a valued member of a loving family. For this continuity of love, we look to our other children, and fix the responsibility on their shoulders. With the exception of one major planning miscalculation (which I discuss later), Mary and I are satisfied that so far we have done a reasonably good job of planning, although we realize it is a job that, almost by definition, can never be completed.

One way to approach the job is to break the problem down into five interrelated questions that you should be able to answer:

- How do you get advice and information in this area? Misinformation or lack of qualified advice can have unfortunate results.
- What is your goal? You must decide what quality of life you can provide for your child.
- What resources will you have available to incorporate into your plan? Governmental programs will probably be one, and there could also eventually be proceeds from your estate, such as bonds, stock, real estate, cash, and life insurance. (It's even possible to give your child a house, or to leave it to him in some way after your death, and make plans with a not-for-profit organization to provide supervision.)
- How can these resources be passed on in the most effective way? Wills, trusts, and nonbinding agreements can be adapted to personal circumstances. Governmental programs and retirement plans may already be in place and need no further adjustment, or they can require continued attention.
- How can you see that your child receives compassionate supervision and decision-making guidance to protect him and yet give him maximal appropriate independence? Various forms of guardianships, trust agreements, and even informal family understandings can be tailored to meet his needs.

I urge you to acquire a basic understanding of long-range planning even if you believe you have adequately provided for your youngster's future or even if you don't feel he is seriously enough disabled to require special services. You could be wrong. For example, if you make no provision at all, your child will receive the total amount of whatever inheritance he may receive from you when he comes of age. Even if he is only mildly retarded, will he be able to handle the money? Will he be susceptible to unwise financial propositions? Do you know that the receipt of even a modest inheritance could make him ineligible for many governmental benefits? A minimal knowledge of estate planning would alert you to such dangers.

Although your child's future happiness will be affected by legal arrangements, governmental programs, and the amount of your estate, factors that influence his emotional life—the human equation—can be equally important. For that reason all planning decisions should be affected by consideration of how they will affect your child's sense of continuity and stability, his contact with happy memories, and relationships from the past. Handicapped kids, whether they be institutionalized, in special education courses, or in sheltered workshops, live in a world that lacks stability and is filled with people who come and go. Owen was moved from one dorm to another three times in one year. Planning decisions should aim toward maintaining stability and encouraging continuity.

Through careful planning, I try to ensure that people working with Owen will see him as a human being and not as a silent, inanimate client. Will they know enough about the details of his life to gauge what environment is most apt to ensure his happiness? When considering wills and trusts, I will discuss ways such concerns can be passed on to future caregivers and can be legally safeguarded. Careful planning can help guarantee that the human factor is taken into consideration.

Obtaining Advice and Information

Fortunately, much excellent material can be obtained to assist your planning effort. First you must learn the basics; for example, how do Social Security and Medicare differ from Supplemental Security Income and Medicaid in the assistance they offer? I have found *How to Provide for Their Future,* prepared by the Association for Retarded Citizens (ARC), and the article "Estate Planning: Providing for Your Child's Future," by Henry A. Beyer, in the December 1986 issue of *Exceptional Parent,* to be excellent resources. The booklet *Estate Planning for Parents of Persons with Developmental Disabilities* (May 1982, available from the Disability Law Center of Massachusetts; a contribution of $1.00 is requested) is also valuable, particularly since it is written in clear, straightforward language free of jargon. (See Resources: Law.)

After you've done some background reading, I suggest you contact someone knowledgeable in the field—an estate planner, an insurance adviser, a lawyer, or a counselor—to discuss your situation in general terms. It's important that the professional have no vested interest, and that he be experienced in dealing with matters affecting the handicapped (don't spend your time and money on a "general practice" professional while he educates himself in "handicap law"). Ask for recommendations of qualified people from the state bar association, the nearest chapter of ARC, a community counseling agency, or the state social service agency or special education department with which you have established a good relationship. Estate planning, since it is so influenced by legislative action and changes in the tax law, is subject to frequent alteration. Therefore, no matter how well-read you think you are, never make irreversible decisions or enter into contractual agreements without first seeking expert advice.

Factors to Secure a Satisfactory Quality of Life

Arriving at the life style you wish to provide involves meeting two quite different needs:

- Making sure that plans are in place so your child will receive the basic necessities of life—food, housing, education, health services (both maintenance and therapeutic), and clothing. For most parents, the basics must be paid for either by some form of insurance, such as Social Security, Medicare, benefits under an employer's private plan, career military retirement programs (veterans' entitlement programs), or by public funds, such as federal assistance (Supplemental Security Income (SSI), Medicaid, and veterans' benefits), and other related benefits, such as Food Stamps and rent subsidies).
- Providing for what might be called the "extras"—leisure activities, jewelry, a VCR, a TV set, cosmetics, magazines, candy, and so forth. These so-called luxuries, which spell the difference in the quality of life that will be provided, are often paid for by the proceeds of the parent's estate passed on to benefit the child. (Life insurance, one way to make more funds available to provide a higher level of funding than you might ordinarily be able to afford, is discussed in detail in the treatment of wills, trusts, and agreements, since insurance is both a resource and a method of passing on resources.) The importance of separating expenditures for basic necessities from payment for luxuries is also discussed later in this chapter.

Some Suggestions on Funding

Although much federal funding is involved in various local programs, under the Constitution the responsibility for protecting the well-being of vulnerable people, those who can't take care of themselves, rests, in the final analysis, with the family or the individual state.

Even when federal monies are involved, programs often differ from state to state, and financial distribution is made through state agencies. The funding process is far too complex to be described here, yet some critical points should be made. In general, although proceeds from insurance and/or entitlement programs are not affected by the income level of the recipient, benefits from an assistance program are. You must know the difference!

Since some benefits vary, depending upon where you live, plan your child's future on the basis of what you predict will be his state of residence and its laws and regulations. State benefits may even influence your decision about the location of residence if you have flexibility. It is your responsibility to see that the options available to you are exercised and programs are taken advantage of. Don't wait for the government or your insurance carrier to contact you. For example, if you are a military retiree with a mentally retarded child, make sure you're paying supplementary contributions to the Survivor Benefit Plan; if you don't, your child's final benefits may be decreased. If you are covered by your employer under any form of life insurance or retirement plan, check with the personnel officer to see what benefits are available for your youngster.

I suggest everyone with a disabled child visit the local Social Security office to find out what benefits the child is, or would be, entitled to under Social Security *if* you (the parent) are covered, and under what conditions he would receive benefits under SSI if you have no coverage. (Under some circumstances he might qualify for both.) Most people who are eligible for SSI because of disability become eligible at age eighteen and may have become eligible for Social Security even earlier. I advise that you establish your child's eligibility under SSI as soon as he qualifies, even if you are currently supporting him, thus avoiding delay and possible complications later if circumstances change and benefits are suddenly needed. The Social Security office should also be able to refer you to local health and social service agencies that can provide information about other sources of income. Much material is available dealing with the subject, for example, *The Social Security Handbook, Federal Benefits for Veterans and Dependents,* and particularly the "Government Benefits" section of the ARC bulletin *How to Provide for Their Future* (see Resources: Law).

Life Insurance Is a Possibility

Having a handicapped child increases the financial vulnerability of a family. For that reason all kinds of insurance—health, fire, theft, public liability—have special significance, but life insurance is of prime importance in planning for the future. It can increase your, or your spouse's, estate as soon as you pay the first premium. It can lessen the financial burden on the remaining spouse, who, in the event of the death of the wage earner, must face increased responsibilities if the youngster is still at home. Or, at a later date, the life insurance benefit can be left to the handicapped child to enhance his life or make him more independent. Life insurance is the quickest and cheapest way to create an estate and is particularly valuable for young parents who have need for protection for their family at the very time they are least apt to have excess funds available.

A good life insurance plan should be coordinated with your long-range plans and reflect the total family picture. Consult with a reputable insurance planner, but only after you have examined your situation and organized your thoughts. He will need certain information, perhaps even before you meet: the ages and earnings of both you and your spouse, the state of your health, and the details of any retirement plan to which you belong. The number and ages of other dependents are important, but the planner will be particularly interested in your handicapped child, in the expenses involved in his care, the prognosis for the future, and any government programs in which he participates now or may qualify for in the future. (If you have chosen your advisor thoughtfully, he should be knowledgeable about benefits for handicapped citizens.)

You should have a good idea of your total assets and liabilities; he will want to know if you own your home and if you have a will and how it is drawn. An insurance plan will depend upon what funds you have available for all your children and how you plan, through your will, to distribute these funds. (Do any of your other children have special needs?) You should be aware that since life insurance is a contract that you as a parent make with the insurance company, it is not affected by your will unless you make your estate the beneficiary of the policy, which may increase probate costs and possibly tax exposure depending upon your state laws. (Alternative ways to channel funds to your special child are discussed when wills are considered.)

Possibly your most important homework before making insurance decisions is deciding precisely what role you expect life insurance to play in the overall picture. Your meeting should help clarify this decision. As a result of your consultation, the insurance expert should provide a plan that includes alternative courses of action and the advantages and disadvantages of each. If the expert attempts to pressure you into buying insurance at the first meeting, perhaps you have made a poor choice of advisor and need a second opinion.

You may find that the proposal involves the use of various kinds of insurance. A group policy, discussed earlier, if it is available, is almost always cheaper than an individual ordinary life policy and is less apt to include pre-existing conditions that can exclude anyone with a known, serious medical problem. Term insurance provides more coverage for the same premium dollar than does whole life insurance but does not build up cash value and may not be renewable. The option for you to renew the policy without undergoing another qualifying physical is a very important consideration. Be sure you understand the advantages and disadvantages of each of the various kinds of protection available. Always read the fine print, and provide yourself as much flexibility as possible. Your needs will change more than those of the ordinary parent; therefore, ask your insurance carrier how you can maintain flexibility so as to adapt your coverage to the changes time brings.

Under various conditions it could be advisable to insure the lives of mother, father, *and* child. Both parents should be insured if they both work and their salaries are vital to family interests or if only one parent works but the other performs responsibilities in the home that will have to be replaced by hiring a professional home-care worker if the parent should die. Although insuring their child might not occur to many parents, it may be a way to reimburse a relative or friend for money he or she has committed to the care of the youngster during his lifetime after you are gone.

Purchasing a family insurance plan may be one of the few ways to insure your child, since most ordinary plans have pre-existing clauses that would exclude the handicapped applicant on physical grounds. ARC, however, sponsors both a group life insurance plan—the ARC Life Plan, specially designed to give parents low-cost life insurance— and the ARC Security Plan, which offers life insurance to people with mental retardation for specified amounts (currently up to $10,000). For information on either of these two programs, contact your nearest ARC chapter.

A Will Is a Necessity

A will is a legal document that serves many important purposes: it can indicate how the person making the will (called the "testator") wishes his personal assets to be distributed after his death; it can create a trust, provide for funds to be moved ("poured over") from the parent's estate to a trust, and nominate a guardian or in some states a limited guardian or conservator. Finally, through a will a parent can pass on his preferences for the type of care he wishes for a handicapped dependent.

Through a properly drawn will, assets will pass from you to those to whom you wish your property distributed (your *beneficiaries*) with minimal tax loss and maximal benefit. The person whom you appoint in your will to see that terms of the will are carried out (called an *executor* or *conservator*) will see that assets are collected, maintained, and distributed according to the will, and that legal requirements are met and taxes paid. The executor, often a friend or family member, need not be an attorney, and he can use estate funds to obtain one's services if he deems it necessary. A will can be amended through what is called a codicil, or changed at any time during your lifetime unless you become legally incompetent, and in no way does it go into effect till your death. You may need a will even if you and your spouse own all your assets together in what is called "joint tenancy."

If you die *intestate* (without a valid will or with no will at all), the results can be extremely unfortunate. The state provides for such a circumstance through a body of laws called intestacy laws, which stipulate, according to a usually inflexible formula, how your assets are to be distributed—such a percentage to a spouse, such a percentage for a child, and so forth. However, this distribution may not be the way you would wish your affairs to be handled or in the best interests of your family. It could make your handicapped youngster liable to the state for taxes and costs of his care, present and past; cause him to be ineligible for SSI or Medicaid benefits; and even result in the appointment of an attorney, under the supervision of the probate court, to administer the property passed on to him. A properly drawn will can avoid all this. If you have no will, I urge you to have one drawn without delay by a competent lawyer, familiar with laws affecting handicapped people and thoroughly instructed by you in your family affairs and your specific goals.

A carefully drawn will can ensure that your child's financial interests (and custodial if necessary) are coordinated with the interests of other family members (remember, it's necessary to nominate a legal guardian for any minor children). The details of will construction are complex, differ from state to state, and change as federal and state laws change, so I include here only the most general observations. Although you should seek expert advice, there are two pivotal and related decisions you and only you should make: (1) the nature of the supervision and support needed to provide for your child, and (2) how you wish to balance the financial needs of your handicapped child with those of other family members. In this chapter I have given priority to the welfare of the disabled child. Obviously, other considerations may and should influence your decisions.

Other Financial Considerations

I know of no circumstances under which it's desirable to leave a lot of money directly to your handicapped youngster. Many factors argue against such a move: He may be incapable of financial management and vulnerable to exploitation (court-supervised guardianship of his estate may, as a result, be required by law and could provide a different management from one you would have preferred). Leaving funds to your child in excess of his needs may make the surplus unavailable for other family members, even in the event of emergencies. (Your will, through a carefully drawn trust, can avoid this problem.) When Owen was two (before we had become veteran campaigners), we established a trust fund to be turned over to him at age twenty-one that provided no such flexibility. By that one well-intentioned but ill-advised legal action, we set a course for his financial future that effectively ruled out his participation in any governmental programs based on need, unless we were to expend all the proceeds of the trust to get under the maximal estate allowed SSI recipients (currently $1,900 for an individual; $2,800 for a couple).

A trust drawn for Owen when he was in his late twenties—we had become more sophisticated about legal matters by that time—provided flexibility so that income not required for his annual maintenance could, at the discretion of the trustee, be distributed ("sprinkled") to his siblings.

Most parents begin by assuming complete financial responsibility for their child, but as time passes, many find they no longer can assume the excessive costs involved and must seek various forms of public and private assistance. Other parents are able to continue full or partial support but find making complete financial provision for their child's lifetime support out of the question. Only a very few well-to-do parents have the financial capability, if they choose, to be completely independent of outside support.

Obviously, the dollar amount committed to the handicapped child through the will depends upon the parent's estate and philosophy, but in almost every instance it is desirable to commit resources so they go to the child indirectly and don't disqualify him from governmental support. One way to accomplish this through your will is to exclude your child completely from participation in your estate—disinherit him—and distribute your estate to the other children, thus depending upon governmental welfare programs to meet your disabled child's needs. Although this approach can be emotionally difficult, parents with very small estates or other significant obligations have limited alternatives and should consider it.

The risk involved in this strategy is that if governmental programs are reduced or eliminated, the child can be left with insufficient resources. One way to minimize the risks involved in disinheritance is to leave a gift (bequest) to a close friend or family member along with a request that the recipient use the funds for the benefit of the child. This action—called a "morally obligated gift"—solves some problems but creates others. Since the recipient becomes the legal owner of the property, he must pay taxes on income generated by the gift, an out-of-pocket expense, and no matter how well-intentioned he may be, changing circumstances could divert the use of the gift from the purposes intended. He could be subject to mental illness, predecease your child, be divorced, or become bankrupt, in which case all his estate, including your gift, could be vulnerable to the claims of his creditors. And if later he has financial problems that adversely affect his immediate family, he could be placed in an unfortunate moral dilemma about whom to give priority.

Trusts

Another, I believe better, way to provide for the future is to create some form of trust, either built into your will or completely independent. A trust is valuable in that it can be extremely flexible and can be tailored to your particular needs. All that is required is that you examine your resources, decide upon priorities, and consult a good lawyer.

A trust is a legal arrangement created by one person, the "settlor" (in this case you, the parent) through which another person (the "trustee") owns and manages property for a third person (the "beneficiary"), in this case your handicapped child. Don't be concerned with the fact that legally the trustee "owns" the property, in that he has legal title to it. He can use the property only for the benefit of your child, the beneficiary, who legally has "equitable title" to the property. The trustee must be chosen carefully, should be fully aware of the responsibilities involved, and, of course, agree to serve. Provision should be included in the trust for the appointment of successor trustees to replace the first trustee were he to become unavailable. It's advisable, if possible, that the primary trustee not be significantly older than the beneficiary, since one of the trustee's responsibilities is to help manage the affairs of the disabled person, and more continuity is possible if the trustee and the beneficiary are of similar age. (Our son Reid, age thirty-six, is successor trustee for Owen, who is twenty-nine.)

If the disabled person is still a child, your spouse, a friend, or a close family member might be a logical selection as first trustee, with an institution as co-trustee. If your disabled child is older when the trust is created, a mature and responsible sibling could be an appropriate selection as either a trustee or a successor trustee.

Equally careful attention should be given to the appointment of an institution as co-trustee if one is thought necessary. This may be the case if the trust is large, or if the primary trustee is not familiar with legal matters or financial management. Provision should be made in the trust so that the individual trustee has the power to replace the institutional trustee (this guarantees performance and reasonable fees). Trust departments of banks as well as other organizations are often selected. For example, local chapters of ARC will serve in such a capacity. The trust, sometimes referred to as the trust instrument, must specify the duties and responsibilities of the trustee, and you, as settlor, should carefully examine the qualifications of the institution, if one is needed, and the fees they charge.

Trusts can be established by the will of the settlor and include direction as to what part of the settlor's estate will fund the trust. Such a trust will not take effect during the lifetime of the settlor (called an inter vivos trust) and can be either revocable or irrevocable by the settlor during his lifetime, depending upon its construction. Parents and other parties may add to the trust with cash or bequests in their wills rather than making gifts directly to the handicapped beneficiary. Other trusts that go into effect during the settlor's lifetime are obviously not controlled by his will and can include procedures by which he can change trustees.

Every trust should state the purposes that it is to serve. For reasons discussed earlier, the purpose of the kinds of trusts with which I am concerned here is to make it possible for the beneficiary to enjoy a higher quality of life than would be possible if only governmental benefits were available, but it should specifically state that the proceeds are to supplement, and not supplant, governmental assistance. Although this type of instrument is often identified as a "luxuries" trust, the document should be careful to *avoid* stipulating that proceeds may never be used to support the beneficiary, since, if government sources ever prove to be unavailable or if unanticipated conditions prevail, it may be necessary for the trust to be used for that very purpose.

The trust should describe the trustee's powers (how he may act) and may be specific in stipulating exactly what the trustee can or can't do and the precise manner in which actions must be taken (these are called "imperative powers"). Or the trustee may be given "discretionary powers," which means he can use his best judgment to see that the stated purposes of the trust are carried out. On the other hand, the trust can stipulate a combination of the two types of powers. Some discretion is often necessary if the trustee is to have the flexibility required to adapt to changing conditions.

In view of my earlier concern that the human factor be included in planning for the future, I suggest the trustee be instructed to perform certain minimal duties at trust expense (requirements or suggestions will depend upon personal circumstances). For example, if the beneficiary is institutionalized, the trustee might be directed to visit the beneficiary's place of residence a certain minimum number of times a year, at which time he might be expected to inspect facilities and eat one meal in the cafeteria. The trust might stipulate that the trustee confer with teachers and sheltered-workshop or supported-employment supervisors concerning educational and vocational progress, that an annual physical and dental examination by an independent physician or dentist be required, that the recreational program be looked into, and, perhaps most important of all, that the trustee discuss how the beneficiary feels about the care he is receiving and those who provide that care. Typical questions could be: Does he have enough spending money? Does he enjoy all the comforts that can reasonably be provided? Does he have any complaints, and, if so, are they justified?

I recommend that you give a copy of your child's profile (see Appendix A) to the trustee (but not make it part of the trust document) and that you request by cover letter that the trustee review the profile annually, share it with staff, and update it regularly with staff assistance. One ingredient of many trusts with which you should be familiar is the "spendthrift" clause. This provision ensures that the beneficiary may not pledge, give, transfer, mortgage, or use assets of the trust and that no creditor, including the state government or a subdivision of it, can secure trust assets or income. This clause indicates that the proceeds of the trust are in no way under the control of the beneficiary and that they will not be used for his basic maintenance. Finally, the trust should name the person, persons, or institution that will receive any assets of the trust in existence at its termination. The termination date (ordinarily at the death of the beneficiary) must be stipulated in the trust document itself. As you can see, trusts are complicated, and I have only begun to scratch the surface. If you have questions, contact an attorney or the nearest branch of ARC.

Guardianship: Is It the Right Answer?

If your child, like Owen, is presently totally incapable of taking care of himself and in all probability will continue to require total care in the future, a legal guardian is necessary when the youngster is no longer a minor. (Fortunately, most handicapped people are not as severely affected as Owen, and they have other, less-restrictive alternatives.) Guardianship is a reasonable possibility if without it your child might harm himself, be abused, be involved in serious crime, be forced into prostitution, be a danger to others, be unable to observe even the most basic safety precautions, or run away from home and be incapable of obtaining the basic necessities of life.

Guardianship is a serious matter, since it involves a major loss of personal rights and freedoms and can result in reducing a handicapped individual's opportunities to grow and gain independence. When you consider guardianship, familiarize yourself with both the rights your child would lose—there's a long list—and the legal responsibilities the guardian must shoulder. Be sure that you have examined and exhausted all other realistic alternatives. Be sure guardianship is not just a convenient way for a caregiver to handle a frustrating situation.

The probate court in the county of residence of the deceased person has jurisdiction over guardianship proceedings. Ordinarily, provision may be made in a will to appoint a guardian for minor children, but it would go into effect only if both parents die before all their children become eighteen, and it would expire when the youngest child reaches eighteen. Requesting guardianship for a child over eighteen generally requires petitioning the appropriate probate court, which will notify you of the procedures required. I retained a lawyer when I acted to become Owen's guardian and strongly suggest you do the same. The petition will certainly require that confirming diagnostic reports be filed from qualified professionals. All interested parties must be notified and a hearing held, at which time the court will decide whether to appoint a plenary (full) guardianship, to appoint some variation of partial guardianship, or to rule that the individual needs no guardian assistance whatsoever.

A total or plenary guardianship must be established by a court and is a legal relationship between a competent adult (the guardian, who may be you or your spouse) and a minor child or handicapped individual (ward), granting the guardian power to act for the ward, who is unable to make competent decisions for himself. In many states limited forms of guardianship are available for less severely handicapped individuals, individuals who are capable of acting on their own in many areas. In these cases no legal finding of total incompetence is required. The terms vary from state to state, but sometimes two guardians may share the responsibility: a "guardian of the estate" is concerned with the financial well-being of the disabled person (paying bills, managing money, paying taxes) while a "guardian of the person" is involved in the management of personal matters and decision making (living and educational arrangements, social relationships).

It may be advantageous for you to serve as guardian during your lifetime, with provision made in your will to have your spouse or another family member take over after your death. As we have seen, one person can serve as guardian both of the person and of the estate, or, in other circumstances, one individual can act as guardian of the person, and an institution—a bank's trust department, for example—can act as guardian of the estate. (Sometimes a trust arrangement can eliminate the necessity of guardianship of the estate.) Ask your lawyer, ARC representative, or contact person with the state agency what forms of limited or partial guardianship are possible in your state and what they involve.

Another way to provide continuing protection and supervision of a child's affairs (if a parent is not assuming that responsibility) is through the opportunity some states now offer for public guardianship and public conservancy (limited guardianship). In this arrangement, after a court has determined that some type of guardianship is needed, the state decides what type of arrangement best meets the needs of the handicapped person, and then assigns the responsibility to the appropriate welfare department. In some states that do not provide complete services, the public guardian's responsibilities are limited primarily to advocacy and decision-making assistance.

Another recent development, which may be more applicable to the needs of a parent who is still involved with his child's welfare, is a kind of collective guardianship effort, which involves a creative use of trusts. The Virginia Beach Community Trust for the Developmentally Disabled is an example. In this plan, participating families who wish to provide for the future of a handicapped family member pool their resources to cover the administrative costs of guardianship and continuing management of the funds left in trust. These proceeds are intended to *supplement* the earnings and governmental benefits of the developmentally disabled participants and not *supplant* them. The trust, which provides continued financial management after families are no longer able to do so, is so worded that money is earmarked for uses "above and beyond" that governmental assistance to which the disabled participant is entitled and will therefore not disqualify him from continued federal aid. The trust describes its benefits to parents as follows:

- Peace of mind and an economical way of providing trust benefits
- An opportunity to learn various ways to plan for and protect the future of their child, both financially and personally

- Relief from the emotional and financial burdens assumed by relatives or friends
- An opportunity to participate in a trust, with all its benefits, which would not be affordable to many families
- Protection of funds designated for the handicapped child

A number of community trusts throughout the country follow this general pattern. You may want to find out if there is a community trust near you, or you may be interested in seeing if a similar trust can be started in your own community. For information on the Virginia Beach enterprise, write Virginia Beach Community Services Board, MR/DD Programs, Pembroke Six, Suite 218, Virginia Beach, VA 23462.

This community approach offers a remarkable solution to the difficult question we all face at one time or another: What happens after we're gone? In this approach a community and the parents in that community join together to ensure that a future with dignity and hope will be provided to the handicapped members of that community.

Dos and Don'ts
for Independent Living

1. *Be willing to let go of your child in his struggle to join society, but don't abandon him.*

2. *Be sure that IEP construction is long-range and practical.* Planning should be directed toward reaching the maximal independence possible.

3. *Skills should be emphasized that are needed for life as it exists in your local community and requirements met that are needed for graduation.*

4. *Push to see that these practical skills are learned as much as possible in the environment in which they will be used.* Community-based programs or school-based (community-referenced) programs that are integrated with the nonhandicapped school population should be encouraged.

5. *See that a vocational rehabilitation counselor and a community linkage person are involved in your IEP meetings as early as possible and a work assessment made.*

6. *Be a force for excellence.* Praise existing special programs that are good, but advocate improvements where needed. Work with the staff to build and maintain a high school whose special education program is integrated, age-appropriate, community-referenced, and future-oriented. (Excuse the jargon, but I believe this shorthand says it all.)

7. *Know the current laws.* Current federal and state statutes as amended, regulations, and programs and eligibility requirements, as well as departmental practices affecting the transition stage and adult life, should be understood.

8. *Don't attempt to hide sex under the carpet (the subject tends to pop up no matter what you do).* Your child is a sexual human being. Understanding his needs in this area is extremely difficult, but making no attempt to understand them is out of the question. Read good books on the subject, discuss your questions and concerns with trusted friends,

your child's caregivers, or knowledgable professionals, and bring it up at the IEP or the IPP meeting.

If problems arise, seek professional advice. If the question is a legal one, talk with your lawyer.

9. *Depending upon your child's condition, see that he receives appropriate sex education.* Ensure that as part of that course attention is given to helping him learn how to protect himself from sexual abuse. (Obviously daughters are as vulnerable as sons.) In selecting a residential placement, find out the institution's position on sexual matters and make it one factor in your decision.

10. *Give emphasis to your child's leisure planning.* The experiences gained during recreation can help him learn social skills that will assist his integration into the community. Too much unfilled time has been the curse of many disabled citizens.

Don't limit your program selection to purely physical activities. Some of the most valuable recreational possibilities can be enjoyed with minimal activity. Urge that the IEP include lifetime leisure skills and encourage your community recreational leaders to be aware of the handicapped population and provide integrated activities in which they can participate. Keep your child occupied.

11. *Learn about financial help.* Become familiar with the private and public financial resources that are involved with supporting recreational activities for the handicapped population and paying for special communication equipment and orthotic devices.

12. *Let go.* Begin with the assumption that your child can do more than you expect he can. If he continues to live at home, treat him as an adult. It you haven't already done so, adapt the house to allow him maximal privacy and independence, and remember that all independence carries with it some risk.

13. *Cooperate with agency staff.* Approach the IPP interdisciplinary team with an attitude of informed cooperation and enlightened self-interest. However, don't hesitate to invoke the appeal process (as a last resort) to protect your child's ultimate best interests. Understand the IPP before you approve it, and approve it only after you have carefully studied all aspects and compared the services proposed with all needs involved.

14. *If you can't find a satisfactory residence, start one.* Many parents have become facility operators primarily to provide suitable placement for their own child. It is difficult, but it can be done.

15. *Give your child ongoing family support.* Physical separation from the family should not mean the severance of emotional support.

16. *Make arrangements for after you're gone.* Financial and appropriate supervisory arrangements should be drawn up to protect your child's interests (see Chapter 27).

17. *Make your church your child's church.* Work to see that every opportunity is taken to include your child in the active church community.

Epilogue

Owen grows older. Time passes more quickly now for Mary and me as another cycle in our family's life picks up steam. Within an eleven-month period, Reid, Tom, and Sarah all were married, and new in-laws begin to get to know Owie. (These are interesting encounters.) The guard has begun to change: Tom substituted for us at a Parents' Weekend in Kentucky, went bowling with Owen, saw the talent show, and met Owen's friends; Reid, his stepson E. J., and his wife Cathy invited Owen home with them over the Christmas holidays when Mary and I were out of the country. Cathy is sure she can solve Owie's digestive problems through a complex regimen of diet, stomach massage, and love that only she understands. (Darned if it doesn't seem to help.)

Our two grandsons are normal, healthy kids, and their normalcy reassures us that Owen's problem is not hereditary, although genetic science has not yet progressed to the point where it can tell us what went wrong or offer complete reassurance.

For the first time, Owen begins to look like a mature man and no longer a gangling teenager. He has put on weight, and when I shave him, I notice his beard is darker and heavier. Signs of the aging process begin to show on Mary and me, too, and we increasingly think of our son's future without us. We are reconciled to the fact that Owen will never develop beyond his present level, and our planning and hopes for his future are focused on ensuring a continuation for the remainder of his life of his current environment, where he seems happy and secure.

Looking back on our life with this "crazy kid," I doubt if we could have done anything that would have substantially altered his future. Despite the heartache and worry that even now remain part of our life, I know Owie has given far more to us than we would have thought possible when we first heard the news so many years ago that day in Albany. The old questions—Why him? and Why us?—remain unanswered, and yet Mary and I have reached a reconciliation with life where the answers are no longer important. We are content with ourselves and with a life that has been strangely made richer since Owen.

Appendix A
The Notebook

Materials

Use a regular, hardcover, 11″ × 9″ loose-leaf notebook to take to meetings and to hold the material you accumulate during any one year. Then, transfer this material, if you wish, to a large cumulative notebook kept permanently at home. Label the outside cover of the larger book to indicate the years included. The smaller book will always be current.

Never paste records in; you will want to make copies (and copies of copies). Get a 3-hole punch so that you can include letters, reports, etc., in your book. Strengthen the holes with self-sticking reinforcements (the notebook will get a lot of use).

Keep outsized materials, pamphlets, etc., separately in a file near your reference books. They will get lost or fall out at inopportune moments if you stuff them into your notebook and then attempt to resurrect them.

Things to Do

- Enter materials promptly.
- *Never* lend your book to anyone, no matter how trustworthy they may appear. Instead, make copies of required material.
- Be sure all material is dated.
- Request that all critical information given to you orally is confirmed in writing and entered.
- Follow up important telephone conversations with confirming letters, with a copy for your book.

Information to Include

Divide both the "cumulative" and the "current" books into categories, such as medical, dental, educational, living arrangements, future planning, financial, miscellaneous. Categories will vary depending upon your child's age and circumstances and many will contain subsections. For example, the medical section might contain a section for tests, another for medication.

Set aside a section at the front to contain vital, quick-reference information on resource people. A simple homemade form, punched for a loose-leaf binder, will make recurring record keeping easier and jog your memory about people

IMPORTANT PEOPLE FOR THE YEAR (19__)*

Name	Title	Address	Phone
	(Fill in)	(Fill in)	(Fill in)

Bureaucratic
Fay White   Dept. Mental Retard.
Jack Ebersol   SS Office
Don Evans   City Budgeting Agency

Educational
Frank Dow   Homeroom Teacher
Lucy Smith   P.E. Teacher
Jim Foley   Super. of Schools
Mary Smith   School Secretary

Financial/Legal
Dot Percy   Attorney
Harry Matty   College Grant Officer

General
Betty White   Safety Engineer
Harry Fuzz   Adapt. Hous. Arch.

Health
Lynn Lacy   Pediatrician
Nat Turner   Phys. Therapist
Adam Clark   Genetic Counselor
Shelly Fay   Dentist

Recreation
Sam Foot   Com. Rec. Dir.
Caty Wogon   Camp Ho-Ho Dir.

Resource
Paul White   Ref. Librarian
Amy Round   Com. Counseling

Support/Advocate
Shelly Now   Head Parents' Gr.
Nelly Fry   State Advocate
Pat Nason   Dir. ARC

*The nature of the categories will differ depending on your child's age and circumstances.

Fig. 2

who have been important to your child. The completed forms should be kept for current and future reference. Figure 2 is a sample form in which I have inserted fictitious names to show how it might look.

A Profile

Another ingredient of your notebook is a thumbnail sketch of your child, copies of which will be helpful to his baby-sitters, camp counselors, sheltered workshop supervisors, respite workers, and so forth. Let's call it "An Introduction to _____," with your youngster's name inserted (although throughout the book I refer to it as the "profile"). Again, a simple homemade form will serve beautifully, as would an anecdotal, running account of important happenings and insights into what makes your child the individual he is. The form that follows is a more structured approach that may help parents remember important considerations.

It is drawn up using Owen as a model to illustrate the things caregivers might be interested in knowing. Each parent will, of course, adapt the form to his own youngster and add whatever other categories will be helpful.

PROFILE

Date _____

An Introduction to _____
(fill in your child's name)

(Recent photo of youngster)

The following information may help you know and understand Owen. Please excuse the dry statistics, but they are part of the picture and are important. What is more helpful are the insights into Owen's personality that we have acquired down through the years.

Owen's full name: <u>Peter Owen Callanan</u> His nickname <u>Owie</u> Birth-date <u>1/3/60</u> Height <u>5'9"</u> Normal weight <u>135</u> Eye color <u>blue</u> Hair color <u>brown</u>

Owen's problem: Owen can neither speak nor understand language. His cognitive age is roughly that of a 3-year-old. He has severe constipation problems (check with me for precautionary actions), and has poor gross-motor reactions but unusually good fine-motor coordination. In general, he has a sunny disposition and is not a disciplinary problem.

Owen loves: Applesauce, flashing lights, jigsaw puzzles, soft ice cream, coffee with lots of sugar and cream, fast cars, and all excessive tactile, visual, and auditory sensation. He likes to watch construction work, trees bending in the wind, and clouds moving in the sky. He also likes to pat people who have bristly hair on the head (they should be forewarned).

Owen's unusual characteristics: He waves his hands, jumps up and down, and makes unusual sounds when excited. He will cross his legs widely and, when standing, has a profile like a pair of scissors standing on end. Sometimes he sits and stares off into space, looking, apparently, at nothing—for hours on end.

Owen hates: Icy, slippery pavements; hard, crunchy food; going to bed early; being made to go to the toilet.

Things to be careful of with Owen: He's not watchful crossing the street (oblivious to traffic). He could easily get lost if unsupervised. Because of his insensitivity to pain, he might scald himself in the shower or bath. His diet needs monitoring to prevent bowel impaction, and not monitoring his personal hygiene means his teeth and body remain perpetually unwashed, and in an unspoiled, natural state.

Things Owen does best: He excels at any kind of puzzle requiring fine-motor manipulation. He gets along with people, walks in long, mile-devouring strides, sleeps soundly, and is a champion smiler.

Things Owen has trouble with: He sometimes soils his underpants, does not keep track of his belongings, and isn't good at nor does he enjoy most active, competitive games.

Appendix B
Aids to Basic Competency

The basic library is divided into categories. (Refer to the Resources section for suggestions. In many instances, materials mentioned in the Resources have been recommended by other parents or have proved helpful to Mary and me.) The categories are:

1. Special dictionaries and/or glossaries, which help you understand the common technical terms you may encounter: medicine and special education are apt to be most important, but law, human services, dentistry, and orthotics are also helpful. To the best of my knowledge, no one glossary covering all areas currently exists.

2. Your updated personal notebook (see Appendix A).

3. One or two magazines; for example, *Exceptional Parent, Accent on Living*, and/or a publication of the national organization concerned with your child's disability. (The September 1989 issue of *Exceptional Parent* contains a comprehensive directory of resources of interest to us; this is an annual feature.)

4. The U.S. Constitution and Bill of Rights (particularly the Fourteenth Amendment). In addition, obtain a book on the rights of and advocacy for handicapped citizens and the names and addresses of public officials (federal, state, and local) who represent you and/or hold positions that might affect people who are handicapped. (Your newspaper, library, or local governmental office should have this information.)

5. Books, pamphlets, and/or articles concerned with your child's particular disability (if it is diagnosed) and a clear and in-depth medical description of it in layperson's language. A personal narrative telling the story of a handicapped person with psychological insights that seem to speak to your own circumstances might also be helpful.

6. A collection of up-to-date federal and state laws and regulations dealing with the handicapped population in matters affecting education (from preschool to postsecondary), the transition from school to independent living and community services, and the legal rights of handicapped people to equal opportunity. (Your local education department and state department of human services should help locate them if you wish to augment material mentioned in the Resources.)

Also, a description of state and federal programs for handicapped citizens that implement these laws, and pertinent information on the state and federal agencies that control them. (Your local librarian should be of help here. Many libraries have the reference manual *Social Service Organizations and Agencies Directory* or a similar reference book.)

7. The following references: a comprehensive directory of national and state resources for citizens with handicaps; a more detailed directory of public and private institutions (residential and day, including summer camps); a directory of 800 (toll-free) telephone numbers (available, free, from the National Information Center for Children and Youth with Handicaps).

8. Materials available as the result of membership in one or two organizations that offer clearinghouses or newsletters in certain areas. Parents may change their membership from time to time as their child develops. For example, for the parents of a handicapped daughter with postsecondary educational potential, the American Association of University Affiliated Programs for Persons with Developmental Disabilities (AAUAP) might be of interest.

9. Finally, the Library of Congress's National Library Service for the Blind and Physically Handicapped's Reference Circular 85-2, *Building a Library Collection on Blindness and Physical Handicaps: Basic Materials and Resources* is an outstanding source of information, useful for construction of your library.

Resources

The listings that follow are selective and represent only a portion of the help available. Where possible, I have included resources that have been useful to our family or our friends, or of which I have some knowledge; however, a listing in this section does not imply my endorsement of the help, since only you and the professionals assisting you are in a position to decide what information is appropriate in your child's care.

Many excellent organizations and print materials are not listed because they relate to a relatively small group of readers, who are concerned with specific medical conditions. You can locate specialized resources by using the bibliographies and directories that follow; you should make every effort to keep your use of these key directories *current*. (See Chapter 8 and Appendix B for ways to build a basic home resource library.) Three excellent general sources are: the "State Resource Sheets" available from the National Information Center for Children and Youth with Handicaps (NICHCY), the *Directory of National Information Sources on Handicapping Conditions and Related Services*, and the current annual Education Issue of *Exceptional Parent*, which includes a "Directory of Organizations." They are broad in their coverage and informative in most areas you may encounter.

Although addresses, phone numbers, and names given here are, to the best of my knowledge, currently accurate, they will change with time. Don't be discouraged if you get a wrong number or a letter is returned. Call directory assistance or contact a national clearinghouse or an appropriate state department of education or health and human services to obtain the up-to-date address. Occasionally, prices for books or services are included here. They, too, will change and my listings should be used only as rough indicators. Ask the supplier for current quotations. In addition, as time passes, items listed as free or available may no longer be either free or available. Even if a book is out of print, it very often is available through interlibrary loan. Certain libraries, called full or partial depositories, contain large collections of government publications. Ask your librarian how she can help you locate out-of-print government material.

Every year more information is stored in electronic retrieval systems or databanks. Ask your local librarian which of these systems might help you and how you can utilize them. Make sure the librarian knows specifically what information you seek.

Accreditation. *See* Facilities, Schools, Institutions, and Clinics.

Adaptive Housing and Equipment. *See also* Independent Living.

The National Rehabilitation Information Center (NARIC) makes available information on assistive devices and rehabilitation-related topics (see Clearinghouses/Databanks/Information).

The National Technology Center maintains a national database and user network. Contact the American Foundation for the Blind (see Associations).

Access for the Handicapped: The Barrier-Free Regulations for Design and Construction in All 50 States, 1984, by Peter S. Hopf and John A. Raeber (New York: Van Nostrand Reinhold).

Accessibility: Designing Buildings for the Needs of Handicapped Persons, 1983, National Library Service for the Blind and Physically Handicapped, Bibliography No. 83-2.

Accessible Environments for the Disabled (available from HUD User, Box 6091, Rockville, MD 20850; tel. 800-245-2691; $8.00). Another manual, *Adaptive Housing: Technical Manual for Implementing Adaptive Dwelling Unit Specifications* ($3.00) is also available from HUD User.

Adaptive Environments (Massachusetts College of Art, 621 Huntington Ave. and Evans Way, Boston, MA 02115-5891; tel. 617-739-0088 (voice or TTY)). This nonprofit organization offers workships, publications, and consultation concerned with the design and construction of settings that meet each person's individual needs.

Housing Interiors for the Disabled and Elderly, 1982, by Bettyann Raschko (New York: Van Nostrand Reinhold). A wonderful sourcebook, with pictures, diagrams, and dimensions.

How to Create Interiors for the Disabled: A Guidebook for Family and Friends, 1978, by Jane Randolph Cary (New York: Pantheon Books).

Ideas for Making Your Home Accessible, 1979, by Betty Garee (Bloomington: Cheever Publishing Inc.; available from Accent Special Publications, P. O. Box 700, Bloomington, IL 61702; $7.45 postpaid). The book offers specific information, which is dated, but its general advice is still helpful.

Advocacy

Your state's protection and advocacy office is identified on your NICHCY State Resource Sheet. *See also* Law; Support Groups.

Advocacy Handbook: A Beginner's Guide to Affecting Change, 1978, prepared by Juliane Dow (Parent Information Center, P.O. Box 1422, Concord, NH 03301; tel. 603-224-7005).

Disability Rights Education and Defense Fund Inc. (2212 6th St., Berkeley, CA 94710; tel. 415-644-2555 [voice and TDD]).

"Effective Advocacy: How to Be a Winner," by Tony Apollini, *Exceptional Parent,* February 1985.

A Guide to Mediation of Special Education Problems, 1985, by Judith Raskin

(Parent Information Center, P.O. Box 1422, Concord, NH 03301; tel. 603-224-7005).

How to Get Services by Being Assertive, 1980, by Charlotte Des Jardins (Coordinating Council for Handicapped Children, 20 East Jackson, Chicago, IL 60604; tel. 312-939-3513).

Rights of Individuals with Handicaps under Federal Law, 1988, from the Office for Civil Rights, U.S. Department of Health and Human Services.

Associations

Alexander Graham Bell Association for the Deaf, Inc. (3417 Volta Place NW, Washington, DC. 20007; tel. 202-337-5220 [voice/TDD]).

Alliance of Genetic Support Groups (38th and R Streets NW, Washington, DC 20057; tel. 202-625-7853).

American Cancer Society, Inc. (1599 Clifton Rd. NE, Atlanta, GA 30329; tel. 404-320-3333).

American Cleft Palate Association (ACPA)/The Cleft Palate Foundation (1218 Grandview Ave., University of Pittsburgh, Pittsburgh, PA 15211; tel. 800-24-CLEFT, 412-481-1376).

American Council on Rural Special Education (ACRES) (Attention: Dr. Doris Helge, National Rural Development Institute, Western Washington University, Bellingham, WA 98225; tel. 206-676-3576).

American Foundation for the Blind, Inc. (AFB) (15 West 16th St., New York, NY 10011; tel. 212-620-2147).

American Society for Deaf Children (ASDC) (814 Thayer Ave., Silver Spring, MD 20910; tel. 301-585-5400 [voice/TDD]).

Arthritis Foundation/American Juvenile Arthritis Organization (AJAO) (1314 Spring St. NW, Atlanta, GA 30309; tel. 404-872-7100).

Association for Persons with Severe Handicaps (TASH) (7010 Roosevelt Way NE, Seattle, WA 98115).

Association for Retarded Citizens of the United States (ARC) (2501 Avenue J, P.O. Box 6109, Arlington, TX 76006; tel. 800-433-5255).

Association for the Care of Children's Health (ACCH) (3615 Wisconsin Ave. NW, Washington, DC 20016; tel. 202-244-1801).

Autism Society of America (ASA) (1234 Massachusetts Ave. NW, Suite 1017, Washington, DC 20005; tel. 202-783-0125).

Council on Cardiovascular Disease in the Young (American Heart Association Center, 7320 Greenville Ave., Dallas, TX 75231; tel. 214-373-6300).

Cystic Fibrosis (CF) Foundation (6931 Arlington Rd., Bethesda, MD 20814; tel. 800-FIGHT CF, 301-951-4422).

Epilepsy Foundation of America (EFA) (4351 Garden City Dr., Landover, MD 20785; tel. 301-459-3700).

Fragile X Foundation (P.O. Box 300233, Denver, CO 80220; tel. 800-835-2246, ext. 58).

Huntington's Disease Society of America, Inc. (HDSA) (140 West 22nd St., New York, NY 10011-2420; tel. 212-242-1968).

Little People of America, Inc. (LPA) (P.O. Box 633, San Bruno, CA 94066; tel. 415-589-0695).

March of Dimes Birth Defects Foundation (MOD) (1275 Mamaroneck Ave., White Plains, NY 10605; tel. 914-428-7100).

Muscular Dystrophy Association (MDA) (810 Seventh Ave., New York, NY 10019; tel. 212-586-0808).

National Association for Sickle Cell Disease, Inc. (NASCD) (4221 Wilshire Blvd., Suite 360, Los Angeles, CA 90010-3503; tel. 800-421-8453, 213-936-7205)

National Down Syndrome Congress (NDSC) (1800 Dempster St., Park Ridge, IL 60068-1146; tel. 800-232-NDSC, 312-823-7550).

National Easter Seal Society (70 East Lake St., Chicago, IL 60601; tel. 312-726-6200 [voice], 312-726-4258 [TDD]).

National Hemophilia Foundation (NHF) (The Soho Building, 110 Greene St., Room 406, New York, NY 10012; tel. 212-219-8180).

National Organization for Rare Disorders, Inc. (NORD) (P.O. Box 8923, New Fairfield, CT 06812; tel. 800-447-6673, 203-746-6518).

National Tuberous Sclerosis Association, Inc. (NTSA) (4351 Garden City Dr., Suite 660, Landover, MD 20785; tel. 800-CAL-NTSA, 301-459-9888).

Prader-Willi Syndrome Association (PWSA) (6490 Excelsior Blvd., Suite E-102, St. Louis Park, MN 55426; tel. 612-926-1947).

Prescription Parents, Inc. (P.O. Box 426, Quincy, MA 02269; tel. 617-479-2463).

Sibling Information Network (University Affiliated Program on Developmental Disabilities, University of Connecticut, 249 Glenbrook Rd., Box U-64, Storrs, CT 06268; tel. 203-486-5035).

Spina Bifida Association of America (SBAA) (343 South Dearborn St., Room 310, Chicago, IL 60609; tel. 312-663-1562, 800-621-3141).

Turner's Syndrome Society (York University Administrative Studies, Building #006, 4700 Keele St., Downsview, Ontario M3J IP3, Canada; tel. 416-736-5023).

United Cerebral Palsy Associations, Inc. (UCPA)/UCP Research and Educational Foundation (66 East 34th St., New York, NY 10016; tel. 800-USA-1UCP, 212-481-6300).

Bibliographies

Many associations, clearinghouses, parents' groups, and governmental organizations offer current bibliographies in their area of interest as part of their regular services (the Association for Persons with Severe Handicaps, for example). Contact them.

Locating reading material for the young reader is very important, and more and more material is becoming available. The Maryland State Planning Council *Reader's Guide,* with its section "For the Younger Reader—Books *for* Children *About* Children with Handicaps," is a good example.

I have found the National Library Service for the Blind and Physically Handicapped particularly helpful and have drawn upon several of their current circulars in the Resources section. I urge you to obtain their current bibliographies and "Reference Circulars." Particularly valuable in establishing a basic library are: *Building a Library Collection on Blindness and Physical Handicaps: Basic Materials and Resources,* April 1985, No. 85-2, and *Reference Books in Special Media,* September 1982, No. 82-4.

If you have trouble with the mechanics of locating resource material, get *How to Find Information about Your Subject: A Guide to Reference Materials in Local Libraries,* 1980, by Merete Gerli (Report No. D-102, Congressional Research Service, Library of Congress, Washington, DC 20542).

Other sources I particularly recommend you monitor on a continuing basis are: *The Health Resource Collection Subject Bibliography,* 1988 (Family Library, Children's National Medical Center, 111 Michigan Ave. NW, Washington, DC 20010; tel. 202-745-4055).

The United States Government Printing Office. Write the Superintendent of Documents (U.S. Government Printing Office, Washington, DC 20402) for a listing of subject bibliographies (for instance, "Children and Youth" and "The Handicapped") or phone their order/information desk (202-783-3238). Ask for their "Subject Bibliography Index."

Children's Literature

The Association for the Care of Children's Health (ACCH) has many excellent print and nonprint resources for children. Send for their "Resource Catalog." I have found their pamphlets extremely helpful in the preparation of this book. Get their excellent annotated and indexed bibliography, *Books for Children and Teenagers about Hospitalization and Disabling Conditions,* 1987.

A Hospital Story: An Open Family Book for Parents and Children Together, 1984, by Sara B. Stein (New York: Walker; also available from ACCH for $7.95).
Feeling Free, 1979, by Brightman M. Sullivan (New York: Harper and Row).
Health, Illness and Disability: A Guide to Books for Children and Young Adults, 1983, by Pat Azarnoff (New York: R. R. Bowker).
Lester's Turn, 1980, by J. Slepian (New York: Macmillan).
Margaret's Moves, 1987, by Berniece Rabe (New York: Dutton).
Pediatric Projects, Inc. (P.O. Box 1880, Santa Monica, CA 90406; tel. 213-828-8963). This organization offers a variety of inexpensive reading materials for children, as well as toys and games.
The Teen-Age Hospital Experience: You Can Handle It, 1982, by Elizabeth Richter. Copies available through Pediatric Projects.
Thursday's Child, 1980, by V. Poole (Boston: Little, Brown).

Clearinghouses/Databanks/Information

American Association of University Affiliated Programs for Persons with Developmental Disabilities (8630 Fenton St., Suite 410, Silver Spring, MD

20910; tel. 301-588-8252). They publish an annual *Resource Guide To Organizations Concerned with Developmental Disabilities.*

Clearinghouse on Disability Information (Office of Special Education and Rehabilitative Services, U.S. Department of Education, Switzer Building, 400 Maryland Avenue, Room 3132, Washington, DC 20202-2524; tel. 202-732-1241).

Council for Exceptional Children (CEC) (1920 Association Dr., Reston, VA 22091; tel. 703-620-3660).

Educational Resources Information Center (Central ERIC, National Institute of Education, U.S. Department of Education, Washington, DC 20208; tel. 202-254-7934).

HEATH Resource Center (Higher Education and Adult Training for People with Handicaps) National Clearinghouse (One Dupont Circle NW, Suite 670, Washington, DC 20036; tel. 202-939-9320 [voice/TDD]).

HUD User (Box 6091, Rockville, MD 20850; tel. 800-245-2691).

Independent Living Research Utilization Project of the Institute for Rehabilitation and Research, 3233 Wesleyan, Suite 100, Houston, TX 77027; tel. 713-960-9961).

Mobility International (228 Burough High Street, London SE1 IJX, England; tel. 01-403-5688).

National Center for Education in Maternal and Child Health (NCEMCH) (38th and R Streets NW, Washington, DC 20057; tel. 202-625-8400).

National Center on Postsecondary Transition for Students with Learning Disabilities (Learning Disability College Unit, University of Connecticut, East Hartford, CT 06108).

National Genetics Foundation, Inc. (555 West 57th St., New York, NY 10019; tel. 212-586-5900).

National Information Center for Children and Youth with Handicaps (NICHCY) (Box 1492, Washington, DC 20013; tel. 703-893-6061, 800-999-5599).

National Information Center on Deafness (Gallaudet University, 800 Florida Ave. NE, Washington, DC 20002; tel. 800-672-6720, 202-651-5000 [voice], 202-651-5052 [TDD]).

National Library Service for the Blind and Physically Handicapped (NLS/BPH) (Library of Congress, 1291 Taylor St. NW, Washington, DC 20542; tel. 202-287-5100).

National Rehabilitation Information Center (NARIC) (c/o MACRO Systems, 8455 Colesville Rd., Suite 935, Silver Spring, MD 20910-3319; tel. 301-589-9284, 800-346-2742).

Counseling (and the Effects of the Emotions)

After the Tears: Parents Talk About Raising a Child with a Disability, 1987, by Robin Simon (The Children's Museum of Denver). A sensitive approach to the pressures involved in raising a child with Down syndrome.

The Chronically Ill Child: A Guide for Parents and Professionals, 1981, by Audrey T. McCollum (New Haven: Yale University Press).

Counseling Parents of the Mentally Retarded: A Sourcebook, 1978, by Robert L. Noland (Springfield, IL: Charles C Thomas).

The Disabled and Their Parents: A Counseling Challenge, 1983, by Leo Buscaglia (Thorofare, NJ: Charles Slack, Inc.).

Families, Professionals and Exceptionality: A Special Partnership, 1986, by Ann P. and H. Rutherford Turnbull III (Columbus, OH: Merrill).

Growing up Handicapped: A Guide for Parents and Professionals to Helping the Exceptional Child, 1977, by Evelyn West (San Francisco: Seabury Press). Many thoughtful psychological insights for those involved with children with physical disabilities.

On Death and Dying, 1970, by Elizabeth Kübler-Ross (New York: Macmillan).

When Bad Things Happen to Good People, 1963, by Harold S. Kushner (New York: Avon).

Dictionaries

Ask your local resource people what glossaries are available locally for special education, law, etc.

Black's Law Dictionary: Definitions of the Terms and Phrases of American and English Jurisprudence Ancient and Modern, 4th ed., 1968, by Henry Campbell Black (St. Paul, MN: West Publishing Co.).

Dictionary of Social Work Terms, by Robert J. Barker (National Association of Social Workers, Publication Sales Department, 7981 Eastern Ave., Silver Spring, MD 20910).

Dictionary of Special Education and Rehabilitation, 2d ed., 1985, by Kelly and Glenn Vergason (Denver, CO: Love Publishing Co.).

Dorland's Illustrated Medical Dictionary, 26th ed., 1985 (Philadelphia: Saunders). Available in Braille.

The Glossary, 1985, by Jeanne Buckovitch, Bonnie Dunham, Carol Kosnitsky, and Judith Raskin (Parent Information Center, P.O. Box 1422, Concord, NH 03302-1422; $6.00).

Webster's Medical Desk Dictionary, 1986 (Springfield, MA: Merriam-Webster Inc.).

Directories

Accent on Living Buyer's Guide, 1988-89 ed. (Accent Special Publications, P.O. Box 700, Bloomington, IL 61702; $10.95 postpaid).

Comprehensive Clinical Genetics Service Centers: A National Directory, 1985 (National Center for Education in Maternal and Child Health, 38th and R Streets NW, Washington, DC 20057; tel. 202-625-8400; free).

Directory of College Facilities and Services for the Disabled, 2d ed., 1986, edited by Carol H. Thomas and James L. Thomas (Phoenix, AZ: Oryx Press).

Directory for Exceptional Children: A Listing of Educational and Training Facilities, 1987 (Porter Sargent Publishers Inc., 11 Beacon Street, Boston, MA 02108).

Directory of Living Aids for the Disabled Person, April 1984, Veterans Administration, Office of Procurement and Supply (Superintendent of Documents, U.S. Government Printing Office, Washington, DC 20402).

Directory of Members of the National Association of Private Residential Resources (6400H Seven Corners Place, Falls Church, VA 22044; tel. 703-536-3311).

Directory of National Information Sources on Handicapping Conditions and Related Services, 1986, U.S. Department of Education (available from Harold Russell Associates, 8 Winchester Place, Suite 304, Winchester, MA 01890; tel. 617-729-9090; $25.00 postpaid).

National Directory of Federally Funded Parent Information and Training Centers (National Information Center for Children and Youth with Handicaps, Box 1492, Washington, DC 20013; free while supplies last).

A National List of Voluntary Organizations in Maternal and Child Care (National Center for Education in Maternal and Child Health, 38th and R Streets NW, Washington, DC 20057; tel. 202-625-8400; free).

National Organizations Concerned with Visually and Physically Handicapped Persons, November 1983, National Library Service for the Blind and Physically Handicapped, Reference Circular 84-2. A more complete list is given in the *Directory of National Information Sources on Handicapping Conditions and Related Services.*

Resource Directory (HEATH Resource Center, One Dupont Circle NW, Suite 800, Washington, DC 20036; tel. 202-939-9320 or 800-54-HEATH [both voice/TDD]). Includes list of toll-free numbers.

Disability

Your health professional should be your primary source of information, but sometimes isn't. The National Information Center for Children and Youth with Handicaps (NICHCY) has available (free) general information "Fact Sheets," recently updated, covering 13 major disabling conditions. The Fact Sheets cover definition, prevalence, characteristics, educational implications, and references and resources for each condition.

Titles mentioned in the main body of this book may also be of interest. I particularly recommend *Books for Children and Teenagers about Hospitalization, Illness and Disabling Conditions*, available from ACCH.

Usually, one of the main concerns of a national organization specializing in a specific disease is to develop materials about that disease, and such an organization should be one of the first sources you contact. One of the most helpful books in the entire literature on disabilities is *Children with Handicaps: A Medical Primer*, 2d ed., 1986, by Mark L. Batshaw, M.D., and Yvonne M. Perret, M.S.W. (Baltimore: Paul H. Brookes Publishing Co.).

ARTHRITIS

The Arthritis Foundation (its membership group is the American Juvenile Arthritis Organization) publishes clearly written pamphlets and books dealing with many aspects of this condition. Write them for *Arthritis: Literature for Patients and the Public*, at their national office (Box 19000, Dept. Pre, Atlanta, GA 30326) or contact a local affiliate.

AUTISM

Autism: A Practical Guide for Parents and Professionals, 1980, by Maria J. Paluszny (Syracuse: Syracuse University Press).
Children with Autism, 1988, by Michael Powers (Kensington, MD: Woodbine House).
Son Rise, 1977, by Barry Neil Kaufman (New York: Warner Books).

CANCER

Young People with Cancer: A Handbook for Parents, 1983 (from the National Cancer Institute, Bethesda, MD 20205), NIH Publication no. 83-2378. For information about cancer, call 1-800-4-CANCER.

CEREBRAL PALSY

Coping with Cerebral Palsy: Answers to Questions Parents Often Ask, 1983, by Jay Schleichkorn (Austin, TX: PRO-ED).
Handling the Young Cerebral Palsied Child at Home, 1975, by Nancie Finnie (New York: Dutton).
Under the Eye of the Clock: The Life Story of Christopher Nolan, 1988, by Christopher Nolan (New York: Dell). A pediatrician friend calls this one of his favorite narratives.

DOWN SYNDROME

An Overview of Down Syndrome, revised 1986, by Siegfried Pueschel, M.D. (Publications, Association for Retarded Citizens, P.O. Box 6109, Arlington, TX 76005).
Babies with Down Syndrome: A New Parents Guide, 1986, edited by Karen Stray-Gunderson (Kensington, MD: Woodbine House). A helpful reading list and glossary.
Our Special Child: A Guide to Successful Parenting of Handicapped Children, 1981, by Bette M. Ross (New York: Walker & Co.).

EPILEPSY

Children with Epilepsy: A Parents Guide, 1988, by Helen Reisner (Kensington, MD: Woodbine House). An excellent reading list.
Does Your Child Have Epilepsy?, 1983, James E. Jan, et al. (Austin, TX: PRO-ED).
Epilepsy: You and Your Child. A Guide for Parents, 1983 (Epilepsy Foundation of America, 4351 Garden City Dr., Suite 406, Landover, MD 20785; free)

FETAL ALCOHOL SYNDROME

The Broken Cord: A Family's Ongoing Struggle with Fetal Alcohol Syndrome, 1989, by Michael Dorris (New York: Harper and Row).

HEARING

The Silent Garden: Understanding the Hearing Impaired Child, 1983, by Paul W. Ogden and Suzanne Lipsett (Chicago: Contemporary Books). A first-rate, clear presentation. Mary and I found it very helpful.

LEARNING DISABILITY

Misunderstood Child: A Guide for Parents of Learning Disabled Children, 1984, by Larry Silver (New York: McGraw-Hill).
Smart but Feeling Dumb, 1984, by Harold N. Levinson (New York: Warner Books).

LEUKEMIA

This Is the Child: A Father's Story of His Young Son's Battle with Leukemia, 1983, by Terry Pringle (New York: Alfred A. Knopf).

LUNG DISEASE

Better Living and Breathing, 3d ed., 1983, by Kenneth Moser, M.D., Carol Archibald, R.N., Patsy Hansen, R.N., Birgitta Ellis, P.T., and Donna Whelan, R.R.T. (St. Louis: C. V. Mosby). This is a good, practical, upbeat book in layman's language with marvelous illustrations.

MENTAL RETARDATION

Helping Your Exceptional Baby: A Practical and Honest Approach to Raising a Mentally Retarded Baby, 1981, by Cliff Cunningham and Patricia Sloper (New York: Pantheon Books). Good developmental checklist.
"The Problem of Mental Retardation," 1979, President's Committee on Mental Retardation (Washington, DC 20201).

MULTIPLE SCLEROSIS

Multiple Sclerosis, A Fact Sheet, 1988, by Richard Lechtenberg, M.D. (Philadelphia: F. A. Davis).

PHYSICAL DISABILITY. *See also* Independent Living; Play, Toys; Recreation.

"Physical Disabilities and Special Health Problems: Fact Sheet," 1982, ERIC Clearinghouse on Handicapped and Gifted Children (Council for Exceptional Children, 1920 Association Dr., Reston, VA 22091; free).
Raising a Handicapped Child: A Helpful Guide for Parents of the Physically Disabled, 1986, by Charlotte E. Thompson, M.D. (New York: Ballantine).

SPINA BIFIDA

Parents' Guide to Spina Bifida, 1988, by Beth-Ann Bloom and Edward Seljeskog, M.D. (Minneapolis: University of Minnesota Press).

VISUAL IMPAIRMENT

Can't Your Child See? A Guide for Parents of Visually Impaired Children, 2d ed., 1985, by Eileen P. Scott, James E. Jan, and Roger D. Freeman (Austin, TX: PRO-ED).

Early Childhood

Early Childhood Special Education: Birth to Three, 1988, by J. B. Jordan, J. J. Gallagher, P. L. Hutinger, and M. B. Karnes (Reston, VA: Council for Special Education). Gives parents and professionals an excellent overview of services available.

A Guide for Parents of Handicapped Children, 1984, by P. J. Winton, A. P. Turnbull, and J. Blacher (Baltimore: University Park Press). Recommended highly by a college professor specializing in the field. Although the publisher is no longer in business, I hope this book is still available through interlibrary loan.

Handicapped Infants and Children: A Handbook for Parents and Professionals, 1983, by Carol Tingey (Austin, TX: PRO-ED).

Implementing Early Intervention, 1989, by Carol Tingey (Baltimore: Paul H. Brookes Publishing Co.).

Infant Education, 1977, edited by Bettye Caldwell and Donald Stedman (New York: Walker & Co.).

Infants and Mothers: Differences in Development, revised ed., 1986, by T. Berry Brazelton, M.D. (New York: Delacorte). Gives good developmental guidelines.

Normal and Handicapped Children: A Growth and Development Primer for Parents and Professionals, 1980, by Wilbur S. Thain, Glendon Casto, and Adrienne Peterson (Littleton, MA: PSG Publishing).

A Parents' Guide to Accessing Programs for Infants, Toddlers, and Preschoolers with Handicaps, edited by Catherine Wetherby (available from the National Information Center for Children and Youth with Handicaps (NICHCY)).

Teaching the Young Child with Motor Delays: A Guide for Parents and Professionals, 1986, by Marci J. Hanson and Susan R. Harris (Austin, TX: PRO-ED).

Yes They Can! A Handbook for Effectively Parenting the Handicapped, 1981, by Renee Mollan (Irvine, CA: Reality Publications).

Education

The resources on this topic are too numerous to catalogue extensively here; however, Reference Circular 85-2 of the National Library Service for the Blind and Physically Handicapped and an appropriate subject bibliography from the HEATH Resource Center and/or the U.S. Government Printing Office should prove helpful. The book that I have found most comprehensive is *Negotiating the Special Education Maze: A Guide for Parents and Teachers*, 1982, by

Winifred Anderson, Stephen Chitwood, and Deidre Hayden (Prentice-Hall Inc., Englewood Cliffs, NJ 07632).

The HEATH Resource Center publishes an annual resource directory, a newsletter, *Information from HEATH,* and fact sheets, all free, which are excellent for information on postsecondary education. The National Information Center for Children and Youth with Handicaps is a first-rate resource for pre-college-age students. (See Clearinghouse section of Resources for addresses.) For more specialized material, consult *Lovejoy's College Guide for the Learning Disabled,* 1985, by Charles T. Straughn II and Dr. Marvelle S. Colby (New York: Monarch Press).

Facilities, Schools, Institutions, and Clinics

Accreditation Council for Services for Mentally Retarded and Other Developmentally Disabled Persons (4435 Wisconsin Ave. NW, Suite 202, Washington, DC 20016; tel. 202-363-2811).

Commission on Accreditation of Rehabilitation Facilities (2500 North Pantano Rd., Tucson, AZ 85715; tel. 602-886-8575).

Gallaudet University (800 Florida Ave. NE, Washington, DC 20002; tel. 202-651-5000 [voice/TDD]).

National Accreditation Council for Agencies Serving the Blind and Visually Handicapped (15 West 65th St., 9th Floor, New York, NY 10023; tel. 212-496-5880).

Shriners Hospitals for Crippled Children (2900 Rocky Point Dr., Tampa, FL 33607; tel. 813-883-2575).

Federal Agencies

Administration on Developmental Disabilities, Office of Human Development Services, U.S. Department of Health and Human Services (Room 348F, HHS Building, 200 Independence Ave. SW, Washington, DC 20201; tel. 202-245-2890).

Architectural and Transportation Barriers Compliance Board (111 18th St. NW, Washington, DC 20036; tel. 202-653-7951).

Crippled Children's Service, Division of Maternal and Child Health (U.S. Department of Health and Human Services, 5600 Fisher's Lane, Room 7-22, Rockville, MD 20857; tel. 301-443-2350).

National Center for Education in Maternal and Child Health (38th and R Streets NW, Washington, DC 20057; tel. 202-625-8400).

National Eye Institute (National Institutes of Health, Building 31, Room 6A32, Bethesda, MD 20892; tel. 301-496-5248).

National Institute on Disability and Rehabilitation Research (Office of Special Education and Rehabilitative Services, Mail Stop 2305, U.S. Department of Education, 400 Maryland Ave. SW, Washington, DC 20202; tel. 202-732-1134).

National Institute of Neurological and Communicative Disorders and Stroke

(National Institutes of Health, Building 31, Room 8A-16, Bethesda, MD 20892; tel. 301-496-5751).

National Park Service (Department of the Interior, 18th and C Streets NW, P.O. Box 37127, Washington, DC 20013-7127; tel. 202-343-4747).

Office for Civil Rights, U.S. Department of Education (400 Maryland Ave. SW, Washington, DC 20202; tel. 202-732-1496, 202-732-1467 [TDD]).

Office for Civil Rights, U.S. Department of Health and Human Services (Room 5514, North Bldg., 330 Independence Ave. SW, Washington, DC 20201; tel. 202-472-2916 [TDD]).

Office of Housing and Urban Development (HUD). *See* HUD User in Clearinghouses/Databanks/Information.

President's Committee on Employment of People with Disabilities (1111 20th St. NW, Washington, DC 20036; tel. 202-653-5044).

President's Committee on Mental Retardation (330 Independence Ave. SW, Washington, DC 20201; tel. 202-245-7634).

Rehabilitation Services Administration (Office of Special Education and Rehabilitative Services, U.S. Department of Education, 330 C Street SW, Washington, DC 20202; tel. 202-732-1294).

Social Security Administration (6401 Security Blvd., Baltimore, MD 21235; tel. 301-594-7700, 800-325-0778 [TDD]).

Special Advisor for Disabilities, U.S. Department of Housing and Urban Development (Room 10184, 451 Seventh St. SW, Washington, DC 20410; tel. 202-426-6030).

Special Education Programs, Office of Special Education and Rehabilitative Services (U.S. Department of Education, Switzer Bldg., Room 3511-2313, 400 Maryland Ave. SW, Washington, DC 20202; tel. 202-732-1007).

U.S. Government Printing Office (Washington, DC 20402; tel. 202-275-2091).

Veterans Administration (810 Vermont Ave. NW, Washington, DC 20420; tel. 202-389-2886 [veterans' benefits], 202-389-5010 [medicine and surgery]).

Finances. *See* Chapter 15 as well as the pages listed under "Finances" in the index.

Genetics

These resources were helpful to me in providing general information for the preparation of this book.

March of Dimes Birth Defects Foundation and the National Genetics Foundation, Inc., both produce excellent materials.

Information and Resource Project, Clinical Genetics and Child Development Center, Dartmouth Medical School (Hanover, NH 03756; tel. 603-646-8467). Provides both general information and individual services.

The Hereditary Factor: Genes, Chromosomes and You, 1976, by W. L. Nyhan (New York: Grosset and Dunlop).

Know Your Genes, 1977, by A. Milunsky (Boston: Houghton Mifflin Co.).

Guides

"Closer Look," a project of the Parents Campaign for Handicapped Children and Youth, is apparently no longer in existence (and I miss it). Among its excellent publications are *One Step at a Time*, 1981, by B. Scheiber, and *Practical Advice to Parents*, 1981, by B. Scheiber and Cory Moore. Both of these publications were helpful to me for background information for this book.

Caring for Your Disabled Child, 1965, by Benjamin Spock and Marion Lerrigo (New York: Macmillan). Factual information—dated, but excellent general advice.

Children with Handicaps: A Medical Primer, 2d ed., 1986, by Mark L. Batshaw, M.D., and Yvonne Perret, M.S.W. (Baltimore: Paul H. Brookes Publishing Co.).

Home Care for the Chronically Ill or Disabled Child, 1985, by Monica Loose Jones (New York: Harper and Row). This is a first-rate resource! If you don't read anything else, this one is a must. Its Suggested Reading list is particularly helpful.

Managing Physical Handicaps: A Practical Guide for Parents, Care Providers, and Educators, 1963, by Beverly A. Fraser and Robert N. Hensinger (Baltimore: Paul H. Brookes Publishing Co.).

Medical Aspects of Developmental Disabilities in Children: Birth to Three, 1984, by James A. Blackman (Rockville, MD: Aspen Systems Corp.).

Pocket Guide to Federal Help for Individuals with Disabilities, Publication No. E-87-22002 (Clearinghouse on Disability Information, Office of Special Education, Washington, DC 20202).

Program Guide for Infants and Toddlers with Neuromotor and Other Developmental Disabilities, 1978, edited by Frances P. Connor, G. Gordon Williamson, and John M. Siepp (New York: Teachers College Press).

A Reader's Guide for Parents of Children with Mental, Physical, or Emotional Disabilities, 1983, by Cory Moore, Kathryn Gorham Morton, and Anne Southard (Maryland State Planning Council on Developmental Disabilities, One Market Center, Box 10, 300 West Lexington St., Baltimore, MD 21201). Although old, with some dated information, this is still one of the best sources available. An updated version is in the works; there will be a charge for it.

Summary of Existing Legislation Affecting Persons with Disabilities, August 1988 (Publication No. E-88-22014, Office of Special Education and Rehabilitative Services, Washington, DC 20202).

Independent Living. *See also* Adaptive Housing; Suppliers and Catalogs.

Design for Independent Living: The Environment and Physically Disabled People, 1979, by Raymond Lifchez and Barbara Winslow (Berkeley: University of California Press).

A Handbook for the Disabled: Ideas and Inventions for Easier Living, 1982, by Suzanne Lund (New York: Charles Scribner's Sons). An outstanding manual covering all aspects of how to live independently. It's a must.

Housing for Deaf Adults with Special Needs (Publication No. 0434, National Information Center on Deafness, Gallaudet University). A resource list for hearing-impaired people with additional handicapping conditions.

Independent Living Research Utilization Project of the Institute for Rehabilitation and Research (3233 Wesleyan, Suite 100, Houston, TX 77027; tel. 713-960-9961).

The Source Book for the Disabled: An Illustrated Guide to Easier and More Independent Living for the Physically Disabled, 1981, edited by Glorya Hale (New York: Bantam). Contains an extremely interesting section on the "disabled parent."

Law (and Estate Planning)

Remember that state laws differ, so consult with your own lawyer (see Chapter 27).

The American Bar Association's Commission on the Mentally Disabled offers many services directed primarily at attorneys, including a free newsletter, and for $13.00 postpaid, a self-selecting list of "disability experts." Your own lawyer or support group may wish to look into the extensive legal services the ABA makes available. Write the Commission on the Mentally Disabled, American Bar Association, 1800 M St. NW, Suite 200, Washington, DC 20036 (tel. 202-331-2240).

Alternatives: A Family Guide to Legal and Financial Planning for the Disabled, 1983, by L. Mark Russell (Evanston, IL: First Publications).

Educating Handicapped Children: The Legal Mandate, 1979, by Read Martin (Champaign, IL: Research Press Co.).

"Estate Planning for Parents of a Handicapped Person," in *Kaleidoscope*, vol. 1, no. 3. (*Kaleidoscope*, a quarterly, is published by Connecticut's University Affiliated Program on Developmental Disabilities, 991 Main St., East Hartford, CT 06108.)

Estate Planning for Parents of Persons with Developmental Disabilities, prepared by the Center for Law and Health Sciences, Boston University School of Law (available from the Disability Law Center Inc. of Massachusetts, 11 Beacon St., Suite 925, Boston, MA 02108; tel. 617-723-8455 [voice/TTY]). A contribution of $1.00 is requested.

Federal Benefits for Veterans and Dependents, from the Veterans Administration ($4.50).

How to Provide for Their Future, revised 1989, by the Association for Retarded Citizens ($8.00). An outstanding resource with an excellent reference section, including some individual state materials.

National Center for Law and the Deaf (Gallaudet University, 800 Florida Ave.

NE, Washingon, DC 20002; tel. 202-651-5000.
The Social Security Handbook, 7th ed., (DHEW No. (SSA) 05-10135).

Nutrition, Dental Health, and Feeding

For feeding equipment, *see* Suppliers in this section.

Breast Feeding the Baby with Down Syndrome, Feb. 1985, by Judy Good (Publication No. 23, La Leche League International, P.O. Box 1209, Franklin Park, IL 60131-8209).

"Day to Day Dental Care, A Parents' Guide," July 1985, by David Starks, Geraldine Market, Christine Black Miller, and Judith Greenbaum in *Exceptional Parent,* vol. 15, no. 4, pp. 10–17.

Dental Health in Children with Phenylketonuria (PKU) (Publication No. HRS-D-MC 84-1, U.S. Department of Health and Human Services).

Helping Persons with Handicaps Clean Their Teeth, revised 1985, by Arthur J. Nowak, D.M.D., National Easter Seal Society, Brochure A-262.

Mealtimes for Persons with Severe Handicaps, 1986, edited by Robert Perske, Andrew Clifton, Barbara M. McLean, and Jean Ishler Stein (Baltimore: Paul H. Brookes Publishing Co.).

Nutrition and Feeding of Infants and Toddlers, 1984, by R. Howard and H. Winter (Boston: Little, Brown). A comprehensive overview of feeding in general, with particular reference to problems faced by handicapped children.

A Nutrition Handbook: Eating for Good Health for Caretakers of the Handicapped Child, by Denise Carp, Jackie Crick, and Connie Webster and edited by Redessa Harris (available for a modest charge from the Nutrition Division, John F. Kennedy Institute for Handicapped Children, 707 North Broadway, Baltimore, MD 21205; tel. 301-522-5441). It's the best of its kind that I have seen.

Pre-Feeding Skills: A Comprehensive Resource for Feeding Development, 1987, by Suzanne Evans Morris and Marsha Dunn Klein (Tucson: Therapy Skillbuilders).

Periodicals

Accent on Living (P.O. Box 700, Bloomington, IL 61702; tel. 309-378-2961; quarterly; $8.00/year).

American Rehabilitation (available from U.S. Government Printing Office, Washington, DC 20402; quarterly).

The Arc (available from the Association for Retarded Citizens; six issues/year; $15.00).

Bulletins on Science and Technology for the Handicapped (published by the American Association for the Advancement of Science, Washington, DC; quarterly; free).

Computer-Disability News: The Computer Resource Quarterly for People with Disabilities (National Easter Seal Society, 70 East Lake Street, Chicago, IL 60601; free).

Disability Rag (P.O. Box 145, Louisville, KY 40201).

Entourage (4700 Keele St., Downsview, Ontario, Canada M3J 1P3; tel. 416-661-9611; quarterly). An upbeat and creative magazine promoting community living, geared to Canadian readers, and written in French and English.

Exceptional Parent (1170 Commonwealth Ave., 3d Floor, Boston, MA 02134; tel. 617-730-5800; eight issues/year; $24.00).

Journal (Association for Persons with Severe Handicaps [TASH], 7010 Roosevelt Way NE, Seattle, WA 98115; tel. 206-523-8446; quarterly).

OSERS News In Print (Office of Special Education and Rehabilitative Services, U.S. Department of Education, Washington, DC 20202-2524).

Paraplegia News (Paralyzed Veterans of America, PVA Publications, 5201 North 19th Ave., Suite 111, Phoenix, AZ 85015; tel. 602-246-9426; monthly; $12.00).

Worklife: A Publication on Employment and People with Disabilities (President's Committee on Employment of People with Disabilities, 1111 20th St. NW, Washington, DC 20036; quarterly; free).

Personal Narratives

After the Tears: Parents Talk about Raising a Child with a Disability, 1987, by Robin Simons (New York: Harcourt Brace Jovanovich). Good advice at the end of each chapter.

Cara: Growing with a Retarded Child, 1982, by Martha Moraghan Jablow (Philadelphia: Temple University Press).

A Child Called Noah, 1972, by Josh Greenfield (New York: Pocket Books). Also by the same author, *A Place for Noah* (same publisher).

The Child Who Never Grew, 1950, by Pearl S. Buck (New York: John Day).

A Difference in the Family: Living with a Disabled Child, 1981, by Helen Featherstone (New York: Penguin).

One Miracle at a Time, 1985, by Irving Dickman with Dr. Sol Gordon (New York: Simon and Schuster).

The Story of My Life, 1954, by Helen Keller (Garden City, NY: Doubleday).

Play, Toys. *See also* Children's Literature; Recreation.

Feeling Free, 1979, by Mary Beth Sullivan, Alan Brightman, and Joseph Blatt (Reading, MA: Addison-Wesley).

Games Children Play: Instructive and Creative Play Activities for the Mentally Retarded and Developmentally Delayed Child, 1980, by Manny Sternlicht and Abraham Hurwitz (New York: Van Nostrand Reinhold).

Games, Sports, and Exercises for the Physically Handicapped, 1982, by Ronald C. Adams et al. (Philadelphia: Lea & Febiger).

Language of Toys: Teaching Communication Skills to Special Needs Children,

1987, by Sue Schwartz and Joan Miller (Kensington, MD: Woodbine House).

Let's Play With Our Children: Ideas for Families of Children with Severe Handicaps, 1986, by Pat Downey, an ACCH booklet. It has an excellent resource section.

Make the Most of Your Baby, 1981, by June Mather (Association for Retarded Citizens).

Medical Toys and Books; Quarterly (Pediatric Projects, Inc., P.O. Box 1880, Santa Monica, CA 90406; tel. 213-828-8963).

Play and Recreation: An Annotated Bibliography, 1988, edited by P. Campione (ACCH).

Publishers

These not-for-profit organizations publish and/or make available print and nonprint materials.

American Foundation for the Blind (15 West 16th St., New York, NY 10011).

Association for the Care of Children's Health (3615 Wisconsin Ave. NW, Washington, DC 20016; tel. 202-244-1801).

Association for Retarded Citizens (2501 Ave. J, P.O. Box 6109, Arlington, TX 76005; tel. 800-433-5255).

Gallaudet University Press (800 Florida Ave. NE, Washington, DC 20002; tel. 202-651-5000 [voice/TDD]).

National Maternal and Child Health Clearinghouse (NMCHC) (38th and R Streets NW, Washington, DC 20057).

PACER Center, Inc. (4826 Chicago Ave., Minneapolis, MN 55417).

The following commercial organizations specialize in topics of interest to handicapped persons. Getting on their mailing lists will keep you posted on recent publications.

Abingdon Press (201 8th Ave. South, Nashville, TN 37202).

Boston University Bookstore, special needs section (660 Beacon St., Boston, MA 02215; tel. 617-236-7461).

Exceptional Parent Press (1170 Commonwealth Ave., Boston, MA 02134).

Paul H. Brookes Publishing Co. (P.O. Box 10624, Baltimore, MD 21285-0624; tel. 301-337-9580).

PRO-ED (8700 Shoal Creek Boulevard, Austin, TX 78758; tel. 512-451-3246).

Woodbine House (10400 Connecticut Ave., Suite 512, Kensington, MD 20895; tel. 800-843-7323).

Recreation and Travel. *See also* Independent Living; Play, Toys.

Access Amtrak: A Guide to Amtrak Services for Elderly Travelers, available from National Railroad Passenger Corp. (400 North Capitol St. NW, Washington, DC 20001).

Access Travel, Airports: A Guide to Accessibility of Terminals, from Airport

Operators Council International (1220 19th St. NW, Washington, DC 20036; free).

American Camping Association (Bradford Woods, Martinsville, IN 46151; tel. 317-342-8456).

Camps for Children with Disabilities: Make the Right Choice for Your Child, a brochure from the National Easter Seal Society (two for $ .35).

Guide to Recreation, Leisure and Travel for the Handicapped, 1985, a two-volume set. Vol. 1, *Recreation and Sports*, and Vol. 2, *Travel and Transportation*, edited by Rod W. Durgin, Norene Lindsay, and Ellen Hamilton, are available from Resources Directories (3361 Executive Parkway, Suite 302, Toledo, OH 43606; tel. 419-536-5353). Extremely comprehensive directories, including a state-by-state travel guide.

"Let's Play to Grow" program. Write Eunice Kennedy Shriver for information at the Joseph P. Kennedy, Jr., Foundation (1350 New York Ave. NW, Suite 500, Washington, DC 20005-4709; tel. 202-393-1250). The foundation also supports and provides information on Special Olympics.

Ocean House, a project of Community Alternatives, Inc. (Summer Holiday Program, Pembroke Six, Suite 218, Virginia Beach, VA 23462; tel. 804-490-7562).

Reference Circular No. 82-3, *Information for Handicapped Travelers*, National Library Service for the Blind and Physically Handicapped.

Special Olympics. *See* "Let's Play to Grow" above.

Religion

Accessibility Audit for Churches: Opening Doors for Persons with Handicapping Conditions, 1983, prepared by Education and Cultivation Division, General Board of Global Ministries, The United Methodist Church, 7820 Reading Rd., Cincinnati, OH 45237.

Congregational Awareness Program: Protestant, Catholic, Jews, 1975, by the Association for Retarded Citizens ($1.25). Includes a listing of materials on religion available from ARC.

Our Special Child, 1981, by Bette M. Ross (New York: Walker & Co.). A sensitive story of a child with Down syndrome offering insights in the area of religion and sexuality.

A Resource Manual for Full Participation, 1983, compiled by the Ecumenical Task Force on the Church and the Disabled, Wisconsin Conference of Churches (1955 W. Broadway, Madison, WI 53173; tel. 608-222-9779).

Resources: Persons with Special Learning Needs, 1982, published by the Division of Education on Ministry, National Council of Churches (Room 706, 475 Riverside Dr., New York, NY 11015).

Safety

In Chapter 14 I list several resources on safety, particularly the magazine articles on fire safety (see note 1 in Chapter 14), which I have found helpful.

Bicycle Safety Tips, 1984, brochure from National Easter Seal Society (three for $ .35).

Buyer's Guide: The Safe Nursery, August 1986, a booklet to help avoid injuries from nursery furniture and equipment (U.S. Consumer Product Safety Commission).

Home Safety Checklist for Older Consumers, 1985 (free from U.S. Consumer Product Safety Commission, OIPA, Washington, DC 20207; tel. 800-638-2772).

The NFPA Catalog: Fire Safety Products and Services, National Fire Protection Association (Battery March Park, Quincy, MA 02269; tel. 800-344-3555).

Medic Alert (P.O. Box 1009, Turlock, CA 95318). Write them about identification bracelet and clearinghouse.

A Safe Home Is No Accident, revised 1985, National Easter Seal Society, Brochure A-210 (two for $ .35).

U.S. Consumer Product Safety Commission (Washington, DC 20207; tel. 800-638-2772, 800-638-8270 [TTY]). Ask for their publications catalog.

Sexuality

Ask the Sex Information and Education Council of the U.S. (SIECUS; New York University, 32 Washington Place, New York, NY 10003) for its annotated publication, *Sexuality and Disability: A Bibliography of Resources Available for Purchase*. It includes books, journals, booklets, pamphlets, bibliographies, and resources organized by disability (e.g., cancer, hearing impairment, kidney disease, mental handicap, multiple sclerosis, ostomy, etc.). SIECUS also publishes a similar bibliography for professionals. Many Planned Parenthood organizations provide resources for handicapped citizens. For information, contact the Planned Parenthood Federation of America (810 Seventh Ave., New York, NY 10019; tel. 212-541-7800). In addition, more and more national organizations concerned with specific disabilities offer guidebooks on sexuality.

Human Sexuality in Health and Illness, 3d ed., 1984, by Nancy Fugate Woods (St. Louis: C. V. Mosby). An excellent, frank book both generally and specifically within the context of various disabilities.

Incurably Romantic, 1985, by Bernard F. Stehle (Philadelphia: Temple University Press).

Sex and the Spinal Cord Injured: Some Questions and Answers, by M. G. Eisenberg and L. C. Rustad (U. S. Government Printing Office, Stock No. 051-000-00081-1).

Sex Education and Counseling for Mentally Handicapped People, 1983, edited by Ann Craft and Michael Craft (Austin, TX: PRO-ED).

Sex Education for Disabled Persons, 1975, by Irving R. Dickman (Public Affairs Pamphlet, Public Affairs Committee, 381 Park Ave., New York, NY 10016). This pamphlet was particularly valuable to me in the preparation of Chapter 25.

Sexual Options for Paraplegics and Quadriplegics, 1975, by Thomas O.
Mooney, Theodore M. Cole, and Richard A. Chilgren (Boston: Little,
Brown).

Suppliers and Catalogs. *See also* Independent Living, particularly
Suzanne Lund's *Handbook for the Disabled,* listed in that section.

Abbey Medical (13782 Crenshaw Blvd., Garden City, CA 90249).

Accent on Living. This magazine has an "Index of Advertisers." It also has
available for sale books dealing with purchasing techniques and product
availability; for example, *Wheelchairs and Accessories* ($8.45 postpaid)
and *Going Places in Your Vehicle* ($7.45 postpaid).

Achievement Products Inc. (P.O. Box 547, Mineola, NY 11501; tel.
516-747-8899).

The Adaptive Equipment Center. This is an information clearinghouse for
custom-made and commercially available equipment and technical devices
for personal care, mobility, seating, communication, and other activities
of daily living. Its ABLEDATA is an updated database. Contact them at
Newington Children's Hospital, 181 East Cedar St., Newington, CT
06111; tel. 800-344-5401 (outside CT) or 203-667-5405 (voice/TDD).
Searches are free for up to 8 pages of information.

Crestwood Company (P.O. Box 04606, Milwaukee, WI 53204-0606; tel.
414-461-9876).

Danmar Products Inc. (221 Jackson Industrial Drive, Ann Arbor, MI 48103;
tel. 313-761-1990).

Exceptional Parent, which annually publishes a "New Products" listing.

Fred Simmons, Inc. (Box 32, Brookfield, IL 60513-0032; tel. 800-323-7305).

Mobility and Mobility Aids for Visually Handicapped Individuals, February
1984, National Library Service for the Blind and Physically Handicapped,
Bibliography No. 94-1.

J. A. Preston Corporation (60 Page Rd., Clifton, NJ 07012; tel. 201-777-2700).

Recording for the Blind (20 Roszcl Rd., Princeton, NJ 08540; tel.
609-452-0606).

Reference Circular 83-3, *Sports, Games, and Outdoor Recreation,* National
Library Service for the Blind and Physically Handicapped. Lists "Sources
of Specially Designed (Sports) Equipment."

Support Groups

The National Information Center for Children and Youth with Handicaps
publishes a national list of federally supported parents' programs.

Advocacy Handbook: A Beginner's Guide to Affecting Change, by Juliane Dow
(Parent Information Center, P.O. Box 1422, Concord, NH 03301; tel.
603-224-7005).

Brothers and Sisters: A Special Part of Exceptional Families, 1985, by Thomas

H. Powell and Peggy Ahrenhold Ogle (Baltimore: Paul H. Brookes Publishing Co.).

Collaboration Among Parents and (Health) Professionals (CAPP), U.S. Department of Health and Human Services, Division of Maternal and Child Health (330 Independence Ave. SW, Washington, DC 20201). For information, contact Federation for Children with Special Needs (95 Berkeley Street, Suite 104, Boston, MA 02116; tel. 617-482-2915).

Coordinating Council for Handicapped Children (20 E Jackson Blvd., Room 900, Chicago, IL 60604; tel. 312-939-3513 [voice], 312-939-3519 [TDD]).

Family Resource Coalition (Suite 1025, 230 North Michigan Ave., Chicago, IL 60601; tel. 312-726-4750). Its *FRC Report,* published three times a year, is excellent.

Learning Together: A Guide for Families with Genetic Disorders, by Debra Haffner, U.S. Department of Health and Human Services, DHHS Publication No. (HSA)80-5131.

Looking Forward: A Guide For Parents of Children with Disabilities, 1980, Maryland State Planning Council on Developmental Disabilities (201 W. Preston St., Baltimore, MD 21201; free). This is an excellent guide, which has been used as a model by several other states. Does your state have something similar? Ask your Developmental Disabilities Council.

Parent Advocacy Coalition for Educational Rights (PACER) (4826 Chicago Ave., Minneapolis, MN 55417-1055; tel. 617-827-2966 [voice/TDD]).

A Parents' Guide to Accessing Parent Groups, Community Services, and to Keeping Records, by Suzanne Ripley and Carol Rewers (available from National Information Center for Children and Youth with Handicaps).

Parents Speak Out: Then and Now, 2d ed., 1985, edited by H. Rutherford Turnbull and Ann P. Turnbull (Columbus, OH: Charles E. Merrill). This is one of several helpful *Parents Speak Out* books by the Turnbulls.

The Self-Help Sourcebook: Finding and Forming Mutual-Aid Self-Help Groups, 1988, compiled and edited by Edward J. Madara and Abigail Meese (Self-Help Clearinghouse, Saint Clares-Riverside Medical Center, Denville, NJ 07834; tel. 201-625-7101, 201-625-9053 [TDD]; $9.00 postpaid). Write for their bibliography.

Shoreline Association for Retarded and Handicapped Citizens, Inc. (SARAH) (55 Park St., Guilford, CT 06437). An excellent example of what one community can do.

Sibling Information Network, Connecticut's University Affiliated Program on Developmental Disabilities (The University of Connecticut, 991 Main St., East Hartford, CT 06105; tel. 203-282-7050). Sample copies of their valuable newsletters are available upon request.

Sibling Support Group Handbook, available from Greater Boston Association for Retarded Citizens (1249 Boylston St., Boston, MA 02215; tel. 617-266-4520; $9.00 postpaid).

Technical Assistance for Parent Programs (TAPP), a project of the National Network of Parent Centers, funded by Office of Special Education and Rehabilitative Services. For information, including the Regional Center nearest you, write TAPP Project, 95 Berkeley Street, Suite 104, Boston, MA 02116 (tel. 617-482-2915).

We Have Been There: Families Share the Joys and Sorrows of Living with Mental Retardation, 1983, compiled by T. Dougan, L. Isbell, and P. Vyas (Nashville: Abingdon Press).

Testing

For details on college entrance, write Services for Handicapped Students (Box 2891, Princeton, NJ 08541) concerning SAT testing, and contact Test Administration (P.O. Box 168, Iowa City, IA 52743) for the "Special Testing Guide," which deals with ACT assessment.

Parents Can Understand Testing, 1980, by Henry S. Dyer (Columbia, MD.: National Committee for Citizens in Education; tel. 301-596-5300; $4.50 postpaid).

Prenatal Tests, 1988, by Robin J. R. Blatt (New York: Vintage Books).

PRO-ED (8700 Shoal Creek Boulevard, Austin, TX 78758) publishes many books on testing.

Work

Job Hunting for the Disabled, 1983, by Edith Marks and Adele Lewis (Barron's Educational Series, Inc., 113 Crossways Dr., Woodbury, NY). Dated, but presents a practical, nuts-and-bolts approach to employment.

Making Job Opportunities for Mentally Retarded People a Reality, 1980 (Publication No. 70-6, Association for Retarded Citizens, 2501 Avenue J, P.O. Box 6109, Arlington, TX 76005).

Planning for a Job: Tips for Disabled Students, by the President's Committee for Employment of People with Disabilities (Washington, DC 20036; tel. 202-653-5044; free).

Transition from School to Work: New Challenges for Youth with Severe Disabilities, 1987, by Paul Wehman, M. Sherril Moon, Jane M. Everson, Wendy Wood, and J. Michael Barcus (Baltimore: Paul H. Brookes Publishing Co.).

Index